Preface

An involvement of the immune system is suspected in various cardiovascular diseases. Recent advances in the fields of molecular biology, genetics, cell biology, and immunology have made it possible to identify several pathomechanisms. However, still more questions arise with regard to the pathophysiology, diagnosis, and treatment of immunologically mediated cardiovascular diseases. In this book, leading scientists and clinicians from different areas of cardiology present the state-of-the-art knowledge on the involvement of the immune system in myocardial and vascular diseases.

In the field of myocarditis, both the virological and the immunological findings are presented, and the interactions between the virus and the immune system are discussed. Since the cellular immune system and its mediators play an important role in the inflammation by bacteria that cause endocarditis and septic shock, studies investigating the underlying pathomechanisms are described. Another major topic in this volume is the involvement of the immune system in arteriosclerosis and coronary heart disease, which represents an important problem in clinical cardiology. The final chapter addresses the question of therapeutic options, presenting new approaches for a specific and effective therapy based on the current knowledge of immunologically mediated cardiovascular diseases.

The volume thereby demonstrates both the common immune mechanisms and the individual differences between the various cardiovascular diseases. The editors therefore hope that the book will serve as a reference for scientists as well as clinicians working in the fields of immunology and cardiology. Finally, the editors would like to thank all the authors for describing their latest findings and sharing their future ideas on the role of immune mechanisms in cardiovascular diseases.

Berlin, July 1996   Heinz-Peter Schultheiss
                                                    Peter Schwimmbeck

Contents

The Immunology of Myocarditis

Immunological Mediators in Inflammation of the Heart

Immunological Mediators in Arteriosclerosis

List of Contributors

Badorff, C.
Department of Internal Medicine/Cardiology,
Benjamin Franklin Hospital, Hindenburgdamm 30,
12200 Berlin, Germany

Baig, M.K.
Department of Cardiological Sciences,
St. George's Hospital Medical School, Cranmer Terrace,
London, SW17 ORE, UK

Barry, W.
Cardiology Division, University of Utah Medical Center,
50 North Medical Drive, Salt Lake City, UT 84132, USA

Becker, A.E.
Department of Cardiovascular Pathology,
Academic Medical Center, University of Amsterdam,
Meibergdreef 9, 1105 AZ Amsterdam, The Netherlands

Cao, Wei
Laboratory for Transplantation Immunology,
Department of Cardiothoracic Surgery,
Stanford University School of Medicine, Stanford,
CA 94305–5247, USA
Current address: Chiron Corp., D-233, Department
of Nucleic Acid Systems, Division of Probe Identification,
4560 Horton Street, Emeryville CA 94608–2916, USA

Chapman, N.
Department of Pathology and Microbiology,
University of Nebraska Medical Center, Omaha, NE 68198, USA

Chin, T.
Pediatric Cardiology Division, University of Utah Medical Center,
50 North Medical Drive, Salt Lake City, UT 84113, USA

Collins, A.D.
National Heart and Lung Institute, Heart Science Centre,
Harefield Hospital, Harefield, Middlesex, UB9 6JH, UK

Cooke, J.P.
Section of Vascular Medicine, Falk Cardiovascular Research Center,
Stanford University School of Medicine, 300 Passteur Drive,
Stanford, CA 94305–5246, USA

Coonar, A.S.
Department of Cardiological Sciences, St. George's Hospital Medical
School, Cranmer Terrace, London, SW17 ORE, UK

Crisp, S.J.
National Heart and Lung Institute, Heart Science Centre,
Harefield Hospital, Harefield, Middlesex, UB9 6JH, UK

Curry, K.
Sudden Infant Death Syndrome and Division of Child Neurology,
Department of Pediatrics, University of Maryland, Baltimore,
MD 21201, USA and Laboratory of Mathematical Biology,
DCBDC, Frederick Cancer Research and Development Center,
National Cancer Institute, Frederick, MD 21702, USA

de Boer, O.J.
Department of Cardiovascular Pathology, Academic Medical Center,
University of Amsterdam, Meibergdreef 9, 1105 AZ Amsterdam,
The Netherlands

Dörner, A.
Department of Internal Medicine/Cardiology, Benjamin Franklin
Hospital, Free University of Berlin, Hindenburgdamm 32,
12200 Berlin, Germany

Dunn, M.J.
National Heart and Lung Institute, Heart Science Centre,
Harefield Hospital, Harefield, Middlesex, UB9 6JH, UK

Entman, M.L.
Department of Medicine, Cardiovascular Sciences, Baylor College
of Medicine, One Baylor Plaza, Houston, TX 77030–3498, USA

Epstein, S.E.
Cardiology Branch, Bldg. 10, Room 7B04, National Institutes
of Health, Bethesda, MD 20892, USA

Fallon, J.T.
Mount Sinai Medical Center, The Cardiovascular Institute,
Department of Medicine and Pathology, Box 1194,
One Gustave L. Levy Place, New York, NY 10029, USA

Frangogiannis, N.
Section of Cardiovascular Sciences, Department of Medicine,
The Methodist Hospital and the DeBakey Heart Center,
Houston, TX 77030, USA

Frei, P.P.
Department of Immunological Diseases, Boehringer Ingelheim
Pharmaceuticals Inc., P.O. Box 368, 900 Ridgebury Road,
Ridgefield, CT 06877, USA

Goldman, J.H.
Department of Cardiological Sciences, St. George's Hospital
Medical School, Cranmer Terrace, London, SW17 ORE, UK

Gregory, C.R.
Laboratory for Transplantation Immunology, Department
of Cardiothoracic Surgery, Stanford University School
of Medicine, Stanford, CA 94305–5247, USA
or Department of Surgery and Radiological Sciences,
School of Veterinary Medicine, University of California, Davis,
Davis, CA 95616–8745, USA

Hamrell, B.B.
Department of Physiology and Biophysics, University of Vermont,
Burlington, VT 05405, USA

Harrison, P.C.
Department of Immunological Diseases, Boehringer Ingelheim
Pharmaceuticals Inc., P.O. Box 368, 900 Ridgebury Road,
Ridgefield, CT 06877, USA

Huang, E.-S.
Lineberger Comprehensive Cancer Center, University
of North Carolina, Chapel Hill, NC 27599, USA

Huang, X.
Laboratory for Transplantation Immunology, Department
of Cardiothoracic Surgery, Stanford University School
of Medicine, Stanford, CA 94305–5247, USA
Current address: Fibrogen, Inc., 772 Lucerne Drive,
Sunnyvale, CA 94086, USA

Huber, M.
Institute for Pathology, Department of Molecular Pathology,
University of Tübingen, 72076 Tübingen, Germany

Huber, S.A.
Department of Pathology, University of Vermont, Burlington,
VT 05405, USA

Hufnagel, G.
Abteilung für Innere Medizin – Kardiologie, Klinikum der Philipps-
Universität, 35043 Marburg, Germany

Hummel, M.
German Heart Institute Berlin, Augustenburger Platz 1,
13353 Berlin, Germany

Johnson, C.M.
Section of Critical Care, Department of Pediatric and Adolescent
Medicine, Mayo Clinic and Mayo Foundation, Rochester,
MN 55905, USA

Kämmerer, U.
Institute for Pathology, Department of Molecular Pathology,
University of Tübingen, 72076 Tübingen, Germany

Kandolf, R.
Institute for Pathology, Department of Molecular Pathology,
University of Tübingen, 72076 Tübingen, Germany

Kelm, M.
Department of Medicine, Division of Cardiology, Pneumology,
Angiology, Heinrich-Heine-University, Moorenstr. 5, 40225
Düsseldorf, Germany

Kerr, W.
Department of Immunological Diseases, Boehringer Ingelheim
Pharmaceuticals Inc., P.O. Box 368, 900 Ridgebury Road,
Ridgefield, CT 06877, USA

Klingel, K.
Institute for Pathology, Department of Molecular Pathology,
University of Tübingen, 72076 Tübingen, Germany

Knowlton, K.U.
Department of Medicine, University of California, San Diego,
CA, USA

Kramer, B.
Institute for Pathology, Department of Molecular Pathology,
University of Tübingen, 72076 Tübingen, Germany

Kühl, U.
Benjamin Franklin Hospital, Department of Internal Medicine/
Cardiology, Free University of Berlin, Hindenburgdamm 30,
12200 Berlin, Germany

Lee, R.T.
Vascular Medicine and Atherosclerosis Unit, Cardiovascular
Division, Brigham and Women's Hospital and Harvard Medical
School, 75 Francis St., Boston, MA 02115, USA

Lefer, D.J.
Department of Medicine, Cardiology Section, Tulane University
School of Medicine, 1430 Tulane Avenue, SL 48, New Orleans,
LA 70112, USA

Lehr, H.-A.
Institute of Pathology, Johannes Gutenberg University,
Langenbeckstr. 1, 55101 Mainz, Germany

Libby, P.
Vascular Medicine and Atherosclerosis Unit, Cardiovascular
Division, Brigham and Women's Hospital and Harvard Medical
School, 75 Francis St., Boston, MA 02115, USA

Lindsey, M.
Section of Cardiovascular Sciences, Department of Medicine,
The Methodist Hospital and the DeBakey Heart Center,
Houston, TX 77030, USA

Liu, P.
GW1-508, The Toronto Hospital, General Division, Toronto,
Ontario M5G 2C4, Canada

Luther, H.-P.
Max Delbrück Centre for Molecular Medicine,
Robert-Rössle-Str. 10, 13125 Berlin, Germany

Madwed, J.B.
Department of Immunological Diseases, Boehringer Ingelheim
Pharmaceuticals Inc., P.O. Box 368, 900 Ridgebury Road,
Ridgefield, CT 06877, USA

McKenna, W.J.
Department of Cardiological Sciences, St. George's Hospital Medical
School, Cranmer Terrace, London, SW17 ORE, UK

Messmer, K.
Institute for Surgical Research, University of Munich,
Marchioninistr. 15, 81377 Munich, Germany

Modali, R.
BioServe Biotechnologies Ltd., Laurel, MD 20707, USA

Moreno, P.R.
Cardiac Catherization Laboratories, Massachusetts General Hospital,
32 Fruit Street, Boston, MA 02114, USA

Morris, R.E.
Laboratory for Transplantation Immunology, Department
of Cardiothoracic Surgery, Falk Cardiovascular Research Building,
Upper Level North, Stanford University School of Medicine,
Stanford, CA 94305–5247, USA

Müller, J.
German Heart Centre, Augustenburger Platz 1, 13353 Berlin,
Germany

Müller-Werdan, U.
Martin-Luther-Universität Halle-Wittenberg, Klinikum Kröllwitz,
Klinik für Innere Medizin III, Ernst-Grube-Str. 40, 06097 Halle/Saale,
Germany

Nair, R.V.
Laboratory for Transplantation Immunology, Department
of Cardiothoracic Surgery, Stanford University School of Medicine,
Stanford, CA 94305–5247, USA or Department of General Surgery,
University of Arizona, College of Medicine, Tucson,
AZ 85724–5058, USA

Noutsias, M.
Department of Cardiology, Benjamin Franklin Hospital, Free
University of Berlin, Hindenburgdamm 30, 12200 Berlin, Germany

Ramsingh, A.
David Axelrod Institute, Wadsworth Center, New York State
Department of Health, Albany, NY 12201, USA

Romero, J.
Combined Division of Pediatric and Infectious Disease,
Creighton University/University of Nebraska Medical Center,
Omaha, NE 68198, USA

Rose, M.L.
National Heart and Lung Institute, Heart Science Centre,
Harefield Hospital, Harefield, Middlesex, UB9 6JH, UK

Rothlein, R.
Department of Immunological Diseases, Boehringer Ingelheim
Pharmaceuticals Inc., P.O. Box 368, 900 Ridgebury Road,
Ridgefield, CT 06877, USA

Schultheiss, H.-P.
Department of Internal Medicine/Cardiology,
Benjamin Franklin Hospital, Free University of Berlin,
Hindenburgdamm 32, 12200 Berlin, Germany

Schulze, K.
Department of Internal Medicine/Cardiology,
Benjamin Franklin Hospital, Free University of Berlin,
Hindenburgdamm 32, 12200 Berlin, Germany

Schwimmbeck, P.L.
Department of Internal Medicine/Cardiology,
Benjamin Franklin Hospital, Free University of Berlin,
Hindenburgdamm 32, 12200 Berlin, Germany

Selinka, H.-C.
Institute for Pathology, Department of Molecular Pathology,
University of Tübingen, 72076 Tübingen, Germany

Shapiro, B.
Laboratory of Mathematical Biology, DCBDC, Frederick Cancer
Research and Development Center, National Cancer Institute,
Frederick, MD 21702, USA

Smith, C.W.
Speros P. Martel Section of Leukocyte Biology, Department
of Pediatrics and Texas Children's Hospital, Baylor College
of Medicine, Houston, TX 77030, USA

Speir, E.
Cardiology Branch, Bldg. 10, Room 7B04, National Institutes
of Health, Bethesda, MD 20892, USA

Theofilopoulos, A.N.
Immunology Department, The Scripps Research Institute,
10666 North Torrey Pines Road, La Jolla, CA 92037, USA

Tracy, S.
Department of Pathology and Microbiology, University
of Nebraska Medical Center, Omaha, NE 68198, USA

van der Wal, A.C.
Department of Cardiovascular Pathology, Academic Medical Center,
University of Amsterdam, Meibergdreef 9, 1105 AZ Amsterdam,
The Netherlands

Wallukat, G.
Max Delbrück Centre for Molecular Medicine, Robert-Rössle-Str. 10,
13125 Berlin, Germany

Werdan, K.
Martin-Luther-Universität Halle-Wittenberg, Klinikum Kröllwitz,
Lehrstuhl für Kardiologische Intensiv medizin an der Klinik für
Innere Medizin III, Ernst-Grube-Str. 40, 06097 Halle/Saale, Germany

Wheeler, C.H.
National Heart and Lung Institute, Heart Science Centre,
Harefield Hospital, Harefield, Middlesex, UB9 6JH, UK

Winquist, R.J.
Department of Immunological Diseases, Boehringer Ingelheim
Pharmaceuticals Inc., P.O. Box 368, 900 Ridgebury Road,
Ridgefield, CT 06877, USA

Witthaut, R.
Martin-Luther-Universität Halle-Wittenberg, Klinikum Kröllwitz,
Lehrstuhl für Kardiologische Intensiv medizin an der Klinik für
Innere Medizin III, Ernst-Grube-Str. 40, 06097 Halle/Saale, Germany

Wollenberger, A.
Max Delbrück Centre for Molecular Medicine, Robert-Rössle-Str.
10, 13125 Berlin, Germany

Yacoub, M.H.
National Heart and Lung Institute, Heart Science Centre,
Harefield Hospital, Harefield, Middlesex, UB9 6JH, UK

Yilmaz, B.
Department of Pharmacology, Ege University, 53100 Bornova,
Izmir, Turkey

Youker, K.A.
Section of Cardiovascular Sciences, Department of Medicine,
The Methodist Hospital and the DeBakey Heart Center,
Houston, TX 77030, USA

Zhao, L.
Cardiology Division, University of Utah Medical Center,
50 North Medical Drive, Salt Lake City, UT 84132, USA

The Immunology of Myocarditis

Mechanisms and Genetics of Autoimmunity

A.N. Theofilopoulos

Introduction

The development of the immune system has been hypothesized to be a three-part process that discards useless cells (death by neglect), retains useful cells (positive selection), and deletes or inactivates dangerous cells (negative selection). Studies in the last few years in mice transgenic for antigen receptors have strongly indicated that this hypothesis is essentially correct (von Boehmer 1994; Nossal 1994). Although substantial information has recently been acquired about the editing process by which self-tolerance is imposed, our understanding of the mechanisms and genetic basis of pathogenic autoimmune syndromes is far from resolved.

The broad spectrum of human and animal diseases believed to be autoimmune in nature have been divided into systemic and organ-specific categories, and can be mediated by humoral and/or cellular mechanisms (Theofilopoulos 1993a). Diseases of the myocardium have been classified on the basis of etiology into those of known and unknown origins, the latter constituting the so-called "cardiomyopathies". As with many diseases of unknown etiology, a role for autoimmune mechanisms in the pathogenesis of cardiomyopathies (hereafter referred to as myocarditis) has received prominent attention (Rose et al. 1993; Caforio 1994). Moreover, several of the classic autoimmune diseases, such as lupus and diabetes, exert profound effects on the myocardium. An illustration of this is provided in lupus strains of mice wherein crosses of BXSB with NZB or NZW develop severe lupus, and approximately 80% of the animals exhibit degenerative coronary vascular disease with arterial immune deposits and myocardial infarcts (Hang et al. 1981).

The most discussed scenario in the pathogenesis of autoimmune myocarditis has been that of antigenic mimicry wherein the initial insult, thought to be a viral infection, is followed by a heart-muscle-specific cellular and/or humoral autoimmune response (Rose et al. 1993; Barry 1994). Other mechanisms have also been considered, and multiple genes appear to contribute to virus-induced myocarditis in experimental animals (Rose et al. 1993).

As described in a recent review (Theofilopoulos 1995a, 1995b), the main issues that need to be resolved with regard to autoimmune diseases, including

Immunology Department, The Scripps Research Institute, 10666 North Torrey Pines Road, La Jolla, CA 92037, USA

autoimmune myocarditis, are: (a) the nature of the inciting antigens; (b) the mechanisms by which autoimmunity is induced; and (c) the number and structure of autoimmunity-predisposing genes.

Nature of Inciting Antigen

The determination of the nature of the inciting antigen is central for an understanding of the pathogenesis of autoimmune diseases. The relative paucity of information about etiologic agents in autoimmunity is compounded by three areas of ambiguity. Firstly, it is not clear whether identified autoantibodies and corresponding antigens have any relation to the inciting agent or have a pathogenic role in a given disease. Although transplacental or experimental transfer of autoantibodies has led to disease in some instances (myasthenia, pemphigous, hemolytic anemia), these situations are the exception and not the rule in experimental models. Moreover, myocarditis induced in mice by cardiac myosin injection is transferrable by T cells but not by associated autoantibodies (Smith and Allen 1993; Neu et al. 1990).

Secondly, the immense diversity of autoantibodies observed in some autoimmune diseases causes considerable difficulty in identifying the potentially inciting antigen. For example, more than 30 different autoantibody specificities have been identified in lupus, autoantibodies against several pancreatic and non-pancreatic antigens have been described in diabetes, and in myocarditis, among others, antibodies against myosin (Alvarez et al. 1987), adenine nucleotide translocator (Schwimmbeck et al. 1993; Schultheiss and Bolte 1985), and β-adrenergic receptors (Limas and Limas 1993) have been observed. Some investigators have attempted to explain this diversity on the basis of structural motifs common to many otherwise diverse molecules, whereas others suggest that this "spreading" of the autoimmune response may be caused by recognition, processing, and presentation of diverse polypeptides which are all associated with a single subcellular unit (the so-called particle hypothesis of autoimmunization; Tan 1989). It is likely that the most important autoantigenic epitopes are recognized by $CD4^+$ T cells, and that experimental models which would enable the identification of these epitopes in most human autoimmune diseases are still lacking. It would appear, however, that these responses may engage several T-cell clones, thereby spreading the response to an extent that makes detection of the original pathogenetic peptide epitopes difficult.

Thirdly, there is uncertainty about the length of time between the initial exposure to the inciting antigen and the onset of human autoimmune disease. In certain situations, a short interval between antigen exposure and disease onset (i.e., rheumatic fever after streptococcal infection) may allow identification of a causal relationship. Even in these situations, the genetic diversity of the human population makes epidemiologic and immunologic studies difficult. Thus, the critical response by T (and B) cells to the environmental epitope is likely to occur only transiently, and probably precedes the clinical onset of symptoms and the appearance of an autoimmune response by many years.

Mechanisms of Autoimmunity

Several non-mutually exclusive mechanisms for the induction of pathogenic autoimmune responses have been proposed (Theofilopoulos 1995a), four of which are applicable to organ-specific autoimmune diseases such as myocarditis. They include: (a) responses to anatomically-sequestered self-antigens; (b) responses to "cryptic" self-antigens; (c) responses to antigens that are normally ignored due to the absence of adequate presentation or co-stimulation, and (d) responses to foreign mimics.

The Anatomic Sequestration Model

A well-known form of autoimmune disease resulting from an absence of self-tolerance is the response to peripheral tissue antigens normally sequestered behind impervious anatomical barriers. Such antigens are not available to the developing immune system inside the thymus and, therefore, tolerance to them does not exist. Sequestration of antigens behind anatomic barriers has clearly been documented in recent experiments with mice transgenic for the hepatitis B surface antigen (HBsAg) (Ando et al. 1994). Intravenous injection of $CD8^+$ cytotoxic T-cell lines and clones specific for this antigen into transgenic animals with widespread tissue expression of HBsAg failed to cause disease or infiltration in any organ but the liver. This indicates that the vascular endothelium and basement membrane constitute an extremely effective barrier that normally precludes access of T cells to most tissue antigens. Any release of such antigens into the general circulation due to inflammation or trauma can incite an autoimmune response. Several examples of autoimmune injury following availability of previously anatomically-sequestered antigens exist, such as sympathetic ophthalmia following eye injury and orchitis after vasectomy.

Recent data have clearly established that experimentally-induced thymic availability of peripheral-tissue-associated antigens leads to tolerance and loss of susceptibility to tissue-specific autoimmune diseases. For example, streptozotocin-induced diabetes in mice is inhibited by prior elimination of mature T cells with anti-CD3 monoclonal antibody and tolerization of the newly-emerging T cells by intrathymic injection of streptozotocin-treated islet cells (Herold et al. 1992). Similarly, intrathymic injection of pancreatic islet cells prevents autoimmune disease in the diabetes-prone BB rat and the NOD mouse (Posselt et al. 1992; Gerling et al. 1992). Diabetes in NOD mice is also inhibited by the intrathymic injection or intravenous administration of glutamic acid decarboxylase (Kaufman et al. 1993; Tisch et al. 1993), which apparently is the major autoantigen in this disease. Moreover, prevention of experimental encephalomyelitis, a model for multiple sclerosis (MS), is achieved by intrathymic injection of myelin basic protein (MBP) or its major encephalitogenic peptide (Khoury et al. 1993), and of experimental gastritis by transgene expression of a major autoantigen associated with this disease in the thymus (Alderuccio et al. 1993).

The available evidence indicates that anatomically-sequestered peripheral tissue antigens may not induce thymic tolerance, and that organ-specific autoimmunity may be eliminated by inducing such tolerance. If this is as important a mechanism as suspected, certain organ-specific autoimmune diseases can be viewed as representing a conventional immunologic response against self-antigens without invoking exogenous mimics as cofactors. Tissue-tropic pathogens, such as viruses, may be important in inducing the initial organ damage that results in the availability or up-regulation of previously sequestered antigens, as well as the production of co-stimulatory factors necessary for the immune response.

The "Crypticity" Model

In the simplest form of the "crypticity" model, a sufficient quantity of the autoantigenic peptide is not presented by the MHC in thymic epithelial or other antigen-presenting cells, and the nascent T cell does not receive a negative signal for elimination by apoptosis (Gammon et al. 1991; Sercarz et al. 1993). Thus, a cohort of potentially self-reactive T cells escape thymic negative selection and enter the periphery. Since the self-peptides are produced at a subthreshold level and/or do not bind avidly to the self-thymic MHC, they have been termed "cryptic" antigens. This crypticity may result from either an insufficient or excessive processing of the antigen peptide, the dominance of a flanking epitope competing for the same MHC molecule (Moudgil et al. 1996), or the inability of the specific MHC to bind the peptide.

Several interesting examples of this mechanism have been demonstrated. In mice, autoreactivity to cytochrome c can be induced by immunization with a specific peptide derived from this protein (Mamula et al. 1992). However, this peptide is not derived from the normal proteolytic cleavage of cytochrome c due to the absence of enzymatic cleavage sites (Mamula 1993). As a result, the antigenic peptide capable of binding to the self-MHC (to induce tolerance) is not generated in the endocytic compartment of antigen-presenting cells, and T cells with this autoreactive potential can escape into the periphery. A second mechanism for the failure of thymic tolerance has been demonstrated in transgenic mice bearing the hepatitis B "e" (core) antigen. Since the transgene-encoded protein is produced throughout preneonatal and neonatal life, thymic tolerance mechanisms should eliminate any T cells reactive with this "self" antigen. However, transgenic mice immunized with a particular peptide (pp 129–140) develop immune responses against the peptide, and also against the entire core antigen (Milich et al. 1991). It appears that this peptide binds weakly to thymic MHC and a sufficient density of MHC/peptide is not generated on the surface of thymic epithelial cells to efficiently eliminate nascent T cells with reactivity to this peptide. As a result, T cells with potential self-reactivity escape into the periphery, where they can be clonally expanded and generate a progressively more polyclonal response against this antigen.

The fundamental question is how epitopes that are normally cryptic become visible to the immune system and elicit a sustained pathogenic response.

Several mechanisms have been postulated including, among others: (a) activation of T and B cells leading to modifications in antigen processing and enhancement of cryptic peptide presentation; (b) increased production of epitopes following uptake of antigen-antibody complexes, and alterations in antigen accessibility to proteases when bound to antibody; (c) increase in class II synthesis or in the expression of adhesion and co-stimulatory molecules following viral infection, and (d) molecular mimicry (Lanzavecchia 1995).

The "Self-Ignorance" Model

A model, somewhat similar to the "crypticity" model that invokes self-ignorance by T cells has been formulated. Based on well-defined in vitro experiments, it has been suggested that mature resting T cells specific for extrathymic antigens presented by non-professional antigen-presenting cells (APCs) are induced to anergy because of the absence of appropriate "second signals" or "co-stimulatory" factors (Schwartz 1990; Janeway and Bottomly 1994). The self-ignorance hypothesis suggests that there is no induction of anergy, but rather that the mature T cells, unable to receive appropriate co-stimulatory signals, simply ignore such antigens and remain quiescent. Thus, if antigen presentation and co-stimulation through professional APC (dendritic cells, M∅) is adequate, these quiescent self-ignoring cells may be activated and cause tissue damage.

The validity of this theory is supported by the results of studies with lymphocytic choriomeningitis virus (LCMV) glycoprotein (GP)-transgenic animals in the induction of diabetes (Ohashi et al. 1991; Oldstone et al. 1991). Using anti-LCMV-GP T-cell antigen receptor (TCR) and pancreas-expressed GP double-transgenic mice, it was shown that the GP-specific T cells were not deleted, modulated or anergized, as documented by their presence in sufficient numbers using appropriate anti-TCR antibodies and by their efficient GP-specific proliferative and cytotoxic responses in vitro. However, these cells did not attack the GP-expressing pancreatic cells. Upon infection with the appropriate LCMV strain, however, attraction to the pancreas and damage thereto ensued, leading to hyperglycemia.

The interpretation of these findings was that extrathymic tissue-reactive helper and cytotoxic T cells were not activated, deleted or rendered anergic because the "self"-antigen-expressing cells (islet β cells) did not display enough MHC class II-GP peptide complexes, or produce appropriate "co-stimulatory" signals for helper T cell engagement. However, when infection occurs with the virus bearing the pancreas-expressed "self"-epitope, effective presentation and co-stimulation by the infected APC occurs, which leads to activation of the previously quiescent helper, and then cytotoxic, T cells. This model may well be applicable to myocarditis, as recent studies suggest (Donermeyer et al. 1995).

Antigenic Mimicry

The theories of cryptic or ignored-self correlate well with the antigen mimicry hypothesis of autoimmunity, particularly with regard to infectious agents (Oldstone 1987; Dyrberg 1993). The constraints imposed upon construction of coding sequences lead to closely related or identical polypeptides often being found in unrelated proteins, and many peptide fragments of infectious agents are homologous to host proteins, including MHC molecules.

It should be noted that although mimicry is often discussed in relation to autoantibodies, it is most likely applicable to T cells, since T cells recognize linear peptide epitopes whereas antibodies recognize epitopes created by discontinuous residues within a macromolecule. In addition, mimicry between T cell epitopes appears not to require complete concordance in sequence between a foreign and a self-epitope but rather a conformational similarity. Thus, when residues on the immunodominant epitope of MBP that are necessary for TCR or MHC contact were substituted with various aliphatic and aromatic amino acids to maintain binding/stimulating capacity and searches for corresponding common viral/bacterial peptides were made in available protein data bases, several (EBV, papilloviruses, herpes simplex) were found that were capable of being presented by the susceptible MHC haplotype and stimulating MBP immunodominant epitope-specific T-cell clones (Wucherpfennig and Strominger 1995). Similar findings have been reported with thyroid peroxidase-specific T-cell clones (Quarantino et al. 1995). These findings are important because they indicate that (a) mimeotopes cannot be predicted on simple sequence alignments; (b) T cells actually recognize not a single peptide, but rather a limited repertoire of structurally-related peptides derived from different antigens, and (c) if applicable in vivo, it is unlikely that a single pathogen is responsible for a specific autoimmune disease. These findings also explain why it is difficult to link autoimmune diseases with a given pathogen.

Genetics of Autoimmunity

Regardless of the actual mechanism, the propensity to develop autoimmune diseases, including autoimmune myocarditis (Rose et al. 1993), is highly dependent on genetic factors. Therefore, concerted efforts are being made in several laboratories to identify and characterize genes which predispose to autoimmune diseases with the premise that, if successful, findings in this area will be instrumental in unraveling their pathogenesis, provide new means for prognosis and an early, accurate diagnosis, and ultimately result in the development of therapies tailored to treat these defects.

Autoimmune diseases appear to have a multigenic or multifactorial basis. As a result, their genetic definition in humans is difficult, unlike the situation with single-gene defects. As recently reviewed by Weissman (1995), the various problems in addressing the genetic basis of polygenic disease include: (a) possible heterogeneity of causation (genetic heterogeneity) such that a different constellation of mutated genes may lead to the same disease phenotype; (b) high incidence of a disease-prone allele in the population wherein an identified allele may not be contributing to the disease process in all affected individuals; (c) small contributions by any given gene to the disease process, so that large numbers of samples may be required, and any biases in patient selection may obscure the contribution by that gene; (d) diagnoses may be based on observations far removed from the basic physiologic process thereby leading to both false-positive and false-negative classifications of individuals; (e) the suspected genomic region may be too large to permit careful analysis of all of the embedded genes within that region; (f) a suspected gene may not be the actual culprit, but may be in linkage disequilibrium with another important gene located in close proximity, and (g) due to statistical and other factors such as race and environmental effects, replication of results may be difficult and erratic.

Because of these difficulties, and despite the possibility that animal models may not fully reflect the human disorders, we and others have attempted to determine the number and the nature of genes predisposing to polygenic autoimmune diseases in appropriate rodent models. These models offer the advantage that large numbers of animals can be studied under well-defined conditions, and congenic, transgenic and gene knockout animals can be created to establish the role of a suspected gene.

Three approaches are commonly used to define genetic defects: candidate or functional cloning, positional cloning, and positional candidate cloning. The candidate cloning approach screens for genes with structural and functional properties that fit the disease phenotype. Positional cloning relies first on mapping the phenotype to a small segment of a chromosome, and then systematically cloning and screening all genes within that region. Although the most laborious, this approach has the advantage of not requiring any prior knowledge of gene identity or function, and of having closure (it permits characterization of every gene within that region). The positional candidate cloning approach is, as its name implies, a combination of the two strategies (positional cloning and candidate cloning) and involves screening for known genes in the delineated chromosomal segment, thereby significantly reducing the effort required.

In our own studies of lupus genetics in spontaneous mouse models, both the candidate and the positional cloning approaches have been used (Theofilopoulos 1995b). The results of these studies are summarized below as an illustration of the strategies followed in attempting to define the genetics of autoimmune syndromes.

The Candidate Cloning Approach to Genetic Dissection of Lupus

The selection of candidate genes for study was based on the fact that lupus is essentially a lymphoid cell defect disease. This was clearly shown in bone marrow and spleen transfer experiments such as those between BXSB male mice with early-life severe lupus and BXSB females with late-life mild lupus (Eisenberg et al. 1980). Transfer of male lymphocytes to lethally irradiated males or females led to an early-life disease as measured by mortality or glomerulonephritis (GN) rates. In contrast, transfer of female cells led to late disease in both types of irradiated recipients. Thus, the sole factor that determines disease phenotype is the genotype of the transferred pluripotent stem or lymphoid cells and not the genotype of the recipient. Accordingly, a search for candidate genes in lupus should consider only those that are intimately associated with immune system functions. Although the number of potential immune-related genes that could conceivably contribute to this disease is very large, cytokines, apoptosis-affecting proteins those coding for MHC, Ig, and TCR, have received special attention.

As in every other autoimmune disease, the most clearly established genetic association with predisposition to lupus is that related to MHC. A specific MHC haplotype is necessary within a particular lupus strain, as shown in BXSB mice, which are free of disease upon conversion of their MHC from H-2^b to H-2^d, and in BxW mice wherein H-2$^{d/z}$ heterozygocity was shown to be conducive. Yet, it is clear that different MHC haplotypes can be permissive. Moreover, the MHC haplotype *per se* is not sufficient. Thus, NZB mice crossed with normal BALB/c mice congenic for H-2^z do not develop disease, indicating that simple H-2$^{d/z}$ heterozygocity is not sufficient, and that additional NZW genes contribute to the F$_1$ disease. Similarly, although H-2^b is necessary for BXSB disease, we have developed a disease-free subline despite maintenance of H-2^b (Kofler et al. 1991). Susceptibility to autoimmune myocarditis has also been shown to be conferred by both MHC and non-MHC genes (Lodge et al. 1987).

Since lupus is an autoantibody/immune complex disease, Ig genes were the next logical class of candidate genes to be assessed. Extensive genomic and autoantibody studies, however, indicated that: (a) there is no association of lupus with particular Ig haplotypes; (b) the germline Ig gene composition in lupus is identical to normal mice; (c) autoantibodies are encoded by genetic elements closely related to those utilized in responses to exogenous antigens, and (d) with few exceptions, the autoantibody genes are unrestricted. Additional studies, however, suggested that autoantibody responses are antigen-driven, as demonstrated by the clonal convergence upon IgM to IgG switching and by the confinement of productive mutations at the complementarity-determining region (Theofilopoulos 1993b).

Since lupus development is highly dependent on T cells (Finck et al. 1994; Mohan et al. 1995), the next class of genes to be investigated was the TCR *Vβ* and *Vα* genes. Apart from a non-disease-contributing large genomic deletion in the *Vβ* locus of the NZW mouse encompassing the *Cβ1*, *Dβ2* and *Jβ2* segments (Noonan et al. 1986; Kotzin et al. 1985), no other defect in the genomic composition and structure of these genes was identified.

We then proceeded to analyze TCR expression patterns and tolerance-related *Vβ* clonal deletions imposed by endogenous mouse mammary tumor (Mtv) provirus-encoded superantigens. Using a *Vβ* multiprobe RNA protection assay that quantifies expression profiles for all *Vβ* genes, we found that none of the lupus mice displayed such a defect, i.e. depending on their Mtv or *Mls* haplotype, all relevant *Vβ* depletions/deletions were observed, and this was applicable to lupus and lymphoaccumulation-manifesting mice with the *lpr* or *gld* mutations (Singer and Theofilopoulos 1990). These early findings with *lpr* and *gld* mice are relevant to the recent finding of Nagata and associates (Nagata and Golstein 1995) that the *lpr* and *gld* lupus mice exhibit abnormalities in the *Fas* and *FasL* genes which play a central role in apoptosis. The *lpr* mutation mapped to chromosome 19 was found to be associated with an intronic insertion of an early retroviral transposon between exons 2 and 3 of the *Fas* gene, leading to abnormal splicing and termination of transcription. The *lpr*^cg mutation was associated with a single point mutation at the intracellular signal domain of this gene, leading to lack of functionality; the *gld* mutation, mapped to chromosome 1, was associated with a single point mutation in the carboxyl terminus of the Fas ligand, leading to normal transcription, but lack of functionality. In spite of this, as our results indicated, *lpr/gld* mice do not exhibit defects in central T cell deletions. The conclusion that central (intrathymic) deletional tolerance mechanisms in these mice are intact is also applicable to conventional peptide-recognizing T cells, as documented in *lpr* mice transgenic for TCR recognizing H-Y antigen in the context of class I MHC or pigeon cytochrome c in the context of class II MHC (Sidman et al. 1992; Singer and Abbas 1994). Nevertheless, in such mice defects in peripheral T cell deletions have been observed, consistent with the primary role of Fas and FasL in activation-induced peripheral T-cell apoptosis (Russell et al. 1993; Mogil et al. 1995). Thus, the rapid development of lupus in *lpr/gld* mice can be attributed to the inefficient deletion of activated self-reactive T cells in the periphery.

Although the discovery of the *Fas/FasL* gene defects is of major importance, these defects obviously do not provide a universal explanation for murine lupus. Moreover, no defects in the structure, expression or function of the *Fas* gene have been uncovered in the vast majority of lupus patients (Mysler et al. 1994), although rare cases of a phenotype resembling the *lpr/gld* phenotype have been identified (Rieux-Laucat et al. 1995; Fisher et al. 1995). Nevertheless, identification of these defects strongly suggests that lupus pathogenesis may be related to other abnormalities within the multiple genes encoding proteins which promote or inhibit apoptosis. Based on these and other considerations, we have recently developed a multiprobe RNase protection assay wherein expression profiles of most apoptosis genes and the mechanistically-coupled cell-cycle-controlling genes can be expeditiously analyzed. We believe that further detailed functional and genetic studies on these processes are likely to provide additional insights into the pathogenesis of lupus.

The Positional Cloning Approach to Genetic Dissection of Lupus

A second avenue of inquiry for broadly defining lupus genetic defects is positional cloning which involves total genome searches using dense chromosomal maps. The obvious advantage of this approach is that it thoroughly addresses the issue without being biased by any preconceived notions. Chromosomal maps can be created using microsatellite markers.

Microsatellites or simple-sequence length polymorphisms (SSLP) are tandem repeats of usually dinucleotides, e.g. (CA), that exhibit a high degree of polymorphism in the number of repeats at a given chromosomal site and from one individual to another (Lander and Schork 1994). SSLP are abundant (>100 000) and randomly dispersed throughout the mammalian genome, thereby providing an enormous pool from which to derive markers. So far, more than 5000 microsatellite markers have been identified within the 1600 cM mouse genome. Specific SSLP can easily be identified by using conserved sequences flanking the repeats as oligonucleotide primers for polymerase chain reaction followed by electrophoresis of the amplified products on agarose or polyacrylamide gels.

About 2 years ago we began applying this approach for the identification of lupus-associated loci in NZBxNZW F_2 intercross mice (Kono et al. 1994). To establish an exclusion linkage map for NZB and NZW mice, 315 microsatellites were screened and 91 markers were selected for maximum coverage and discernable separation in agarose gels. With the condition that distances between markers did not exceed 20 cM, 97% of the genome was covered.

Using these markers, we then analyzed 150 female F_2 mice for segregation with early mortality, GN (the major cause of death in lupus), anti-chromatin autoantibody and splenomegaly. We identified eight loci, designated Lbw-1 to -8 (Lbw, lupus BxW) on chromosomes 17, 4, 5, 6, 7, 18, 1, and 11, respectively, that contributed to BxW lupus susceptibility and two for splenomegaly, designated Sbw-1 and Sbw-2 on chromosomes 1 and 4, respectively (Sbw, splenomegaly BxW). Four of these loci were NZB dominant, two were NZB recessive, one was NZW dominant and two were NZW recessive. Three loci, Lbw-1 (corresponding to the MHC locus), -7, and -8 on chromosomes 17, 1, and 11, respectively, were linked to increased anti-chromatin response. GN was linked to three loci, Lbw-1, -2, and -6 on chromosomes 17, 4, and 18, respectively, all of which also had linkage to mortality consistent with GN being the major cause of death.

The two non-MHC GN-predisposing loci had no linkage to autoantibody production, suggesting that their contribution to GN involves a stage beyond the initial autoantibody formation. Six loci, Lbw-1 to -6 on chromosomes 17, 4, 5, 6, 7, and 18, respectively, were linked to early mortality, three of which were also associated with GN. The loci which are unlinked to GN may play a role in other pathologic conditions such as vascular disease, neoplasias and others that might contribute to the overall mortality susceptibility. The Lbw-2 locus on chromosome 4 was also identified in similar studies by others (Drake et al. 1994; Morel et al. 1994). This locus appears to exert pleiotropic effects (splenomegaly, mortality, GN) and to be absolutely necessary for early mortality. We have proposed that the basic defect produced by this locus may be lymphocyte hyperactivity/hyperplasia, which then gives rise to autoantibody production, immune complex formation, GN, and death. Such a model would tie together several of the major abnormalities observed in New Zealand lupus mice and provides hope that interruption of single gene functions may have profound effects on lupus development.

Based on our findings to date, we conclude that the genetics of murine lupus follow a multiplicative model of inheritance in which specific combinations of genes acting additively are required for phenotype expression. Moreover, it appears that each susceptibility locus contributes to specific stages of lupus immunopathology, suggesting that each stage has a separate threshold determined by different sets of susceptibility genes. We can speculate that these findings suggest a rationale for combination treatment regimens tailored to affect genetic contributions at different stages.

The chromosomal locations of BW-susceptibility loci have only been approximately defined, and investigations with additional microsatellite markers as well as studies in congenic mice will be required to more precisely localize these genes. Nevertheless, several previously mapped candidate genes of interest are located in chromosomal regions identified in these studies, and we are currently analyzing the structure and expression of some of them. If such efforts fail, we intend to obtain maps for these loci at 0.5 cM intervals, which then may permit gene identification by constructing yeast artificial chromosome (YAC) libraries and employing positional cloning techniques. After identifying genes which are associated with the disease phenotype in lupus mice, a search can then be undertaken to determine the relevance of these findings to the human disease by examining for syntenic relationships between mouse and human chromosomes. Our prediction is that some of these mouse lupus susceptibility loci will also be relevant to human lupus. The strategies outlined for the study of lupus genetics should also be applicable to studies on the genetics of autoimmune myocarditis.

Acknowledgements. This is publication number 9988-IMM from The Scripps Research Institute, 10666 North Torrey Pines Road, La Jolla, CA 92037. The work of the authors cited herein was supported, in part, by United States National Institutes of Health Grants AR39555 and AR31203.

References

Alderuccio F, Toh B-H, Tan S-S, Gleeson PA, van Driel IR (1993) An autoimmune disease with multiple molecular targets abrogated by the transgenic expression of a single autoantigen in the thymus. J Exp Med 178: 419–426

Alvarez FL, Neu N, Rose NR, Craig SW, Beisel KW (1987) Heart-specific autoantibodies induced by coxsackievirus B3: Identification of heart autoantigens. Clin Immunol Immunopathol 43: 129–139

Ando K, Guidotti LG, Cerny A, Ishikawa T, Chisari FV (1994) CTL access to tissue antigen is restricted in vivo. J Immunol 153: 482–488

Barry WH (1994) Mechanisms of immune-mediated myocyte injury. Circulation 89: 2421–2432

Caforio ALP (1994) Role of autoimmunity in dilated cardiomyopathy. Br Heart J 72(Suppl): S30–S34

Donermeyer DL, Beisel KW, Allen PM, Smith SC (1995) Myocarditis-inducing epitope of myosin binds constitutively and stably to I-A^k on antigen-presenting cells in the heart. J Exp Med 182: 1291–1300

14   A.N. Theofilopoulos

Drake CG, Babcock SK, Palmer E, Kotzin BL (1994) Genetic analysis of the NZB contribution to lupus-like autoimmune disease. Proc Natl Acad Sci USA 91: 4062–4066

Dyrberg T (1993) Antigenic Mimicry. In: Bona C, Siminovitch KA, Zanetti M, Theofilopoulos AN (eds) Molecular Pathology of Autoimmune Diseases. Harwood Academic, Langhorne, Pennsylvania, pp 257–261

Eisenberg RA, Izui S, McConahey PJ, Hang LM, Peters CJ, Theofilopoulos AN, Dixon FJ (1980) Male determined accelerated autoimmune disease in BXSB mice: Transfer by bone marrow and spleen cells. J Immunol 125: 1032–1036

Finck BK, Linsley PS, Wofsy D (1994) Treatment of murine lupus with CTLA4Ig. Science 265: 1225–1227

Fisher GH, Rosenberg FJ, Straus SE, Dale JK, Middelton LA, Lin AY, Strober W, Lenardo MJ, Puck JM (1995) Dominant interfering Fas gene mutations impair apoptosis in a human autoimmune lymphoproliferative syndrome. Cell 81: 935–946

Gammon G, Sercarz E, Benichou G (1991) The dominant self and the cryptic self: Shaping the autoreactive T-cell repertoire. Immunol Today 12: 193–195

Gerling I, Serreze D, Christianson S, Leiter E (1992) Intrathymic islet cell transplantation reduces B-cell autoimmunity and prevents diabetes in NOD/Lt mice. Diabetes 41: 1672–1676

Hang LM, Izui S, Dixon FJ (1981) (NZBxBXSB)F$_1$ hybrid: A model of acute lupus and coronary vascular disease with myocardial infarction. J Exp Med 154: 216–221

Herold KC, Montag AG, Buckingham F (1992) Induction of tolerance to autoimmune diabetes with islet antigens. J Exp Med 176: 1107–1114

Janeway CA Jr, Bottomly K (1994) Signals and signs for lymphocyte responses. Cell 76: 275–285

Kaufman DL, Clare-Salzler M, Tian J, Forsthuber T, Ting GSP, Robinson P, Atkinson MA, Sercarz EE, Tobin AJ, Lehmann PV (1993) Spontaneous loss of T-cell tolerance to glutamic acid decarboxylase in murine insulin-dependent diabetes. Nature 366: 69–72

Khoury SJ, Sayegh MH, Hancock WW, Gallon L, Carpenter CB, Weiner HL (1993) Acquired tolerance to experimental autoimmune encephalomyelitis by intrathymic injection of myelin basic protein or its major encephalitogenic peptide. J Exp Med 178: 559–566

Kofler R, McConahey PJ, Duchosal MA, Theofilopoulos AN, Dixon FJ (1991) An autosomal recessive gene that delays expression of lupus in BXSB mice. J Immunol 146: 1375–1379

Kono DH, Burlingame RW, Owens DG, Kuramochi A, Balderas RS, Balomenos D, Theofilopoulos AN (1994) Lupus susceptibility loci in New Zealand mice. Proc Natl Acad Sci USA 91: 10168–10172

Kotzin BL, Barr VL, Palmer E (1985) A large deletion within the T-cell receptor beta-chain gene complex in New Zealand mice. Science 229: 167–171

Lander ES, Schork NJ (1994) Genetic dissection of complex traits. Science 265: 2037–2048

Lanzavecchia A (1995) How can cryptic epitopes trigger autoimmunity? J Exp Med 181: 1945–1948

Limas CJ, Limas C (1993) Immune-mediated modulation of β-adrenoceptor function in human dilated cardiomyopathy. Clin Immunol Immunopathol 68: 204–207

Lodge PA, Herzum M, Huber SA (1987) Coxsackie B-3. Acute and chronic forms of the disease by different immunopathogenic mechanisms. Am J Pathol 128: 455–463

Mamula MJ (1993) The inability to process a self-peptide allows autoreactive T cells to escape tolerance. J Exp Med 177: 567–571

Mamula MJ, Lin J, Janeway C, Hardin J (1992) Breaking T-cell tolerance with foreign and self-co-immunogen: A study of autoimmune B- and T-cell epitopes of cytochrome. J Immunol 151: 789–799

Milich DR, McLachlan A, Raney AK, Houghten R, Thornton GB, Maruyama T, Hughes JL, Jones JE (1991) Autoantibody production in hepatitis B e antigen-transgenic mice elicited with a self-T-cell peptide and inhibited with nonself-peptide. Proc Natl Acad Sci USA 88: 4348–4352

Mogil RJ, Radvanyi L, Gonzalez-Quintial R, Miller R, Mills G, Theofilopoulos AN, Green DR (1995) Fas (CD45) participates in peripheral T cell deletion and associated apoptosis in vivo. Int Immunol 7: 1451–1458

Mohan C, Shi Y, Laman JD, Datta SK (1995) Interaction between CD40 and its ligand gp39 in the development of murine lupus nephritis. J Immunol 154: 1470–1480

Morel L, Rudofsky UH, Longmate JA, Schiffenbauer J, Wakeland EK (1994) Polygenic control of susceptibility to murine systemic lupus erythematosus. Immunity 1: 219–229

Moudgil KD, Grewal IS, Jensen PE, Sercarz EE (1996) Unresponsiveness to a self-peptide of mouse lysozyme owing to hindrance of T cell receptor-major histocompatibility complex/ peptide interaction caused by flanking epitopic residues. J Exp Med 183: 535–546

Mysler E, Bini P, Drappa J, Ramos P, Friedman SM, Krammer PH, Elkon KB (1994) The apoptosis-1/Fas protein in human systemic lupus erythematosus. J Clin Invest 93: 1029–1034

Nagata S, Golstein P (1995) The Fas death factor. Science 267: 1449–1456

Neu N, Ploier B, Ofner C (1990) Cardiac myocin-induced myocarditis: Heart autoantibodies are not involved in the induction of the disease. J Immunol 145: 4094–4100

Noonan DJ, Kofler R, Singer PA, Cardenas G, Dixon FJ, Theofilopoulos AN (1986) Delineation of a defect in T cell receptor beta genes of NZW mice predisposed to autoimmunity. J Exp Med 163: 644–653

Nossal GJV (1994) Negative selection of lymphocytes. Cell 76: 229–240

Ohashi PS, Oehen S, Buerki K, Pircher H, Ohashi CT, Odermatt B, Malissen B, Zinkernagel RM, Hengartner H (1991) Ablation of "tolerance" and induction of diabetes by virus infection in viral antigen transgenic mice. Cell 65: 305–317

Oldstone MBA (1987) Molecular mimicry and autoimmune disease. Cell 50: 819–820

Oldstone MBA, Nerenberg M, Southern P, Price J, Lewicki H (1991) Virus infection triggers insulin-dependent diabetes mellitus in a transgenic model: Role of anti-self (virus) immune response. Cell 65: 319–332

Posselt AM, Barker CF, Friedman AL, Naji A (1992) Prevention of autoimmune diabetes in the BB rat by intrathymic islet transplantation at birth. Science 256: 1321–1324

Quarantino S, Thorpe CJ, Travers PJ, Londei M (1995) Similar antigenic surfaces, rather than sequence homology, dictate T-cell epitope molecular mimicry. Proc Natl Acad Sci USA 92: 10398–10402

Rieux-Laucat F, LeDiest F, Hivroz C, Roberts IAG, Debatin KM, Fischer A, deVillartay JP (1995) Mutations in Fas associated with human lymphoproliferative syndrome and autoimmunity. Science 268: 1347–1349

Rose NR, Herskowitz A, Newmann DA (1993) Autoimmunity in myocarditis: Models and mechanisms. Clin Immunol Immunopathol 68: 95–99

Russell JH, Rush B, Weaver C, Wang RD (1993) Mature T-cells of autoimmune lpr/lpr mice have a defect in antigen-stimulated suicide. Proc Natl Acad Sci USA 90: 4409–4413

Schultheiss HP, Bolte HD (1985) Immunological analysis of autoantibodies against the adenine nucleotide translocator in dilated cardiomyopathy. J Mol Cell Cardiol 17: 603–617

Schwartz RH (1990) A cell culture model for T lymphocyte clonal anergy. Science 248: 1349–1356

Schwimmbeck PL, Schwimmbeck NK, Schultheiss H-P, Strauer B-E (1993) Mapping of antigenic determinants of the adenine-nucleotide translocator and coxsackie B3 virus with synthetic peptides: Use for the diagnosis of viral heart disease. Clin Immunol Immunopathol 68: 135–140

Sercarz EE, Lehmann PV, Ametani A, Benichou G, Miller A, Moudgil K (1993) Dominance and crypticity of T cell antigenic determinants. Ann Rev Immunol 11: 729–766

Sidman CL, Marshall JD, VonBoehmer H (1992) Transgenic T cell receptor interactions in the lymphoproliferative and autoimmune syndromes of lpr and gld mutant mice. Eur J Immunol 22: 499–504

Singer GG, Abbas AK (1994) The Fas antigen is involved in peripheral but not thymic deletion of T lymphocytes in T cell receptor transgenic mice. Immunity 1: 365–371

Singer PA, Theofilopoulos AN (1990) T cell receptor V-beta repertoire expression in murine models of SLE. Immunol Rev 118: 103–127

Smith SC, Allen PM (1993) The role of T cells in myocin-induced autoimmunity myocarditis. Clin Immunol Immunopathol 68: 100–106

Tan EM (1989) Antinuclear antibodies: Diagnostic markers for autoimmune diseases and probes for cell biology. Adv Immunol 44: 93–151

Theofilopoulos AN (1993a) Molecular Pathology of Autoimmunity. In: Bona C, Siminovitch KA, Zanetti M, Theofilopoulos AN (eds) Molecular pathology of autoimmune diseases. Harwood Academic, Langhorne, Pennsylvania, pp 1–12

Theofilopoulos AN (1993b) Immunologic Genes in Mouse Lupus Models. In: Bona CA, Siminovitch K, Zanetti M, Theofilopoulos AN (eds) Molecular Pathology of Autoimmune Diseases. Harwood Academic, Langhorne, Pennsylvania, pp 281–316

Theofilopoulos AN (1995a) The basis of autoimmunity: Part I, Mechanisms of aberrant self-recognition. Immunol Today 16: 90–98

Theofilopoulos AN (1995b) The basis of autoimmunity: Part II, Genetic predisposition. Immunol Today 16: 150–159

Tisch R, Yang X-D, Singer SM, Liblau LS, Fugger L, McDevitt HO (1993) Immune response to glutamic acid decarboxylase correlates with insulitis in non-obese diabetic mice. Nature 366: 72–75

von Boehmer H (1994) Positive selection of lymphocytes. Cell 76: 219–228

Weissman SM (1995) Genetic bases for common polygenic diseases. Proc Natl Acad Sci USA 92: 8543–8544

Wucherpfennig KW, Strominger JL (1995) Molecular mimicry in T cell-mediated auto-immunity: Viral peptides activate human T cell clones specific for myelin basic protein. Cell 80: 695–705

Molecular Pathogenesis of Myocarditis and Cardiomyopathy: Analysis of Virus–Receptor Interactions and Tyrosine Phosphorylation Events

H.-C. Selinka, K. Klingel, M. Huber, B. Kramer, U. Kämmerer, and R. Kandolf

Introduction

Enteroviruses of the human *Picornaviridae* are common agents of viral myocarditis. Various members of the enterovirus group, e.g. coxsackieviruses and echoviruses, have been associated with viral heart disease. Human enterovirus myocarditis is most often caused by group B coxsackieviruses (CVB) [1–3]. The genetic material of CVB is encoded in a single-stranded RNA molecule of positive polarity and about 7500 nucleotides in length [4, 5]. During replication, the genomic viral plus-strand RNA serves as a template for transcription of minus-strand RNA, an intermediate in the life cycle of enteroviruses, which is transcribed again into large amounts of infectious plus-strand RNA [6].

Molecular diagnostic techniques have allowed the detection of enteroviruses in various tissues, such as heart muscle, pancreas, and lymphoid organs [7–10]. Myocardial enterovirus infections are detectable by in situ hybridization and PCR gene amplification not only in acute but also in chronic enterovirus-induced myocarditis, indicating the possibility of enterovirus persistence in the human heart [11–13]. In addition, such infections are observed in patients with "idiopathic" dilated cardiomyopathy, indicating that enterovirus myocarditis may predispose to the development of chronic congestive cardiomyopathy [13–15]. Progress is currently being made in unraveling the molecular mechanisms of enterovirus persistence, the diversity of host and virus genetics and their impact on the nature and severity of the disease. Here we summarize the current knowledge of myocardial enterovirus infection and persistence with regard to the molecular mechanisms of pathogenesis, focussing on CVB-specific virus-binding proteins and virus-induced tyrosine phosphorylation events.

Molecular Mechanisms of Persistent Enterovirus Infection

In order to understand the pathogenic mechanisms of enterovirus myocarditis, murine models have been developed which exhibit histopathologic features

Institute for Pathology, Department of Molecular Pathology, University of Tübingen, 72076 Tübingen, Germany

resembling heart muscle lesions observed in humans. Factors such as age, sex, and as yet unknown genetic determinants have been shown to influence the development of enterovirus myocarditis [12, 16–19]. The discovery of enterovirus persistence in the human heart was substantiated by the observation of coxsackievirus persistence in different murine models of chronic myocarditis. This demonstrates that coxsackievirus B3 (CVB3), typically a cytolytic enterovirus, is capable of evading immunological surveillance in a host-dependent fashion [12]. Patterns of acute and persistent myocardial infection were quantitatively assessed in different immunocompetent mouse strains and directly related to the extent of myocardial tissue damage and inflammation. Acute and chronic myocardial lesions were consistently found to be associated with infected myocardial cells, demonstrating the importance of viral replication in the pathogenesis of ongoing heart muscle disease. No inflammatory lesions developed in the absence of virus replication in the course of the disease. Thus, it can be concluded that virus replication plays a major role in the development and maintenance of target organ disease. CVB3 was found to be capable of inducing a persistent infection in A.CA/SnJ, A.BY/SnJ, and SWR/J mice. In contrast, DBA/1J or C57BL/6 mice were found to be able to eliminate the virus after the acute infection. The different course of the disease in SWR/J (H-2^q) and DBA/1J mice (H-2^q), as well as in A.BY/SnJ (H-2^b) and C57BL/6 (H-2^b) mice indicates that resistance to the development of persistent heart muscle infection is not linked to the H-2 locus of the host.

Regarding the molecular mechanisms of myocardial enterovirus persistence, in situ hybridization with strand-specific RNA probes revealed that persistent enterovirus infection is restricted at the level of genomic plus-strand RNA synthesis [12, 20]. In contrast to the acute infection of myocardial cells, which is characterized by the synthesis of viral plus-strand RNA in great excess, persistently infected cells were found to contain plus- and minus-strands of viral RNA in approximately similar amounts. Viral capsid protein expression was studied by immunohistochemistry with polyclonal antisera raised against two non-overlapping bacterially synthesized structural fusion proteins of CVB3 [21]. The results indicate that the amount of enteroviral capsid protein synthesis is decreased in persistently infected cells, thus reflecting restricted viral RNA synthesis. Altered replication and transcription of the virus, in addition to an immune response insufficient to recognize and clear infected cells entirely, are essential mechanisms for the initiation and maintenance of a persistent infection. Restricted replication with a decreased synthesis of enteroviral plus-strand RNA may explain the common failure to isolate infectious virus from heart muscle after the acute phase of virus replication, which, however, does not exclude the presence of very low infectivity titers.

Besides the strategy of restricted replication, viruses are known to establish persistence by infecting cellular constituents of the immune system itself [22–24]. A multiorgan study of infected animals indicated persistent infection of lymphoid cells from spleen and lymph nodes, in addition to heart muscle cells [25]. Acutely and persistently infected spleen cells were identified by the concurrent in situ detection of viral RNA and cell-specific antigens. During acute myocarditis, the majority of infected spleen cells which are primarily located within spleen follicles, were found to express CD45R/B220 (pre-B and B lymphocytes). Whereas viral RNA was also detected in some CD4$^+$ T-lymphocytes and CD11b-expressing macrophages, no enteroviral genomes were identified in CD8$^+$ T-cells. During chronic myocarditis, enteroviral infection was found to be restricted mainly in B lymphocytes of the germinal center of secondary spleen follicles. Thus, predominantly B lymphocytes may be involved in the dissemination of the virus and maintenance of a non-cardiac viral reservoir.

Virus–Receptor Interactions

Considering the complexity of organ systems, it is not surprising that molecular studies on virus–receptor interactions focus on in vitro models. Although cultured cells may express other surface proteins than tissue cells, almost all receptors for pathogenic viruses have been identified in cell culture models first and later proven to be expressed in human tissues. In contrast to in vivo studies, homogenous cell lines of human and animal origin allow the dissection of the various critical steps of virus–receptor interactions, such as virus binding, uptake of virus, replication, and virus release.

Several attempts have been made to identify putative cellular receptor proteins with a specificity for CVB. From infected HeLa cells, a virus–receptor complex was purified containing virus capsid proteins and a cellular protein of 50 kDa, which was suggested to be responsible for the recognition and binding of CVB [26]. Recently, Shafren et al. [27] reported that decay-accelerating factor (DAF/CD55), a membrane protein of 70 kDa, might be a cell attachment receptor for serotypes B1, B3, and B5 but not for serotypes B2, B4, and B6 of CVB. DAF-transfected murine fibroblast cells, however, did not support CVB infection, suggesting that the cell and tissue tropism of CVB is governed by the presence or absence of additional proteins [27]. These data suggest that the six serotypes of CVB may use several different membrane proteins for specific binding to the surface of host cells. However, competition assays with enteroviruses revealed that all six serotypes of CVB also compete for binding to a common CVB-specific receptor protein [28].

By using virus-overlay protein binding assays (VOPBA), we have identified a putative common CVB receptor protein of 100 kDa in CVB-permissive HeLa cells which is recognized by all six serotypes of CVB [29, 30]. Detergent-solubilized membrane proteins were separated on 7.5% SDS-polyacrylamide gels, electrotransferred onto membranes, partially renatured and exposed to ^{35}S-methionine-labeled CVB3 to detect CVB-specific binding proteins. Autoradiographs of CVB-VOPBAs with membrane proteins of cultured cell lines and human heart tissue are depicted in Fig. 1. As shown in Fig. 1A, the 100 kDa CVB-binding protein is not expressed on the cell surface of CVB-nonpermissive mouse fibroblast cells (LTK), but is expressed on human HeLa cells and mouse YAC-1 T-lymphoma cells, both of which are permissive towards CVB infection. Further studies on different cell lines revealed that productive infection with CVB strictly correlated with expression of this 100 kDa protein, in

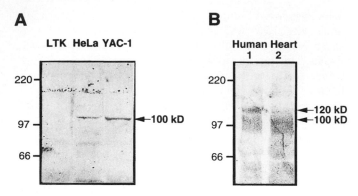

Fig. 1. Autoradiographs of two virus overlay protein binding assays (VOPBA) with ^{35}S-methionine-labeled CVB3. **A** Membrane proteins from CVB-permissive human (*HeLa*) and murine (*YAC-1*) cell lines and from CVB-nonpermissive mouse fibroblasts (*LTK*) were separated by SDS-PAGE, blotted onto PVDF membrane and subjected to a VOPBA. A CVB-specific receptor protein of 100 kDa was identified in the membrane fractions of HeLa and YAC-1 cells. **B** VOPBA with membrane proteins extracted from human myocardial tissue. *Lane 1,* Tissue of a donor heart; *Lane 2,* myocardial tissue of an autopsy heart. Specific binding of CVB was observed to membrane proteins in the range of 100 kDa to 120 kDa

contrast to the 50 kDa CVB-binding protein [26], which was observed only occasionally. Other radiolabeled enteroviruses, such as polioviruses and echoviruses, did not recognize this 100 kDa cell surface protein, whereas CVB3 competed with the other five CVB serotypes for binding. CVB-binding proteins similar to the 100 kDa CVB-specific protein present in CVB-permissive cell lines were detected in human heart muscle tissue (Fig. 1B).

Protein preparations of myocardial tissue from a human donor heart assigned but not used for heart transplantation revealed binding of radiolabelled CVB3 to a distinct protein of 120 kDa as well as to one or several proteins in the range of 100 kDa (Fig. 1B, lane 1). CVB-binding proteins with molecular weights of around 100 kDa were also detected among membrane proteins of myocardial tissue prepared from human autopsy hearts (Fig. 1B, lane 2), whereas binding of CVB to the 120 kDa protein was not observed with this protein preparation. Experiments are underway to determine the identity of these putative CVB receptor proteins from human heart muscle compared with the CVB-binding proteins identified in cultured cell lines of human and non-primate origin.

The functional activity of putative receptor proteins for human pathogenic enteroviruses can be measured by monitoring the products of specific virus–receptor interactions. Binding of CVB to specific cellular receptor proteins leads to a receptor-mediated conformational transition of the 160S virus particles and results in the formation of altered particles (135S-particles or A-particles) [31]. Such 135S A-particles, representing virus particles which have lost the viral capsid protein VP4 in the first step of virus uncoating, were detected in the cell culture supernatant of CVB3-infected HeLa and YAC-1 cell lines (Fig. 2) as well as after incubation of CVB3 with membrane proteins in the

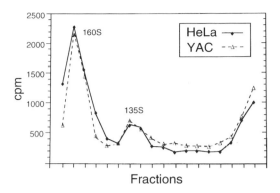

Fig. 2. Functional activity of CVB-specific cell surface receptors. HeLa and YAC-1 cell lines were infected with CVB3 at 37 °C, and cell culture supernatants containing virions and receptor-modified virus particles were overlaid onto a sucrose density gradient and fractionated from the bottom. Specific interactions of CVB virions (*160S* particles) with cellular receptor proteins resulted in the formation of receptor-modified CVB A-particles (*135 S* particles) in both CVB-permissive cell lines

range of 100 kDa. This confirms the presence of functional CVB receptor proteins with a molecular weight of about 100 kDa in human and murine CVB-permissive cell lines.

Tryptic fragments of the purified CVB-receptor protein from HeLa cells, subjected to an amino acid analysis, revealed consensus sequences between the 100 kDa CVB-binding membrane protein and a nuclear protein, nucleolin. Several different cell surface expressed homologues of nucleolin have recently been identified (summarized in [30]), and the 100 kDa CVB-binding protein is apparently a member of this protein family. Moreover, nucleolin-specific antibodies were able to immunoprecipitate the CVB-specific binding protein from membrane fractions of HeLa and YAC-1 cells, suggesting that a nucleolin-related membrane protein acts as a common receptor protein for the six serotypes of CVB.

The permissiveness of YAC-1 T-lymphoma cells towards infection with all six serotypes of CVB shows that not only myocardial cells but also a sub-population of cells of the immune system are potential targets for this group of viruses. Moreover, recent data indicate that the latter cells are involved in the dissemination of the virus in the organism and maintenance of a viral reservoir [25]. Since the 100 kDa CVB-binding protein is present on murine YAC-1 T-lymphoma cells, in human cell lines, and in murine as well as human myocardial tissue, these model systems facilitate the dissection of the various steps of virus–receptor interactions at the molecular level.

Tyrosine Phosphorylation Events in CVB3-Infected Cells

In order to study cellular and viral determinants of pathogenicity, we investigated the influence of CVB3 replication on tyrosine-phosphorylated proteins in cultured cell lines. During CVB3 infection of HeLa cells, certain proteins are either phosphorylated or dephosphorylated on tyrosine residues. These changes can be monitored by using anti-phosphotyrosine antibodies to probe Western blots.

Virus-induced tyrosine phosphorylation comprises early phosphorylation events, as a result of immediate signalling after virus–receptor interaction, as well as protein phosphorylation at later stages during infection. Binding of HIV gp120 protein to galactosyl-sulfatide receptors on CD4-negative brain cells, for example, leads to a rapid induction of tyrosine phosphorylation of proteins within seconds after virus–receptor interaction [32]. Such early signalling events, triggered by the virus–receptor interaction, were not observed with the enterovirus CVB3. Therefore, signals possibly leading to cellular dysfunction may require not only binding of CVB to surface receptors but also uptake of virions into the cell in addition to efficient virus replication.

To address the question of whether CVB infection impairs intracellular communication at later stages of infection, we examined the state of tyrosine phosphorylation of proteins during the course of CVB infection (Fig. 3). Up to 3 h post infection (p.i.), only subtle changes in the pattern of phosphorylated proteins were observed. A protein of about 100 kDa exhibited increased phosphorylation 1 h p.i., as did a protein of 65 kDa, which was hyperphosphorylated in the first 2 h p.i. Four hours p.i., the level of tyrosine-phosphorylated proteins was remarkably reduced as a result of the virus-induced shut-off of host cell protein synthesis; 6 h p.i., tyrosine-phosphorylated proteins were reduced to almost undetectable levels. In contrast to other phosphorylated proteins, the expression of two proteins of 70 kDa and 200 kDa was not impaired during the first 5 h p.i., suggesting that these proteins may be advantageous for early virus replication. However, 6 h p.i., when virus repli-

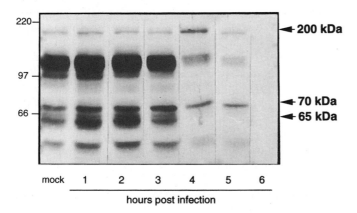

Fig. 3. Kinetics of tyrosine phosphorylation events during CVB3 infection of cultured human cells. To monitor the virus-induced host cell protein shut-off, postnuclear supernatants from CVB3- and mock-infected HeLa cells were prepared 1–6 h p.i. and subjected to SDS-PAGE and anti-phosphotyrosine immunoblotting. Phosphoproteins with molecular masses of 65 kDa, 70 kDa, and 200 kDa, which might be involved in viral pathogenesis, are indicated by *arrows*

cation reached maximum levels, these proteins were also targets of the virus-induced protein shut-off. Analysis of these tyrosine-phosphorylated proteins will allow the identification of cellular or viral proteins with regulatory functions involved in the pathogenesis of acute and chronic heart muscle infections.

Conclusions and Perspectives

Recombinant DNA techniques have allowed important breakthroughs to be made in the study of enterovirus genetics and have provided a basis for an etiologic diagnosis of myocardial enterovirus infection. In situ hybridization studies of endomyocardial biopsy specimens of patients have demonstrated that enterovirus infection is detectable in all stages of acute and chronic enterovirus myocarditis, indicating the possibility of enterovirus persistence in the human heart. In patients with acute onset of heart dilatation, the most dramatic manifestation of myocarditis apart from sudden death, the incidence of myocardial enterovirus infection was found to be approximately 30% [14]. Particularly intriguing is the discovery of a possible enterovirus persistence in chronic dilated cardiomyopathy, which may evolve from acute and chronic myocarditis.

Based on the finding in humans, we followed the natural course of CVB3-induced myocarditis in different immunocompetent mouse strains. The importance of viral replication in the pathogenesis of ongoing disease was underlined by the observation of a strong spatial and temporal correlation between viral replication and the development of myocardial lesions. Persistent heart muscle infection was found to be restricted at the level of genomic plus-strand RNA synthesis. Importantly, we found that the development of persistent heart muscle infection is not linked to the H-2 locus of the host. Despite prominent cell-mediated immune responses, the virus was found to be capable of evading the immunological surveillance in a host-dependent fashion, indicating that as yet unknown genetic determinants control the outcome of the disease. In addition to heart muscle cells, lymphoid cells, such as B lymphocytes, were identified as cellular targets of acute and persistent enterovirus infection. Infected cells of the immune system may represent a non-cardiac enteroviral reservoir.

At the molecular level of virus–receptor interactions, infection of cells of the immune system was studied in CVB-permissive murine YAC-1 T-lymphoma cells. As shown in this paper, similar cellular receptor proteins with molecular weights of 100 kDa were detected in murine YAC-1 and human HeLa cell lines. In HeLa cells, this CVB receptor protein was shown to serve as a common cellular receptor protein for all six serotypes of CVB and was identified as a nucleolin-related membrane protein. Evidence for a specific interaction of CVB with these CVB receptor proteins on HeLa and YAC-1 cells was provided by monitoring receptor-induced conformational changes of the virion leading to the first steps of virus uncoating.

Identification and characterization of CVB-specific receptors on the surface of cardiac myocytes is a major goal which has to be achieved to allow studies on the pathogenesis of enterovirus myocarditis, e.g. with regard to proposed receptor polymorphisms. Recently obtained results of experiments with human myocardial tissue indicate that CVB-infection of human cardiac myocytes is mediated by receptor proteins similar or identical to those detected in CVB-permissive cell lines. Further investigations are underway to determine if the putative receptor proteins of 100 kDa and 120 kDa in human hearts are differentially glycosylated forms of a single receptor protein or two independent virus-binding proteins.

In addition to adsorption of CVB to specific receptor proteins and receptor-mediated modification of the viral surface structure, internalization and replication of the virus are further prerequisites for infection by this group of viruses. Concerning virus replication, the state of tyrosine-phosphorylation of cellular proteins was used as a parameter to identify cellular proteins involved in the process of pathogenicity. Most prominent changes in tyrosine phosphorylation were observed with two proteins of 70 kDa and 200 kDa. Tyrosine phosphorylation events can only be studied in homogenous cell populations in vitro and the data obtained with human HeLa cells will have to be verified with isolated and cultured cardiomyocytes. However, subtle differences in phosphorylation events, either virus-induced or cell-mediated, may be crucial for the switch of acute to chronic stages of enterovirus myocarditis and dilated cardiomyopathy.

Apart from providing an etiologic diagnosis of myocardial infection, the in situ demonstration of myocardial enterovirus infection also has therapeutic implications. Clearly, corticosteroids are contraindicated in the presence of myocardial infection since increased viral replication and inhibition of the endogenous interferon system may follow their use. It is hoped that antiviral agents such as interferon may provide protection against the effects of myocardial enterovirus infection. The protective role of natural fibroblast interferon (IFN-β) in CVB3-infected cultured human heart cells has been described [33]. In addition, we have assessed the synergistic interaction between IFN-β and IFN-γ in persistently infected cultured human myocardial fibroblasts with regard to a low-dose combination treatment [34]. The relationship between the in vitro effects of interferons and their potential in vivo activities is currently being addressed in the murine model of chronic myocarditis to provide further information on the correct therapeutic use of exogenous interferons in this infection.

Acknowledgements. The work discussed in this paper was supported in part by the Fritz Thyssen Foundation, the Deutsche Forschungsgemeinschaft (DFG) and the "fortüne-Programm des Universitätsklinikums Tübingen".

References

1. Kandolf R (1988) The impact of recombinant DNA technology on the study of enterovirus heart disease. In: Bendinell M, Friedman H (eds) Coxsackieviruses - A general update. Plenum, New York, pp 293–318
2. McManus BM, Kandolf R (1991) Evolving concepts of cause, consequence, and control in myocarditis. Curr Opin Cardiol 6: 418–427
3. Martino T, Liu P, Sole MJ (1994) Viral infection and the pathogenesis of dilated cardiomyopathy. Circ Res 74: 182–188
4. Klump WM, Bergmann I, Müller C, Ameis D, Kandolf R (1990) Complete nucleotide sequence of infectious coxsackievirus B3 cDNA: Two initial 5 uridine residues are regained during RNA synthesis. J Virol 64: 1573–1583
5. Kandolf R, Hofschneider PH (1985) Molecular cloning of the genome of a cardiotropic coxsackie B3 virus: Full-length reverse-transcribed recombinant cDNA generates infectious virus in mammalian cells. Proc Natl Acad Sci USA 82: 4818–4822
6. Rückert RR (1990) Picornaviridae and their replication. In: Fields BN, Knipe DM (eds) Virology. Raven, New York, p 507
7. Kandolf R, Ameis D, Kirschner P, Canu A, Hofschneider PH (1987) In situ detection of enteroviral genomes in myocardial cells by nucleic acid hybridization: an approach to the diagnosis of viral heart disease. Proc Natl Acad Sci USA 84: 6272–6276
8. Kandolf R, Kirschner P, Ameis D, Canu A, Erdmann E, Schultheiss HP, Kemkes B, Hofschneider PH (1988) Enteroviral heart disease: Diagnosis by in situ hybridization. In: Schultheiss HP (ed) New concepts in viral heart disease. Springer, Berlin Heidelberg New York, pp 337–348
9. Tracy SM, Chapman NM, McManus BM, Pallansch MA, Beck MA, Carstens J (1990) A molecular and serologic evaluation of enteroviral involvement in human myocarditis. J Mol Cell Cardiol 22: 403–414
10. Foulis AK, Farquharson MA, Cameron SO, McGill M, Schönke H, Kandolf R (1990) A search for the presence of the enteroviral capsid protein VP1 in pancreas of patients with type 1 (insulin-dependent) diabetes and pancreases and hearts of infants who died of coxsackieviral myocarditis. Diabetologia 33: 290–298
11. Kandolf R, Hofschneider PH (1989) Viral heart disease. Springer Semin Immunopathol 11: 1–13
12. Klingel K, Hohenadl C, Canu A, Albrecht M, Seemann M, Mall G, Kandolf R (1992) Ongoing enterovirus-induced myocarditis is associated with persistent heart muscle infection: Quantitative analysis of virus replication, tissue damage, and inflammation. Proc Natl Acad Sci USA 89: 314–318
13. Jin O, Sole MJ, Butany JW, Chia WK, McLaughlin PR, Liu P, Liew CC (1990) Detection of enterovirus RNA in myocardial biopsies from patients with myocarditis and cardiomyopathy using gene amplification by polymerase chain reaction. Circulation 82: 8–16
14. Kandolf R, Klingel K, Zell R, Selinka H-C, Raab U, Schneider-Brachert W, Bültmann B (1993) Molecular pathogenesis of enterovirus-induced myocarditis: Virus persistence and chronic inflammation. Intervirology 35: 140–151
15. Kämmerer U, Kunkel B, Korn K (1994) Nested PCR for specific detection and rapid identification of human picornaviruses. J Clin Microbiol 32: 285–291
16. Huber SA, Job LP, Auld KR, Woodruff JF (1981) Sex-related differences in the rapid production of cytotoxic spleen cells active against uninfected myofibers during coxsackievirus B3 infection. J Immunol 126: 1336–1340
17. McManus BM, Gauntt CJ, Cassling RS (1987) Immunopathologic basis of myocardial injury. Cardiovasc Clin 18: 163–184
18. Tracy S, Chapman NM, Beck MA (1991) Molecular biology and pathogenesis of coxsackie B viruses. Rev Med Virol 1: 145–154
19. Gauntt C, Higdon A, Bowers D, Maull E, Wood J, Crawley R (1993) What lessons can be learned from animal model studies in viral heart disease? Scand J Infect Dis Suppl 88: 49–65

20. Hohenadl C, Klingel K, Mertsching J, Hofschneider PH, Kandolf R (1991) Strand-specific detection of enteroviral RNA in myocardial tissue by in situ hybridization. Mol Cell Probes 5: 1120
21. Werner S, Klump WM, Schönke H, Hofschneider PH, Kandolf R (1988) Expression of coxsackievirus B3 capsid proteins in Escherichia coli and generation of virus-specific antisera. DNA 7: 307–316
22. Matteuci D, Paglianti M, Giangregorio M, Capobianchi MR, Dianzani F, Bendinelli M (1985) Group B coxsackieviruses readily establish persistent infection in human lymphoid cell lines. J Virol 56: 651–654
23. Oldstone MBA (1989) Viral persistence. Cell 56: 517–520
24. Pomeroy C, Hilleren PJ, Jordan MC (1991) Latent murine cytomegalovirus DNA in splenic stromal cells of mice. J Virol 65: 3330–3334
25. Klingel K, McManus BM, Kandolf R (1995) Enterovirus-infected immune cells of spleen and lymph nodes in the murine model of chronic myocarditis: A role in pathogenesis? Eur Heart J 16 (Suppl O): 42–45
26. Mapoles JE, Krah DL, Crowell RL, Philipson L (1985) Purification of a HeLa cell receptor protein for group B coxsackieviruses. J Virol 55: 560–566
27. Shafren D, Bates RC, Agrez MV, Herd RL, Burns GF, Barry RD (1995) Coxsackievirus B1, B3, and B5 use decay accelerating factor as a receptor for cell attachment. J Virol 69: 3873–3877
28. Lonberg-Holm K, Crowell RL, Philipson L (1976) Unrelated animal viruses share receptors. Nature 259: 679–681
29. Selinka H-C, Raab de Verdugo U, Homann H, Zell R, Klingel K, Hofschneider PH, Kandolf R (1993) Molekulare Charakterisierung viraler Rezeptoren: Nachweis Coxsackievirus B3-bindender Proteine. Verh Dtsch Ges Path 77: 431
30. Raab de Verdugo U, Selinka H-C, Huber M, Kramer B, Kellermann J, Hofschneider PH, Kandolf R (1995) Characterization of a 100-kilodalton binding protein for the six serotypes of coxsackie B viruses. J Virol 69: 6751–6757
31. Crowell RL, Philipson L (1971) Specific alterations of coxsackievirus B3 eluted from HeLa cells. J Virol 8: 509–515
32. Schneider-Schaulies J, Schneider-Schaulies R, Brinkmann R, Tas P, Halbrügge M, Walter U, Holmes HC, TerMeulen V (1992) HIV-1 gp120 receptor on CD4-negative brain cells activates a tyrosine kinase. Virology 191: 765–772
33. Kandolf R, Canu A, Hofschneider PH (1985) Coxsackie B3 virus can replicate in cultured human foetal heart cells and is inhibited by interferon. J Mol Cell Cardiol 17: 167–181
34. Heim A, Canu A, Kirschner P, Simon T, Mall G, Hofschneider PH, Kandolf R (1992) Synergistic interaction of interferon-beta and interferon-gamma in coxsackievirus B3-infected carrier cultures of human myocardial fibroblasts. J Infect Dis 166: 958–965

Coxsackievirus Genetics and the Cardiovirulent Viral Phenotype

N. Chapman[1], S. Tracy[1], A. Ramsingh[2], J. Romero[3], K. Curry[4,5], B. Shapiro[5], W. Barry[6], T. Chin[7], and G. Hufnagel[8]

Introduction

The coxsackie B viruses are a group of typical human enteroviruses (family *Picornaviridae*) that are comprised of six serotypes (CVB1-6). The CVBs are common etiologic agents of childhood disease including inflammatory diseases of the heart muscle and of the central nervous system and are the cause of a significant amount of adult inflammatory heart muscle disease (Martino et al. 1995). Dilated cardiomyopathy (DCM) has been linked to enterovirus infection of the heart through a variety of evidence, including serological data as well as molecular detection of viral RNA in diseased heart tissue samples (Keeling and Tracy 1995). A survey of results from a variety of studies suggest that, on average, about 20%–25% of DCM hearts show enteroviral involvement on the basis of polymerase chain reaction (PCR) or in situ hybridization data (Martino et al. 1995). Thus, many cases of both acute myocarditis as well as DCM may be considered as infectious viral diseases.

DCM occurs about 5–8/100 000 in the population worldwide (Manolio et al. 1992). Thus, approximately 1–2 cases per 100 000 likely have an enteroviral (most likely CVB) etiology. In a country the size of the United States, this translates to approximately 2500–5000 cases per year of enteroviral DCM. Inclusion of the number of childhood enteroviral heart disease cases as well as the number of adult acute myocarditis cases would increase this number substantially. This number may be better put in perspective by comparison to

[1]Department of Pathology and Microbiology, University of Nebraska Medical Center, Omaha, NE 68198, USA
[2]David Axelrod Institute, Wadsworth Center, New York State Department of Health, Albany, NY 12201, USA
[3]Combined Division of Pediatric and Infectious Disease, Creighton University/University of Nebraska Medical Center, Omaha, NE 68198, USA
[4]Sudden Infant Death Syndrome and Division of Child Neurology, Department of Pediatrics, University of Maryland, Baltimore, MD 21201, USA
[5]Laboratory of Mathematical Biology, DCBDC, Frederick Cancer Research and Development Center, National Cancer Institute, Frederick, MD 21702, USA
[6]Cardiology Division, University of Utah Medical Center, Salt Lake City, UT 84132, USA
[7]Pediatric Cardiology Division, University of Utah Medical Center, Salt Lake City, UT 84113, USA
[8]Abteilung für Innere Medizin – Kardiologie, Klinikum der Philipps-Universität, 35043 Marburg, Germany

another infectious agent, HIV. The Director of the President's Office of National AIDS Policy reported in 1995 that about 71 000 new HIV infections occur per year in the United States. The number of enteroviral heart disease cases in the United States thus approaches 5%–10% of this case load.

There are at present no vaccines against any human enterovirus other than the polioviruses. It is vital to bear in mind that coxsackieviral heart disease is an infectious disease. Because of the similarity of the CVBs to the polioviruses, and due to the precedent of the highly effective anti-poliovirus vaccines, CVB diseases could be eradicated through a concerted vaccination effort. However, anti-CVB vaccines are not likely to be developed in the near future, due primarily to cutbacks in health care funding worldwide as well as the widespread perception in the vaccine industry of an insufficient market. While deemed a potentially more profitable avenue for development by industry, efficacious anti-enteroviral drugs are as yet in developmental infancy. We have been working to understand the genetics behind, and mechanisms of, the expression of the viral cardiovirulence phenotype of the CVBs in order to lay the groundwork on which it is hoped the rapid development of anti-enteroviral vaccines and/or drugs may occur in the future.

Coxsackievirus B3

Coxsackievirus B3 (CVB3) is one of the CVBs which has been demonstrated to be a cause of human heart disease. Furthermore, much effort has been expended to provide elegant murine models of CVB3 infection to study both acute and chronic CVB3 inflammatory heart disease (Gauntt et al. 1989, Leslie et al. 1989). To date, three published reports exist of infectious cDNA copies of CVB3 genomes have been cloned, sequenced and characterized (Klump et al. 1990, Tracy et al. 1992, Chapman et al. 1994). The viral genome is typical of human enteroviruses (Fig. 1). The genome is a single molecule of linear, positive (or message) sense RNA 7,400 nucleotides long, polyadenylated at the 3′ terminus. The 5′ terminus is not capped but is covalently bound with a small virus encoded protein called VPg (protein 3B, Fig. 1). The single long open

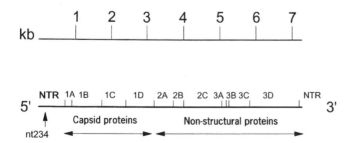

Fig. 1. Schematic outline of a CVB genome. Location of coding regions are shown approximately to scale. Approximate location of the nucleotide 234 is indicated by an arrow. *kb*, kilobase; *NTR*, non-translated region

reading frame (ORF) is flanked by a 5' non-translated region (NTR) comprising 10% of the genome and a much shorter 3' NTR. The ORF codes for 11 viral proteins, four of which are capsid proteins. Replication of the virus is cytoplasmic. CVBs have been demonstrated to replicate in fibroblasts, endothelial cells and myocytes of the heart.

The structure of the virion has been solved to a resolution of 3.5 Å (Muckelbauer et al. 1995) showing many features now known to be typical of the enterovirus capsid, including very evident five-, three-, and two-fold symmetries and the presence of a deep depression which surrounds each of the 12 five-fold axes of symmetry. These depressions, termed canyons, are the likely site for the binding of the cellular receptor; this has been demonstrated for both the related polio- and human rhinoviruses (Chapman and Rossman 1993). As yet, the nature and identity of the CVB receptor is not known; reports have suggested the receptor is variously 50–55 kDa (Mapoles et al. 1985) or 100 kDa (de Verdugo et al. 1995). Human CD55 has been shown able to bind virus but not act as a true receptor (Bergelson et al. 1995).

Attenuation of a Cardiovirulent Phenotype via a Transcriptional Mechanism

Comparing the sequences of two infectious clones of a cardiovirulent CVB3 strain and a non-cardiovirulent CVB3 strain (Klump et al. 1990, Tracy et al. 1992, Chapman et al. 1994), we identified ten genetic sites which changed as a function of the cardiovirulence phenotype (Chapman et al. 1994). To determine which of these sites determined the phenotype, we constructed chimeric viruses by replacing segments of the non-cardiovirulent CVB3 cDNA clone with the homologous segments from the cardiovirulent CVB3 genome containing the different genetic sites. The chimeric cDNA genomes were used to generate progeny virus through transfection of cell cultures. The progeny chimeric CVB3 strains were then assayed in a well-characterized murine model of CVB3 acute inflammatory heart disease (Tracy et al. 1992) to determine which of the substitutions had resulted in switching the non-cardiovirulent parental phenotype to a cardiovirulent phenotype. Of the ten sites originally identified as potential effectors of the cardiovirulence phenotype, only one showed any effect upon the phenotype. The one site was nucleotide 234 (where nucleotide [nt] 1 is the 5' terminal nt of the genome; Figs. 1 and 2) in the 5' NTR. Nucleotide 234 was U in the cardiovirulent strain CVB3/20 and C in the non-cardiovirulent strain CVB3/0. Reconstruction of the chimeric virus back to the parental non-cardiovirulent strain restored the parental non-cardiovirulent phenotype, confirming the site's importance to the phenotype determination.

We then asked whether this single transition affected the higher order structure of the viral RNA. Examination of the location of nt234 in consensus structures (Le and Zucker 1990) of the viral 5 NTR showed nt234 to be between two significant secondary (stem/loop) structures but not within any significant higher-order structure as had been well demonstrated for the single sites which affect poliovirus neurovirulence (Minor 1993). We looked more specifically at this site using two different RNA folding algorithms (Tu et al. 1995) and

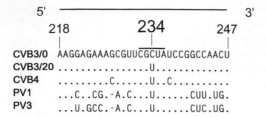

Fig. 2. Alignments of enteroviral sequences across the region encompassing nucleotide 234. Shown are nucleotides 218–234 in 5' to 3' orientation using nomenclature described in the text and in Chapman et al. 1994 and Tracy et al. 1992. The five nucleotide conserved sequence surrounding nucleotide 234 is demarcated by a line. Periods signify identical sequence to reference sequence on first line (CVB3/0). Dashes are deletions relative to reference sequence. CVB4, PV1 and PV3 sequences abstracted from GenBank listings

determined that the site could be involved in transient base-pairing at frequencies more than 50% of the time. Although these findings have to be tested biochemically, they nonetheless suggested grounds for the effect of the C/U transition.

How does the transition effect the phenotype switch? Using murine fetal heart fibroblasts and murine adult cardiomyocytes (Tu et al. 1995) as well as human heart fibroblasts in cell culture (S. Tracy, T. Chin, unpublished data), we inoculated cells either with viruses expressing nt234U or C and determined virus yields, and assayed viral translation and transcription. In heart cells, yields of non-virulent strains (nt234C) were lower than those of virulent strains (nt234U). Viral translation was indistinguishable by SDS-PAGE analysis. However, and to our surprise, the effect of the transition was evident at the level of viral RNA transcription (Tu et al. 1995). Nucleotide 234C caused slower rates and lower yields of viral RNA in heart cells than nt234U.

Attenuation Elsewhere in the CVB3 5' NTR

The mechanism of transcriptional attenuation of CVB3 cardiovirulence was not complete, however, with this work (Tu et al. 1995). We examined RNA sequences numerous wild-type CVB3 strains, both cardiovirulent and avirulent in mice, and noted that all strains, regardless of the phenotype, expressed nt234U. Figure 2 shows such an alignment using for illustrative purposes just a few enterovirus sequences. Furthermore, all other enteroviruses expressed nt234U. Nucleotide 234 was never seen as C. Sequence comparison analysis demonstrated as well a highly-conserved 5mer surrounding nt234, suggesting some grounds for its conservation in all enteroviruses (Fig. 2). If all CVB3 strains expressed nt234U, the finding of nt234C in the genome of CVB3/0 (Tu et al. 1995) must mean that CVB3/0 strain was a mutant, attenuated for cardiovirulence through a transcriptional mechanism based on the expression of nt234C. It also implied that another mechanism(s) determining the virulence phenotype must be in play in nature.

Is this other site in the 5' NTR or elsewhere? To begin to answer this question, wild type strains of CVB3 were tested in murine heart fibroblasts cultures. As before, we observed that yields of virus varied as a function of the phenotype, with lower yields associated with the avirulent strains of virus. Examination of protein translation and RNA transcription as before also showed no difference at the level of translation but a significantly lower transcriptional efficiency for avirulent strains. Even though all strains expressed nt234U, there was still a transcriptional phenotype observed. In experiments still in progress, we have demonstrated that the construction of a chimeric virus by the substitution of the 5' NTR from a non-cardiovirulent CVB3 strain (nt234U) into the CVB3/0 genome results in a non-cardiovirulent phenotype in mice with a lowered transcriptional efficiency in heart cell cultures. As we know that there are not sites downstream of the 5' NTR substitution which control the phenotype, the phenotype must be affected by some site(s) within the 5' NTR of the non-cardiovirulent donor CVB3 strain. This is now being mapped.

Other Studies on CVB3 Cardiovirulence

One other report has investigated the genetics of CVB3 cardiovirulence (Zhang et al. 1993). A cardiovirulent strain of CVB3 was passaged in cell culture numerous times. The resultant virus was significantly attenuated for cardio virulence in a mouse model. The 5' NTR of this attenuated virus strain was sequenced and the single difference which was found was located at 690. This 5' NTR was then substituted for the parental 5' NTR in a chimeric cDNA construct, and progeny virus obtained. When tested in mice, these progeny viruses were as virulent as the parental strain. Thus, these experiments suggest that in this system, the site(s) affecting cardiovirulence do not lie in the 5' NTR but must be somewhere downstream.

In unpublished data discussed at this Symposium (S. Huber), an attenuated CVB3 strain has been sequenced along with the genome of the parental cardiovirulent strain. The single significant difference has been mapped to a region of the capsid protein 1B (VP2) which is exposed on the virion surface, called the E-F loop or VP2 puff. These authors have shown that the attenuated strain induces a Th2 type cytokine response in murine macrophages whereas the cardiovirulent strain induces a Th1 type cytokine response (Huber et al. 1994).

Coxsackievirus B4 Cardiovirulence

Also an established agent of human inflammatory heart disease, coxsackievirus B4 (CVB4) serves more as a model for enteroviral pancreatitis and possibly type 1 diabetes. Chimeric CVB4 strains containing sequences from a pancreovirulent CVB4 strain have been used to locate and identify the viral genetic determinants of murine pancreovirulence (Caggana et al. 1993). Amino acid position 129 (methionine in the avirulent parental strain genome, threonine in the virulent) lies within the exterior D-E loop of capsid protein 1D and is to date the primary site which determines CVB4 pancreatic virulence (Caggana et al. 1993). It is possible that this site is in a location which represents an antigenic epitope recognized by the host cell-mediated immune (CMI) or is presented to B cells as an antigen for an antibody response.

In preliminary studies (S. Tracy, A. Ramsingh, unpublished data), these same chimeric CVB4 strains were used to determine the cardiovirulence phenotype in C3H/HeJ mice, an inbred strain of mouse which is exquisitely sensitive to CVB-induced heart disease. The pancreovirulent CVB4 strain causes significant inflammatory lesions in mouse hearts, while the CVB4 parental strain is non-cardiovirulent. The pancreovirulent chimeric virus, containing thr-129 in the capsid protein 1D on the avirulent background, also is cardiovirulent, thus mapping a site which influences the viral cardiovirulence phenotype in mice. It is intriguing to consider the possibility that these data show a common viral genetic site which operates via a common mechanism to induce inflammatory disease in different organs in mice.

Summary

The CVBs are clearly established etiologic agents of human inflammatory heart disease. This confirmation has been derived primarily from cases of pediatric or neonatal myocarditis in which the virus has been actually isolated from the diseased heart and grown in the laboratory. Recently, a limited outbreak of CVB2 occurred in Omaha NE, which was responsible for the death of one infant, necessitated heart transplantation in another, and seriously involved either liver or the central nervous system in five other children. In this outbreak alone, two hearts were effectively destroyed, resulting in one death and necessitating one transplant. Adult myocarditis and dilated cardiomyopathy is more difficult to pin on the CVBs as infectious virus is rarely isolated from these tissues. However, the evidence is clear from numerous molecular studies that enteroviruses infect approximately 20%–25% of hearts with biopsy-proven myocarditis or DCM.

It is well worth noting that adenoviruses as well have recently been shown to be a significant etiologic presence in pediatric heart disease (Martin et al. 1994). In this study, adenoviruses were detected more frequently than enteroviruses. It will be very interesting to follow this story as it is confirmed and extended.

To date, the mechanisms by which CVBs induce disease have been shown to be related to viral transcription as well as to the expression of specific amino acids on external loops of the viral capsid proteins. These mechanisms are by no means mutually exclusive but do suggest that further work is needed to determine whether primarily a single mechanism is employed by the CVBs, as has been demonstrated for polioviruses and neurovirulence (Minor 1993), or whether more than one primary mechanism is at work. At present, we can only speculate. In the cases where capsid protein changes have been demonstrated to effect virulence phenotype changes (Caggana et al. 1993, Huber et al. 1994), both virus systems have employed either cell culture or mouse passage to derive a phenotype change in the parental virus. In the case where viral RNA transcription has been demonstrated (Tu et al. 1995), the viruses were different isolates and our early work also suggests the phenotypes of other wild type strains vary with the efficiency of viral RNA transcription. Again, further work now in progress in several laboratories will clarify this question.

Enteroviral inflammatory heart muscle disease is defined by the cell-mediated immune response to the viral insult. Work from Huber's group has demonstrated that CMI response plays a key role in causing and determining the extent of disease. However, scid mice also develop raging myocarditis following inoculation with a cardiovirulent CVB3 strain (Chow et al. 1992). This inflammation is dominated by macrophagic infiltration as might be expected in a functional T and B cell deficient host. These results strongly suggest that virus-induced lysis of cardiomyocytes plays the significant role in this case. A pathogenic mechanism which involves both the lysis of target cells by the virus and a vigorous host immune response against such infected target cells is clearly indicated. The questions which now must be addressed are the steps which occur during the infection and subsequent inflammatory response. These are important issues, for from such answers may well come modalities by which enteroviral heart disease might be treated.

The murine model of CVB3 acute myocarditis and dilated cardiomyopathy has also demonstrated the effect of the host genetic background in development of specific diseases as well as in the severity of the disease induced by the virus. In addition, gender has been shown to play a role, with males affected somewhat more than females. Age, too, comes into play, with younger mice more susceptible to severe disease, even death, caused by CVB3. It is likely these factors are in large part immunologically-based as well.

Viral inflammatory heart disease is a significant infectious disease with a complicated pathogenesis. Understanding of the viral genetics which form the primary insult to the host is key to the understanding of how the virus induces the disease.

References

Bergelson JM, Mohanty JG, Crowell RL, St. John NF, Lublin DM, Finberg RW (1995) Coxsackievirus B3 adapted to growth in RD cells binds to decay-accelerating factor (CD55). J Virol 69: 1903–1906

Caggana M, Chan P, Ramsingh A (1993) Identification of a single amino acid residue in the capsid protein VP1 of coxsackievirus B4 that determines the virulent phenotype. J Virol 67: 4797–4803

Chapman MS, Rossmann MG (1993) Comparison of surface properties of picornaviruses: strategies for hiding the receptor site from immune surveillance. Virology 195: 745–756

Chapman NM, Tu Z, Tracy S, Gauntt CJ (1994) An infectious cDNA copy of the genome of a non-cardiovirulent coxsackievirus B3 strain: its complete sequence analysis and comparison to the genomes of cardiovirulent coxsackieviruses. Arch Virol 135: 115–130

Chow LH, Beisel KW, McManus BM (1992) Enteroviral infection of mice with severe combined immunodeficiency. Evidence for direct viral pathogenesis of myocardial injury. Lab Invest 66: 24–31 de Verdugo UR, Selinka HC, Huber M, Kramer B, Kellerman J, Hofschnieder PH, Kandolf R (1995) Characterization of a 100-kilodalton binding protein for the six serotypes of coxsackie B viruses. J Virol 69: 6751–6757

Gauntt CJ, Godeny EK, Lutton CW, Arizpe HM, Chapman NM, Tracy SM, Revtyak GE, Valente AJ, Rozek MM (1989) Mechanism(s) of coxsackievirus-induced acute myocarditis in the mouse. In: de la Maza, Peterson EM (eds) Medical virology 8. Plenum, New York, London, p 161

Huber SA, Polgar J, Schultheiss P, Schwimmbeck P (1994) Augmentation of pathogenesis of coxsackievirus B3 infections in mice by exogenous administration of interleukin-1 and interleukin-2. J Virol 68: 195–206

Keeling PJ, Tracy S (1995) Link between enteroviruses and dilated cardiomyopathy: serological and molecular data. Br Heart J 72: S25–S29

Klump WM, Bergmann I, Muller BC, Ameis D, Kandolf R (1990) Complete nucleotide sequence of infectious Coxsackievirus B3 cDNA: two initial 5' uridine residues are regained during plus-strand RNA synthesis. J Virol 64: 1573–1583

Le SY, Zuker M (1990) Common structures of the 5' non-coding RNA in enteroviruses and rhinoviruses. Thermodynamical stability and statistical significance. J Mol Biol 216: 729–741

Leslie K, Blay R, Haisch C, Lodge A, Weller A, Huber S (1989) Clinical and experimental aspects of viral myocarditis. Clin Microbiol Rev 2: 191–203

Manolio TA, Baughman KL, Rodeheffer R, Pearson TA, Bristow JD, Michels VV, Abelmann WH, Harlan WR (1992) Prevalence and etiology of idiopathic dilated cardiomyopathy. Am J Cardiol 69: 1458–1466

Mapoles JE, Krah DL, Crowell RL (1985) Purification of a HeLa cell receptor protein for group B coxsackieviruses. J Virol 55: 560–566

Martin AB, Webber S, Fricker FJ, Jaffe R, Demmler G, Kearney D, Zhang YH, Bodurtha J, Gelb B, Ni J, Bricker JT, Towbin JA (1994) Acute myocarditis. Rapid diagnosis by PCR in children. Circulation 90: 330–339

Martino TA, Liu P, Petric M, Sole MJ (1995) Enteroviral myocarditis and dilated cardiomyopathy: a review of clinical and experimental studies. In: Rotbart HA (ed) Human enterovirus infections. ASM, Washington D.C., p 291

Minor P (1993) Attenuation and reversion of the Sabin vaccine strains of poliovirus. Develop Biol Stand 78: 17–26

Muckelbauer JK, Kremer MK, Minor I, Diana G, Dutko FJ, Groarke J, Pevear DC, Rossmann MG (1995) The structure of coxsackievirus B3 at 3.5 Å resolution. Structure 3: 653–667

Tracy S, Chapman NM, Tu Z (1992) Coxsackievirus B3 from an infectious cDNA copy of the genome is cardiovirulent in mice. Arch Virol 122: 399–409

Tu Z, Chapman NM, Hufnagel G, Tracy S, Romero JR, Barry WH, Zhao L, Currey K, Shapiro B (1995) The cardiovirulent phenotype of coxsackievirus B3 is determined at a single site in the genomic 5' nontranslated region. J Virol 69: 4607–4618

Zhang HY, Yousef GE, Cunningham L, Blake NW, OuYang X, Bayston TA, Kandolf R, Archard LC (1993) Attenuation of a reactivated cardiovirulent coxsackievirus B3: The 5'-nontranslated region does not contain major attenuation determinants. J Med Virol 41: 129–137

Lessons from Animal Models of Viral Myocarditis

S.A. Huber[1], B.B. Hamrell[2], and K.U. Knowlton[3]

Introduction

Enteroviruses have been identified through in situ hybridization techniques in biopsies from up to 50% of myocarditis and 30% of dilated cardiomyopathy patients [1–3]. The prevalence of viral genomic material in the heart implies an etiological role for enteroviruses in the disease process. A major controversy, however, is whether the virus is the predominant pathogenic element in the disease, or whether the virus acts primarily as a trigger for the induction of immunopathogenic (either autoimmune or virus-immune) myocyte injury. The answer to this question impacts directly on the development of effective therapies for myocarditis and dilated cardiomyopathy.

Murine models of coxsackievirus and encephalomyocarditis virus-induced myocarditis have been developed over the last 30–40 years in an attempt to elucidate the major pathogenic mechanisms in myocarditis and dilated cardiomyopathy [4–10]. These models are additionally used to identify therapies with potential clinical relevance for these diseases [11–15]. Many clinicians reviewing the experimental myocarditis literature might feel that the results are both disappointing and confusing. Although most studies primarily implicate one or more immunopathogenic disease processes, several impressive studies conclude that virus infection of cardiac myocytes results in cellular necrosis and the host immune response is primarily protective [16, 17]. Furthermore, a single therapy, such as immunosuppression, may be both beneficial and highly detrimental to the animal host depending upon either the experimental model used or the time the therapy is initiated relative to infection [12].

Why Develop Animal Models of Human Diseases?

Studying myocarditis and dilated cardiomyopathy in humans is complicated. Myocarditis is difficult to distinguish from other types of cardiac disease since the symptoms are relatively nonspecific. Indeed, the high incidence (usually

[1]Department of Pathology, University of Vermont, Burlington, VT 05405, USA
[2]Department of Physiology and Biophysics, University of Vermont, Burlington, VT 05405, USA.
[3]Department of Medicine, University of California, San Diego, CA, USA.

2%–5%) of "myocarditis" in large, sequential autopsy studies implies that the disease may be relatively common but largely subclinical [4]. Even when myocarditis can be clearly documented, it is difficult to establish the precise onset of the disease, or the relevant etiological agent since many different agents, including a variety of DNA and RNA viruses, protozoa, bacteria and drugs (hypersensitivity reactions), might be involved [4]. Adding to these problems is the genetic and physiological complexity of the patient population. Sex, age, pregnancy and exercise are all factors that may influence either the incidence, severity or outcome of clinical myocarditis [4]. For these reasons, animal models have been established in order to evaluate pathogenic mechanisms and potential therapies.

Animal models are also open to criticism, however. To establish a model, investigators restrict the number of variables and purposely select only a limited number of factors to study at any one time. Restricting the number of variables makes it easier to evaluate how any one factor influences the disease, but also makes it difficult to determine how well the carefully-selected animal model reflects the processes occurring in the far more complex human population. Another reality is that the experimental scientist may be most interested in elucidating basic scientific concepts in immunology, virology or physiology in an animal model. A basic understanding of cellular and intracellular pathophysiology of disease eventually results in important advances in clinically relevant knowledge [18]. The basic scientists' emphasis on potential long-term results and clinicians' interest in more immediate useful information may make it appear that the goals of the basic and clinical scientists are dissimilar. Despite the above problems, animal models can still be powerful tools for understanding clinical myocarditis, provided proper caution is used in evaluating animal-based studies.

Animal Models of Coxsackieviral Myocarditis

The most thoroughly, and frequently studied animal models of myocarditis employ coxsackievirus B3 as the etiological agent. For this reason, the discussions will center on these models.

The Coxsackieviruses

Nearly all experimental CVB3 models use the "Nancy" strain of the virus. While this means that, originally, all such CVB3 must have had a common ancestor isolated from the patient "Nancy", the history of the various virus variants, when they separated, and how often they were passaged in the different experimental laboratories during the time from separation until now is often obscure. Yet, these details can have profound effects on how the various CVB3 variants cause myocarditis in experimental models. RNA viruses are known to have a very high mutation rate and, up to 1 in 100 picornavirus particles may contain a mutation [19]. This means that picornaviruses may quickly develop "genetic drift" and alter characteristics of the virus within even one or two virus passages. In unpublished studies, we compared CVB3 passaged through either HeLa, Hep-2 or Green Monkey kidney cells and found that the type of cell line used to grow the virus could impact the incidence and severity of myocarditis induced in Balb/c mice and whether there was immune or direct virus-mediated myocyte lysis. Similarly, the organ source of the cells used to isolate the virus can dramatically affect both the tissue tropism of CVB3 and pathogenesis of the infection [20]. The "Woodruff" CVB3 Nancy has been cloned and sequenced in the laboratory of one of the authors (K.U.K.) and compared to the published sequence of the CVB3 Nancy virus cloned and sequenced in the laboratory of Kandolf [21]. The number of nucleotide differences between these two CVB3 Nancy strains for each region of the genome is given in Table 1. Clearly, substantial nucleotide differences exist between these two CVB3 variants that may influence how these viruses cause disease. Currently, comparisons are being done of this virus variant with other published CVB3 sequences.

These observations indicate that not all CVB3 Nancy viruses are the same. Care needs to be taken in comparing studies among laboratories since genetic drift in the CVB3 viruses may explain any divergent results. This difficulty should be largely eliminated once infectious cDNAs of the major CVB3 Nancy variants are available, due to the substantially greater genetic stability of the cDNA clones.

Table 1. Comparison of nucleotide changes between Kandolf and Woodruff CVB3 Nancy variants[a]

Genomic region	Nucleotide number	Number of nucleotides	Number of nucleotide changes between Woodruff and Kandolf CVB3 Nancy variants[b]	
5'NTR	1–779	779	25	(3)
VP4	780–948	168	9	(5)
VP2	949–1738	789	32	(4)
VP3	1739–3452	713	30	(4)
VP1	2453–3304	851	33	(4)
2A	3305–3475	440	13	(3)
2B	3746–4042	296	15	(5)
2C	4043–5029	986	137	(14)
3A	5030–5296	266	35	(13)
3B	5297–5362	65	8	(12)
3C	5363–5911	548	76	(14)
3D	5912–7297	1385	201	(15)
3' NTR	7298–7400	102	10	(10)

[a]All base sequence changes. These data do not show whether the change results in an amino acid difference or whether any amino acid differences would be conserved.
[b]Percent of nucleotides for each region of the genome which differ between Kandolf and Woodruff variants.

The Relationship Between Myocarditis and Dilated Cardiomyopathy

Myocyte injury may result from either direct virus infection of the cells or the host defense responses resulting from the infection [4, 22–28]. Immunopathogenic mechanisms can be further divided into killing of infected cardiocytes through recognition of viral antigens expressed on the cardiocyte surface, inadvertent myocyte injury/death/dysfunction due to mediators (cytokines, nitric oxide, etc.) released in the heart during the inflammatory response, and induction of autoimmunity to cellular or extracellular matrix proteins as a consequence of the infection. Several excellent reviews [22–28] are available delineating the different immunopathogenic mechanisms in experimental myocarditis and therefore, an additional review of this literature will not be attempted here. Rather, we wish to discuss (a) what the relative contributions of virus and immune-mediated myolysis in experimental and clinical myocarditis are, and (b) are any of the experimental myocarditis models also models for dilated cardiomyopathy?

Woodruff and Woodruff [29] reported that T-cell-depletion of CVB3-infected mice substantially reduced myocardial inflammation and necrosis. Woodruff [30], using the same model, showed that CVB3-infected mice treated with cortisone developed severe myolysis accompanied by 100 to 10,000-fold increases in cardiac virus titers without evident myocardial inflammation. Selective elimination of T lymphocytes in this model had little effect on viral titers in the heart, presumably because various host defense mechanisms, such as virus-neutralizing antibody, activated macrophage and natural killer (NK) cells, remain active in the T-cell-deficient mice [29, 31]. In cortisone treated mice and in CVB3-infected SCID mice, which also develop severe myolysis with exacerbated cardiac virus titers [16], these virus-controlling host defense responses would be compromised, and could result in far more direct virus pathogenesis than in animals with intact virus-regulating defense mechanisms. Further studies by both Herzum et al. [32] and Knowlton et al. (unpublished observations) have shown that CVB3 infection of cultured myocytes also results in cell death. Again, in tissue culture, many of the infection-controlling responses of "normal" mice will be absent. Therefore, while there is little doubt that CVB3 infections can be highly pathogenic both in vivo and in vitro under specific circumstances, there remains the question of how much of the myocardial damage occurring during myocarditis in immunocompetent mice is virally mediated.

This question is very difficult to answer. Virus-induced myocyte injury can be subtle and not easily seen histologically while elimination of inflammatory cells is far more obvious. One possible indicator of direct virus-mediated myolysis in the heart is the presence of hypereosinophilic myocytes, which might represent necrotic myocytes [4, 16, 29–31]. Woodruff felt that these hypereosinophilic myocytes must be viewed with a certain amount of caution since such hypereosinophilic myocytes can also result from fixation artifact (personal communication). Myocytes that are weakened and damaged by infection might normally still survive in the body, but succumb more easily to ischemic death during tissue retrieval and fixation than uninfected, neighboring cells. Nonetheless, these hypereosinophilic myocytes are at least one indication that both virus and host factors probably contribute to tissue damage in viral myocarditis.

The virus, through its effects on cellular metabolism, might also disrupt myocyte function without requiring myolysis. Various laboratories have demonstrated that sera from myocarditis/dilated cardiomyopathy patients can cause physiological changes in cultured myocytes [33–39]. We investigated whether the virus altered the velocity of sarcomere shortening of isolated papillary muscles from both immunocompetent and T-cell-depleted Balb/c mice infected with CVB3 (Table 2) [40, 41]. Infected immunocompetent mice showed dramatic reductions in shortening velocities with a shift in myosin isoform expression from the fast to slow forms and the expression of atrial natriuretic factor (ANF) mRNA in left ventricular myocardium whereas, T-cell-deficient mice showed apparently normal function [41]. Although these results confirm a role of T-cell-dependent mechanisms in pathogenesis, they cannot disprove a role for direct virus-mediated injury. Other experimental approaches measuring different aspects of myocyte function, or employing different CVB3 variants, may show direct virus-mediated pathogenicity in vivo.

An important concern about the various experimental models of myocarditis relates to how well they mimic the functional and molecular alterations that occur with dilated cardiomyopathy in humans. Since clinical myocarditis is a relatively rare disease, identification of an experimental model of CVB3 infection with characteristics of well-documented dilated cardiomyopathy would be quite useful. Several groups report apparent cardiac hypertrophy with increases in heart:body weight ratios [42]. However, the hallmark of cardiomyopathy is a decrease in ventricular contractility. This is usually accompanied by a shift toward the embryonic program of gene expression in the ventricle. This can be seen in humans and rodents as an increase in ANF mRNA, and in rodents as a shift in myosin isoforms [43]. As shown above, we find decreased Vo in myocarditic hearts with a dramatic shift in ventricular myosin isoform expression, and an increase in ANF mRNA. All of these

Table 2. Changes in unloaded shortening velocity, predominant myosin isozyme and ventricular atrial natriuretic factor expression with virus infection in differing immunological settings

	Normal	Infected, immunocompetent Balb/c	Infected, T-Cell depleted Balb/c	Infected, immunocompetent DBA/2
V_0 (Tm/s, "1SD)	4.14"0.84	1.70"0.33	4.75"0.96	4.74"1.49
Predominant myosin isozyme	Fast	Slow	ND	ND
Ventricular ANF mRNA expression	Absent	Present	ND	Absent

ANF, atrial natriuretic factor; ND, not determined; Tm/s, "1SD

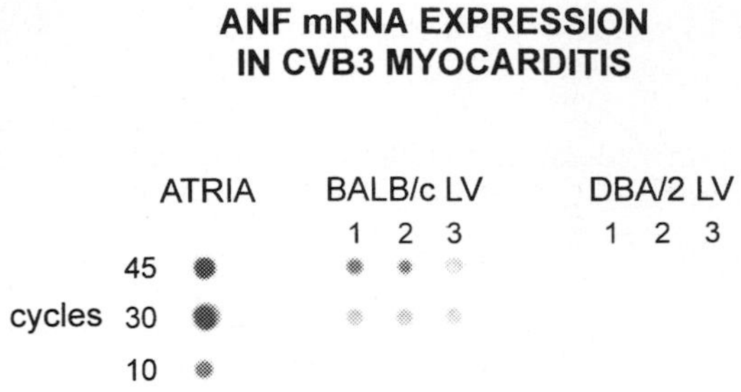

ANF mRNA EXPRESSION
IN CVB3 MYOCARDITIS

Fig. 1. ANF mRNA expression in left ventricle of CVB3-infected Balb/c and DBA/2 mice. Male mice were injected ip with 10^4 PFU CVB3 and killed 7 days later. RNA was extracted from the left ventricles of individual animals and subjected to RT-PCR amplification using 3' and 5' ANF nucleotide primers and the Gibco BRL superscript preamplification system for first strand cDNA synthesis and Taq polymerase (Gibco BRL) for amplification. Aliquots of the amplification product were removed after various cycles, blotted onto nylon membranes (Durolon-UV membranes, Stratagene), fixed with UV light and hybridized with the ANF cDNA probe labelled with Fluor-12-dUTP using the Illuminator nonradioactive detection system and the Prime-It Fluor fluorescent labeling kit from Stratagene according to manufacturer's directions

findings are consistent with a CVB3-induced impairment and ventricular function similar to that seen in cardiomyopathy in humans and in other models of heart failure. One interesting observation is that not all murine myocarditis models show these signs. We have previously published that different inbred strains of mice may develop myocarditis through distinct pathogenic mechanisms [44]. Thus, Balb/c and DBA/2 mice develop equivalent amounts of cardiac inflammation, but myocarditis, in the former strain, is exclusively due to cellular immunity and, in the latter strain, is exclusively due to humoral immunity. Preliminary studies shown in Table 2 and Fig. 1 demonstrate that myocarditis in DBA/2 mice does not result in decreased V_o or increased ANF mRNA expression. The difference in physiological injury produced by myocarditis in Balb/c and DBA/2 mice may reflect the induction of apoptosis in Balb/c myocytes, as shown by staining for fragmented DNA using the TdT-TUNEL assay [45]. Such apoptosis is notably absent in inflamed DBA/2 hearts [Fig. 2]. Selective drop-out of substantial numbers of myocytes through apoptosis might produce sufficient left ventricular dysfunction to induce a hypertrophic/cardiomyopathic phenotype in the remaining cardiocytes.

Conclusions

There are a large number of experimental models of myocarditis and each model can produce distinct results. Any differences among models may reflect a number of factors, including the genetics of the virus variant used as well as genetic characteristics of the host animal strain. Just as each individual in the human population will have characteristics unique to that individual, inbred

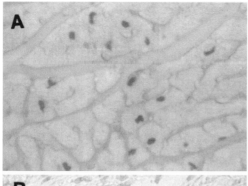
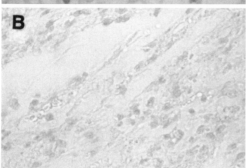

Fig. 2A,B. TdT-TUNEL identification of apoptosis in Balb/c but not DBA/2 hearts. DBA/2 and Balb/c male mice were infected later. A Substantial numbers of apoptotic myocyte nuclei were evident in Balb/c myocardium (dark red staining nuclei) 7 days after infection, both in inflammatory lesions and at distances from these lesions. B In contrast, no apoptotic cells were seen in the hearts of DBA/2 mice, even in areas of intense inflammatory lesions

strains of mice will differ from other strains and many of these differences may impact on whether and how that strain develops myocardial disease. If the clinician thinks that the animal models presently under investigation are complex and confusing, the complexity of the human patient population is likely to be far more substantial. It is unlikely that there is a single animal model which accurately reflects all of clinical myocarditis and dilated cardiomyopathy. Rather, the animal models suggest that the clinical "disease" most likely represents multiple "diseases" with common presenting symptoms and histology but with different pathogenic mechanisms. Future therapeutic regimens may have to be designed to treat the specific pathogenic mechanisms responsible for a given patient's disease.

References

1. Kandolf R (1988) The impact of recombinant DNA technology on the study of enterovirus heart disease. In: M Bendinelli, H Friedman, (eds) Coxsackieviruses: a general update. Plenum, New York, pp 293–318
2. Bowles NE, Richardson PJ, Olsen EGJ, Archard LC (1986) Detection of coxsackie-B-virus-specific RNA sequences in myocardial biopsy samples from patients with myocarditis and dilated cardiomyopathy. Lancet 1: 1120–1123
3. Jin O, Sole MJ, Butany JW (1990) Detection of enterovirus RNA in myocardial biopsies. Circulation 82: 8–16
4. Woodruff JF (1980) Viral myocarditis – A review. Am J Pathol 101: 425

5. Seko Y, Yagita H, Okumura K, Yagaki Y (1994) T-cell receptor V beta gene expression in infiltrating cells in murine hearts with acute myocarditis caused by coxsackievirus B3. Circulation 89: 2170-2175
6. Rabausch-Starz I, Schwarger A, Grunewald K, Muller-Hermelink KH, New N (1994) Persistence of virus and viral genome in myocardium after coxsackievirus B3-induced murine myocarditis. Clin Exp Immunol 96: 69-74
7. Neumann DA, Rose NR, Ansari AA, Herskowitz A (1994) Induction of multiple heart autoantibodies in mice with coxsackievirus B3 and cardiac myosin induced autoimmune myocarditis. J Immunol 152: 343-350
8. Ilback NG, Fohlman J, Friman G (1994) Changed distribution and immune effects of nickel augment viral-induced inflammatory heart lesions in mice. Toxicology 91: 203-219
9. Gauntt CJ, Arizpe HM, Higdon AL, Rosek MM, Crawley R, Cunningham MW (1991) Anti-coxsackievirus B3 neutralizing antibodies with pathogenic potential. Eur Heart J 12 (Suppl D): 124-129
10. Henke A, Huber S, Stelzner A, Whitton JL (1995) The role of CD8+ T lymphocytes in coxsackievirus B3-induced myocarditis. J Virol 69: 6720-6728
11. Sato Y, Maruyama S, Kawai C, Matsumori A (1992) Effect of immunostimulant therapy on acute viral myocarditis in an animal model. Am Heart J 124: 428-434
12. Kishimoto C, Kuroki Y, Hiraoka Y, Ochiai H, Kurokawa M, Sasayama S (1994) Cytokine and murine coxsackievirus B3 myocarditis. Interleukin 2 suppressed myocarditis in the acute stage but enhanced the condition in the subsequent stage. Circulation 89: 2836-2842
13. Herzum M, Huber SA, Weller R, Grebe R, Maisch B (1991) Treatment of experimental murine coxsackie B3 myocarditis. Eur Heart J 12 (Suppl D): 200-202
14. Frizelle S, Schwarz J, Huber SA, Leslie K (1992) Evaluation of the effects of low molecular weight heparin on inflammation and collagen deposition in chronic coxsackievirus B3-induced myocarditis in A/J mice. Am J Pathol 141: 203-209
15. Weller AH, Hall M, Huber SA (1992) Polyclonal immunoglobulin therapy protects against cardiac damage in experimental coxsackievirus-induced myocarditis. Eur Heart J 13: 115-119
16. Chow LH, Beisel KW, McManus BM (1992) Enteroviral infection of mice with severe combined immunodeficiency: evidence for direct viral pathogenesis of myocardial injury. Lab Invest 66: 24
17. Sherry B, Li XY, Tyler KL, Cullen JM, Virgin HW IV (1993) Lymphocytes protect against and are not required for reovirus-induced myocarditis. J Virol 67: 6119-6124
18. Comroe JH, Dripps RD (1976) Scientific basis for the support of biomedical science. Science 192: 105-111
19. Holland J, Spindler K, Horocyski F, Grabau B, Nichols S, Vandepol S (1982) Rapid evolution of RNA genomes. Science 215: 1577-1585
20. Huber SA, Haisch C, Lodge PA (1990) Functional diversity in vascular endothelial cells: role in coxsackievirus tropism 64: 4516-4522
21. Klump MW, Bergmann I, Muller BC, Amers D, Kandolf R (1990) Complete nucleotide sequence of infectious coxsackievirus B3 cDNA: two initial 5' uridine residues are regained during plus-strand RNA synthesis. J Virol 64: 1573-1583
22. Herzum M, Maisch B (1992) Humoral and cellular immune reactions to the myocardium in myocarditis. Herz 17: 91-96
23. Barry WH (1994) Mechanisms of immune-mediated myocyte injury. Circulation 89: 2421-2432
24. Kandolf R, Klingel K, Zell R, Selinka HC, Raab U, Schneider-Brachert W, Bultmann B (1993) Molecular pathogenesis of enterovirus-induced myocarditis: virus persistence and chronic inflammation. Intervirology 35: 140-151
25. Lange LG, Schreiner GF (1994) Immune mechanisms of cardiac disease. N Engl J Med 330: 1129-1135
26. Martino TA, Liu P, Soule MJ (1994) Viral infection and the pathogenesis of dilated cardiomyopathy. Circ Res 74: 182-188
27. Rose NR, Neumann DA, Herskowitz A (1992) Coxsackievirus myocarditis. Adv Intern Med 37: 411-429
28. Huber SA (1993) Animal models: immunological aspects. In: JE Banatvala (ed) Viral infections of the heart. Arnold, London, pp 82-109

29. Woodruff JF, Woodruff JJ (1974) Involvement of T lymphocytes in the pathogenesis of coxsackievirus B3 heart disease. J Immunol 113: 1726–1734
30. Woodruff JF (1979) Lack of correlation between neutralizing antibody production and suppression of coxsackievirus B3 replication in target organs: evidence for involvement of mononuclear inflammatory cells in host defense. J Immunol 123: 31–36
31. Huber SA, Job LP (1983) Cellular immune mechanisms in coxsackievirus group B, type 3-induced myocarditis in Balb/c mice. In: JJ Spitzer (ed) Myocardial injury. Plenum, New York, pp 491–507
32. Herzum M, Rupert V, Kuytz B, Jomau H, Nakamura I, Maisch B (1994) Coxsackievirus B3 infection leads to cell death of cardiac myocytes. J Mol Cell Cardiol 26: 907–913
33. Drude L, Wiemers F, Maisch B (1991) Impaired myocyte function in vitro incubated with sera from patients with myocarditis. Eur Heart J 12 (Suppl D): 36–38
34. Kuhl U, Melzner B, Schafer B, Schultheiss HP, Strauer BE (1991) The Ca-channel as cardiac autoantigen. Eur Heart J 12 (Suppl D): 99–104
35. Sharaf AR, Narrila J, Nieol PD, Southern JF, Khau BA (1994) Cardiac sarcoplasmic reticulum calcium ATPase, an autoimmune antigen in experimental cardiomyopathy. Circulation 89: 1217–1228
36. Wallukat G, Wallenberger A, Morwinski R, Pitschner HF (1995) Anti-beta 1-adrenoceptor autoantibodies with chronotropic activity from the serum of patients with dilated cardiomyopathy mapping of epitopes in the first and second extracellular loops. J Mol Cell Cardiol 27: 397–406
37. Schultheiss HP (1989) The significance of autoantibodies against the ADP/ATP carrier for the pathogenesis of myocarditis and dilated cardiomyopathy – clinical and experimental data. Springer Semin Immunopathol 11: 15–30
38. Schultheiss HP, Schwimmbeck P (1986) Autoantibodies to the adenine-nucleotide translocator (ANT) in myocarditis (MC) – prevalence, clinical correlates and diagnostic value. Circulation 74: 142
39. Schultheiss HP, Kuhl U, Schauer R, Schulze K, Kemkes B, Becker BF (1988) Antibodies against the ADP/ATP carrier alter myocardial function by disturbing cellular energy metabolism. In: HP Schultheiss (ed) New concepts in viral heart disease. Springer, Berlin Heidelberg New York, pp 243–258
40. Hamrell BB, Huber SA, Leslie KO (1994) Reduced unloaded sarcomere shortening velocity and a shift to a slower myosin isoform in acute murine coxsackievirus myocarditis. Circ Res 75: 462–472
41. Hamrell BB, Huber SA and Leslie KO (1995) Depressed unloaded sarcomere shortening velocity in acute murine coxsackievirus myocarditis: myocardial remodelling in the absence of necrosis or hypertrophy. Eur Heart J 16 (Suppl O): 31–35
42. Reyes MP, Ho KL, Smith F, Lerner AM (1981) A mouse model of dilated type cardiomyopathy due to coxsackievirus B3. J Infect Dis 144: 232–236
43. Chien KR, Knowlton KU, Zu H, Chien S (1991) Regulation of cardiac gene expression during myocardial growth and hypertrophy: molecular studies of an adaptive physiological response. FASEB J 5: 3037–3046
44. Huber SA, Lodge PA (1986) Coxsackievirus B3 myocarditis: identification of different pathogenic mechanisms in DBA/2 and Balb/c mice. Am J Pathol 122: 284–291
45. Gavrieli Y, Sherman Y, Ben-Sasson SA (1992) Identification of programmed cell death in situ via specific labeling of nuclear DNA fragmentation. J Cell Biol 119: 493–501

The Role of Cytokines in the Pathogenesis of Myocarditis

P. Liu

Overview of Cytokines

Cytokines are multipurpose low molecular weight "pleotropic" intercellular signaling peptides that are the major mediators of inflammation, cellular growth, cellular transformation, nuclear activation, matrix repair, gene regulation and cell death. They have been best identified with the immune system, to bring about the coordinated response following injury in all tissues (Lange and Schreiner 1994). At low doses, cytokine fine tune the body system for maintenance function. The cytokines regulate host cell function through autocrine (self-regulation) or paracrine (regulation of neighbouring cells) pathways. In cases of severe stimulation, high doses of cytokines are released into the blood stream to produce a potentially endocrine effect. This high level of cytokines may be toxic to target cells. The teleological purpose of this action is to eliminate potentially sources of harm for the organism (such as infected cells), but it ultimately can cause the destruction of the host cell.

A classification based on the increasing information on the molecular structure of these compounds divides cytokines into three broad families: (1) the *growth factor family,* including tumour necrosis factor, epidermal growth factors, which coordinates the response to injury; (2) the *interleukin family,* with the receptors all sharing an immunoglobulin domain; and (3) the *interferon family,* which are produced by all known cell types in defense to foreign gene introduction, and have wide ranging host cellular effects. Almost all the tissues examined so far have receptors for cytokines (including the heart), and multiple tissue types are capable of producing cytokines on their own when stimulated.

The current understanding of the pathogenesis of myocarditis involves the triad of virus immune system and the myocyte acting in concert (Sole and Liu 1993; Martino et al 1994). Cytokines are the key intermediaries in regulating the immune–myocyte interaction. Cytokines likely orchestrate the recognition of viral antigen by the immune system, up regulation of adhesion molecules to attract the immunocytes, the activation of the immune cell in a cascade at the inflammatory foci, the regulation of local vascular flow and angiogenesis, the stimulation of fibroblasts to lay down matrix and collagen, the trigger for hypertrophy and gene expression changes in the myocytes, and the release of

GW1-508, The Toronto Hospital, General Division, Toronto, Ontario M5G 2C4, Canada

oxidative radicals causing direct cellular injury and deaths when cytokines become unregulated (Lange and Schreiner 1994). Thus, it is easy to appreciate how cytokines may play a key regulatory role in the pathogenesis of myocarditis leading to dilated cardiomyopathy (Neumann et al. 1993).

Growth Factor Family

The growth factor family of cytokines are the most actively investigated group at the present time due to their almost universal presence and availability of the biological tools to quantitate them in the serum and tissues. There is family homology to nerve growth factors, which includes tumour necrosis factor α (TNF-α), TNF-β (lymphotoxin), transforming growth factor β (TGF-β) and the FAS antigen. The latter is associated with cellular apoptosis.

TNF can be thought as a master cytokine that coordinates and up regulates many other cytokines, in addition to its own independent action on a wide variety of cells (Buetler and Cerami 1987). It was first discovered as a factor elaborated by the body against endotoxin with unusual tumour killing properties. Later the same compound was found to cause cachexia in cancer patients (cachexin). It is now known that TNF has very wide ranging cell signalling effects, and every cell type has receptor to TNF. TNF-α is elaborated by macrophages and endothelial cells under conditions of immune recognition or stress. TNF-β is elaborated by activated lymphocytes as part of its signalling mechanism to up regulate other immune effectors such as adhesion molecules, interleukins and nitric oxide synthase (NOS).

There are two types of TNF receptors in cells: TNF-R1 and TNF-R2. TNF-R1 (55 kDa) is likely activated intracellularly through a phosphotidylcholine specific phospholipase C, producing 1, 2-diacylglycerol. This in turn activates sphingomyelinase, breaking down sphingomyelin to ceramide. Ceramide in turn can activate nuclear transcription factors such as NF-κB, AP-1, IRF-1, etc., intracellularly with potent effects (Dressler et al. 1992; Schutze et al. 1992). On the other hand, TNF-R2 (75 kDa) receptor is similar in structure to TNF-R1, but has an extra domain, and is activated through a completely different intracellular signalling mechanism, possibly through phosphorylation of p91. TNF-R2 is likely specifically responsible for DNA fragmentation observed in cells (Higuchi and Aggarwal 1993). It may also potentiate the effect of TNF-α/β through alteration of the ligand binding affinity onto TNF-R1 (Tartaglia et al. 1993). Both TNF-R1 and TNF-R2 are expressed in the myocytes, and are elevated in human failing hearts (Torre-Amione et al. 1995). The TNF-R2 also become solubilized in the serum, and is an excellent predictor of cardiac prognosis in patients with heart failure (Ferrari et al. 1995).

Interleukin Family

Interleukins (IL) are cytokines that are important for leukocyte intercellular signalling. The family is constantly expanding, and consists of leukocyte activating factors, such as interleukin (IL)-1,2,4,6 and others, as well as negative modulators, such as IL-10. IL profiles are helpful in identifying T-lymphocyte subtypes that may enhance different aspects of immunity. For example, CD4+ helper T cell type Th1 elaborates IL-2 and interferon γ (IFNγ) that preferentially stimulates cell-mediated immunity. On the other hand, Th2 cell type secretes IL-4 and IL-6 and facilitates antibody production.

The IL receptors, such as the prototype IL-2 receptor (IL-2R) have common extracellular immunoglobulin domains, and four conserved cystein residues that are found across the family members. They appear to be once related during evolution, and have important costimulatory function through intracellular signalling in activating the immune cell following antigen presentation.

Interferon Family

IFNs were first characterized by antiviral assays, but they are also potent immunoregulators and growth factors in their own right. The IFNs are generated by almost every cell in the organism as part of an immediate response to injury. IFNs recently have been found to utilize the unique and newly described JAK-STAT pathway for signal transduction. In this process, there is actual translocation of the receptor intracellularly for nuclear signal trafficking.

Classically IFNα is the largest and is made by leucocytes in response to viruses or nucleic acids. This is a family of about 20 structurally related polypeptides of approximately 18 kDa each, encoded by different genes. IFNβ is a single glycoprotein of 20 kDa, classically made by fibroblast in response to viruses or nucleic acids. However, as mentioned earlier, many cell types are known to make these interferons. Both the IFNα and IFNβ bind to the same receptor, and are known as type I IFNs. They in general have properties of antiviral effects, inhibits cell proliferation, and modulates major histocompatibility complex (MHC) molecule expression by enhancing cell-mediated immunity.

IFNγ on the other hand is made by lymphocytes in response to immune stimuli, and uses a different set of receptor signalling system, and is often known as type II IFN. IFNγ in general activates macrophages, and enhances their ability to act as antigen-presenting cells. The IFNs all have antiviral activity, and has also anti-proliferative effects on non-immune target cells.

Evidence of Cytokine Elevation in Myocarditis and Dilated Cardiomyopathy

The presence of increased cytokine levels in myocarditis has been demonstrated both in animal models and clinical populations with inflammatory heart disease.

In animal models of myocarditis, Yamada et al. followed cytokine levels serially in a murine model produced by inoculating encephalomyocarditis (EMC) virus in DBA/2 mice. They have documented elevated levels of TNF-α soon after viral inoculation. The TNF-α levels became significant elevated by day 3, peaked on day 5, and thereafter declined slowly in the serum during the next 7–14 days (Yamada et al. 1994). Furthermore, our laboratory has observed that tissue expression of TNF-α may indeed persist well into the late stages of myocarditis progressing to dilated cardiomyopathy. This is accompanied by the induction of cytokine-sensitive genes such as that of inducible nitric oxide synthase (iNOS) in the tissues.

Clinically, patients with acute myocarditis and heart failure due to dilated cardiomyopathy also have significantly elevated cytokine levels. Matsumori and coworkers have documented in group of patients with acute myocarditis, that IL-1α was elevated in 23%, TNF-α was elevated in 46%, and macrophage colony stimulating factor (MCSF) was elevated in most patients studied (Matsumori et al. 1994). This degree of cytokine elevation was also found in patients with dilated and hypertrophic cardiomyopathies, but not in patients with coronary artery disease or hypertension.

These studies documenting elevated circulating cytokines are also echoed by studies looking for evidence of cytokine activation in the actual heart tissue. This can be identified potentially by examining for the presence of inducible downstream genes from cytokines such as (iNOS). DeBelder et al. have shown recently that biopsy taken from patients with inflammatory heart disease all showed elevated inducible NOS activity (DeBelder et al. 1993, 1995). This finding was more recently confirmed by a larger sample of patients from the Stanford heart transplant group (Haywood et al. 1996). The most plausible explanation for the high levels of inducible form of NO synthase in these hearts is that there was prior exposure to local cytokines, which are potent inducers of iNOS in these hearts due to recent inflammation (Schulz et al. 1992).

These observations are also confirmed by other studies where patients with dilated cardiomyopathy and possible prior myocarditis have been identified to have increased levels of mRNA for the cytokine IL-1 and the IL-1 receptor (IL-1R) directly within the myocardium, in comparison to controls (Han et al. 1991).

Therefore, there is gathering evidence to suggest that both circulating and direct tissue levels of cytokines are elevated in patients with myocarditis, dilated cardiomyopathy and inflammatory heart disease in general. This is compatible with the concept that the cytokines are potentially important co-ordinators and contributors to the pathogenesis of myocarditis and dilated cardiomyopathy.

Potential Impact of Cytokines on the Heart

The elaboration and persistence of cytokines in the heart can have a multitude of effects on the myocardium. After viral invasion of the myocyte during myocarditis, there is an immediate response by the immune, endothelial and myocytes to elaborate cytokines such as IFN, TNF, and possibly IL. As a result, there is an immediate up-regulation of cell surface molecules such as the MHC and vascular and cellular adhesion molecules to bring in immunocytes. In myocarditis, intercellular adhesion molecule (ICAM-1) has been shown to be up-regulated under the influence of cytokines such as IFN or TNF (Seko et al. 1993). These molecules help to further mobilize immunocytes to the injury area to remove the damaged or toxin/virus-contaminated cells. The ICAM-1 up-regulation can further lead to coupling of T-cells with expressed LFA-1 ligand, leading to killing of the infected host cell by natural killer cells via the perforin mechanism (Seko et al. 1993).

The presence of cytokines in myocarditis is also a potent inducer to up-regulate the iNOS, which can produce nitric oxide (NO) in very large quantities locally (Lowenstein and Snyder 1992). The NO produced from the iNOS is important in directly defending the host tissue from the pathogenic organisms and attenuate viral proliferation. The NO thus produced react vigorously with the iron-sulphur centres of their target molecules, causing denaturation and dysfunction of viral proteins.

Cytokines are also important for the initiation of the repair process. These processes require the generation of new blood vessels through angiogenesis (domains of TGF-β, TGF-α and IL-1), and laying down of scar tissue through fibroblast activation and secretion of collagen and other matrix proteins (function of TNF-α and TGF-β).

To facilitate the repair process, TNF also help to mobilize nutritional resources from peripheral protein sources such as skeletal muscle into central organs, such as the heart, liver and brain under stressful conditions (Hoshino et al. 1991; Matsui et al. 1993). In extreme cases, this can lead to cachexia (Levine et al. 1990; McMurray et al. 1991) However, this is potentially important as nutritional sources are scarce when the organism is injured or ill, and central organ preservation is more important for the organism's long-term survival.

To protect the heart further, cytokines such as TNF and IL are also known to down-regulate cardiac function through multiplicity of pathways (Sobotka et at. 1990), including attenuation of the response to β-1 adrenergic receptor stimulation (Gulick et al. 1989). This appears to involve the down regulation of β-adrenergic receptor number as well as a decrease in receptor affinity, via both NO-dependent and NO-independent pathways. Finkel et al. have demonstrated most of the TNF-α- or IL-2,6-induced decrease in contractility in hamster papillary muscle is blockable by iNOS inhibitors (Finkel et al. 1992). On the other hand, Yokoyama and colleagues have demonstrated the ability of cytokines to depress myocardial function independent of NO, with a concomitant decrease in calcium release, but this was not blockable by NOS inhibitors (Yokoyama et al. 1993). Both of these pathways serve to decrease cardiac contractility and demand for oxygen consumption.

Unfortunately, all the potential beneficial and protective effects of cytokines are generally short term. When the cytokines are stimulated to affect the local tissues long term and at high quantities, the cytokines together with the high level of NO produced can lead to paradoxical tissue damage. This can consist of local peroxynitrite production due to NO and free radical production, or direct cytokine induced cell injury and apoptosis. These are in addition to the persistence of immune cells that can lead to both cell-mediated and antibody-produced tissue injury.

The Specific Role of Interferons in Myocarditis

The IFNs are produced by both immune cells and host cells during the acute phases of myocarditis immediately after viral inoculation, and are important coordinators for the immediate cell defense against the invading pathogen. An overview of the interferon trails in both animals and man is listed in Table 1.

Lutton et al. were the first to demonstrate that IFN may play an important role in myocarditis, and the potential dual nature of the treatment (Lutton and Gauntt 1985). Early treatment of murine IFN (IFN-β), when given within 1 day of inoculation, was able to significantly ameliorate the disease. On the other hand, in later stages of the disease (3–7 days post viral inoculation), the use of IFN-blocking antibodies was actually found to be more beneficial than treating the animals with more IFN itself.

Matsumori et al. have also found that in an EMC model of myocarditis in DBA/2 mice, the administration of IFN-α A/D acutely, in doses ranging between 10^2 to 10^4 U/g/day, was able to produce less viral titres in the host heart, and less myocardial necrosis and cellular infiltration. There was definitely a dose–response effect, and the most effective regimen was when IFN was given to the animals either 1 day before or on the day of viral inoculation. When IFN was given at a much lower dose or on the day of viral inoculation, the effect was marginal and indistinguishable from untreated controls (Matsumori et al. 1987, 1988).

Table 1. Summary of the role of interferons in myocarditis

Investigator	Model	Time with respect to virus infection	Benefit	Harm	Reference
Figulla	CVB2/patients + rhINFα-2a	Late	++		Figulla et al. (1995)
Aitken	IRF-1$^{-/-}$ knockout (decr IFN and absent iNOS)	Since birth (transgenic)		+++	Aitken et al. (1994)
Smith	Myosin in A/J IFNγ removal	N/A (autoimmune)		++	Smith and Allen (1992)
Kanda	EMC / C3H/He + rhINFα A/D	+ 1 day	++		Kanda et al. (1995)
Kishimoto	CVB3 / C3H/H3 + rhINFα A/D	– 1 day	++		Kishimoto and Abelmann (1988)
Matsumori	EMC / DBA/2 + rhINFα A/D	– 1 or 0 days	++		Matsumori and Abelmann (1987)
Lutton	CVB3 / CD-1 + early mINF β	– 1 to 1 day	++		Lutton and Gauntt (1985)
Lutton	CVB3 / CD-1 + late INF-Ab	3–7 days	++		Lutton and Gauntt (1985)

CVB, coxsackievirus; rhINF, recombinant human interferon; decr, decreased; iNOS, inducible nitric oxide synthase; IFN, interferon; N/A, not applicable; EMC, encephalomyocarditis virus; mIFN, murine interferon; Ab antibodies.

Similarly, and almost simultaneously, Kishimoto et al. demonstrated in a CVB3 model of myocarditis that recombinant human IFN-α A/D given within 1 day prior to viral inoculation conferred significant protection against myocarditis (Kishimoto et al. 1988). The IFN-α treated animals again showed lower viral titres and improved histology.

Smith et al. used a non-viral but an autoimmune model of myocarditis produced by myosin inoculation in A/J mice showed that decreasing IFN-γ early during the course of the disease severely worsened the disease. This suggests that interferon, even in the absence of a viral pathogen, plays an important early modulatory role of the immune system, leading to a more balanced response to the antigenic challenge (Smith and Allen 1992).

Kanda et al. made similar observation using recombinant human IFN-α A/D together with an immunomodulator OK432. They have found also a significant amelioration of myocarditis, with additional evidence of reduction of atrial natriuretic peptide protein and mRNA levels during follow-up (Kanda et al. 1995).

We have also documented the importance of iNOS in myocarditis through the use of transgenic knockout models. In animals with the nuclear factor interferon regulatory element (IRF-1) knocked out, there is a partial reduction of IFN levels, as well as complete absence of inducible nitric oxide synthase. The animals homozygous for the IRF-1 knockout mutations have dramatically increased mortality and elevated viral titres in the myocardium (Aitken et al. 1994). This confirms the importance of host–defense mechanisms such as interferons and inducible nitric oxide synthase in the role of viral attenuation and tissue repair.

Figulla and colleagues have used IFN-α in four patients with chronic myocarditis and biopsy positive for enteroviral genome (Figulla et al. 1995). They administered IFN-α subcutaneously every other day for 6 months, and found significant haemodynamic improvement in all patients treated. Two of the four patients also reverted to negative status for viral genome during treatment.

Thus overall, there is both basic and clinical evidence to suggest that the initial role of interferon is very important in myocarditis. It is probably one of first major lines of defence against the pathogenic organism. It also play an important coordinating and modulating role in later stages of the disease.

The Role of Interleukins in Myocarditis

ILs also play an important role in myocarditis. They interestingly demonstrate an important duality of action depending on the stage of the disease, and produces divergent responses in the host following its administration (Table 2).

Lane et al. studied the role of cytokines in myocarditis in the otherwise myocarditis resistant B10.A mice. However, when these animals were concomitantly treated with lipopolysaccharide (LPS), TNF, or IL-1 together with CVB3 viral inoculation, these resistant animals actually developed actual myocardial inflammation and poor clinical outcome (Lane et al. 1992). This demonstrates the facilitatory role of cytokines in the setting of low background levels of immune activation.

Table 2. Summary of the role of interleukins in myocarditis

Investigator	Model	Time with respect to virus infection	Benefit	Harm	Reference
Kishimoto	CVB3 / BALBc + Early IL-2	0–7 days	++		Kishimoto et al. (1994)
Kishimoto	CVB3 / BALBc + late IL-2	7–14 days		++	Kishimoto et al. (1994)
Schwimmbeck	Human lymphocytes/ SCID mice	Since birth		++	Schwimmbeck et al. (1994)
Huber	H310A1 / BALBc +IL-1			++	Huber et al. (1994)
Neumann	CVB3 / A/J +IL-1R	0 day	++		Neumann et al. (1993)
Lane	CVB3 / B10.4 +IL-1 or LPS	0 day		++	Lane et al (1992)

CVB, coxsackievirus; IL, interleukin; SCID, severe combined immune deficiency; IL-1R, soluble interleukin-1 receptor; LPS, bacterial lipopolysaccharide.

On the other hand, A/J mice are generally susceptible to CVB3, and will develop fulminant myocarditis when exposed to the virus. However, if antagonist to IL-1R is given concomitantly with the virus, the animals will develop markedly diminished myocardial injury, less clinical myocarditis and also decreased circulating antibody levels (Neumann et al. 1993). This suggests again that cytokines such as IL-1 can significantly modulate the disease between the virus and the host. This may also offer an attractive target for future intervention.

Huber has determined the potential differential effects of different IL on the phenotype of myocarditis. They observed that if H3 virus was inoculated in BALB/c mice, the animals will demonstrate increased inflammatory cell infiltrate with IL-1 elaboration leading to the production of Th1 cells. On the other hand, if H310A1 virus was inoculated instead into BALB/c mice, the animals had minimal myocarditis, with a minimal IL-1 or Th1 response. Instead, these animals elaborated IL-2 and increased Th2 cell population. The addition of IL-1 to the latter mice will essentially restore the myocarditic response and recapture the Th1 population (Huber et al. 1994).

Schwimmbeck et al performed an intriguing experiment, in which they isolated lymphocytes from five patients with myocarditis and antibodies to the adenine nucleotide translocator. When they injected the lymphocytes into immune deficient mice (SCID mice), they developed lymphocytic infiltrations of the heart (Schwimmbeck et al. 1994). This was associated with significant elevations of IL-2R in the serum, suggesting effective cytokine elevation. This suggests that IL-2 was potentially instrumental in reproducing the phenotype of lymphocytic activation in the heart.

Kishimoto interestingly studied the differential effects of early versus late IL-2 administration. He found that in murine model of CVB3 inoculated into BALB/c mice, early administration of IL-2 in less than 7 days is beneficial, but late administration at 7–14 days was much more harmful (Kishimoto et al. 1994). This confirms the duality of ILs at different stages of the disease. Therefore, cytokine manipulation in the future in the treatment setting will have to take the underlying stage of the disease into account.

The Role of Tumour Necrosis Factor in Myocarditis

To investigate the potential role of TNF-α in myocarditis, Yamada et al. studied a model of myocarditis induced by EMC virus inoculation in young 4-week-old DBA/2 mice, leading to acute inflammation and necrosis is 7–14 days. The animals were randomized to receive recombinant human TNF-α 1 day prior and continued for 2 days after viral inoculation, and it was found that the viral titres were higher and the histopathology worse for the TNF-treated group (Yamada et al. 1994). The administration of TNF-α monoclonal antibodies was somewhat protective if given one day prior to the inoculation. This was ineffective if given 1 day following viral inoculation. Thus, in this model, where the cytokine levels are already elevated, additional cytokine administration will further activate the immune system causing worse disease (Table 3).

Similarly, Lane et al. found that in another model of otherwise mild myocarditis induced in B10.A mice inoculated with CVB3 virus, there was a significant increase in mortality and exuberant pathological lesions in those who received concomitant TNF-α. Presumably these experiments showed that acute elevation of cytokines can indeed lead to significantly greater degree of immune activation, leading to more extensive host damage (Lane et al. 1992).

As may thus be predicted, Smith et al. in a non-viral autoimmune model of myocarditis induced by myosin sensitization in A/J mice found that pretreatment with anti-TNF-α antibody was able to significantly ameliorate the outcome of these animal models (Smith and Allen 1992). However, administration of anti-TNF-α antibody after immunization had no effect on the course of the disease.

Table 3. Summary of the role of tumour necrosis factor in myocarditis

Investigator	Model	Time with respect to virus infection	Benefit	Harm	Reference
Smith	Myosin / A/J + TNF-α Ab	– 1 day	++		Smith and Allen (1992)
Yamada	EMC / DBA/2 + TNF-α Ab	– 1 day	+/–	–	Yamada, Sasayama (1994)
Yamada	EMC / DBA/2 + rhTNF-α	– 1 to 2 days		++	Yamada, Sasayama (1994)
Lane	CVB3 / B10.A + TNF-α	0 day		++	Lane et al. (1992)

TNF, tumour necrosis factor; Ab, antibodies; decr, decreased; EMC, encephalomyocarditis virus; rh, recombinant human; CVB, coxsackievirus.

Preliminary results from our laboratory suggested that in animals which have the TNF-α 55-kda receptor (TNF-R1) knocked out, there is a more exuberant myocarditis in the animals. This may indicate that the signaling process of TNF-α through its receptors is important in triggering host–defense mechanisms. Therefore, when this process is disabled in the knockout animals, the virus has the opportunity to proliferate unchecked. However, during late stages of the disease, there is still extensive presence of TNF-α in the tissues. The continued elaboration of TNF-α in the tissues can lead to abnormal gene regulation, down regulate ventricular function and potential myocyte death via necrosis or apoptosis. This is another example of the duality of cytokines in the pathogenesis of myocarditis.

Potential Therapeutic Role of Cytokines in Myocarditis

As mentioned previously, cytokines are important modulators of inflammation and repair, and may offer tremendous opportunities as therapeutic targets to modulate the natural history of diseases such as myocarditis and dilated cardiomyopathy. However, one will need to keep in mind the paradoxical nature of the cytokines, depending on the stages of the disease where they are found.

Cytokines are likely very important for host protection during the acute viral phase of myocarditis. In patients who are potentially immune compromised or are in the very acute phase of the disease, the administration of cytokines may provide an extra degree of protection. This may supplement the use of antiviral agents to be tested in the future for this condition. However, the proper dose and route of administration, timing and type of biological agents to be used is still yet to be determined.

On the other hand, during the chronic phases of the disease, where immune activation is part of the tissue destructive phase, the use of inhibitors of activating cytokines, or the use of cytokines that are intrinsically inhibitory may have an important therapeutic role. Currently in disease processes such as rheumatoid arthritis or other immunologically mediated conditions, many of the new agents that attenuate cytokine production, such as soluble TNF-R2 or TNF antibodies have been found to be very effective in disease remission. These are exciting opportunities for exploration of these strategies in myocarditis and dilated cardiomyopathy in the future, especially in the chronic setting.

Summary

Cytokines are intercellular signalling molecules that are elaborated at high levels by a variety of cells during the acute phase of myocarditis. They serve as important mediators of immune response, inflammation, cellular growth, and tissue repair. The cytokines are currently classified into the three families of IFNs, ILs, and growth factors.

Acutely, cytokines are important as up-regulators of adhesion molecules, costimulatory signals for host immune cell activation, and potent inducers of NO production via iNOS. Cytokines such as TNF and ILs also help to mobilize nutrients, initiate the repair process, and down regulate myocardial function to decrease oxygen consumption. However, when this activation is excessive, or prolonged beyond the presence of the virus, as determined often by host genetic factors, tissue destruction and chronic disease such as cardiomyopathy will ensue.

A variety of studies have addressed the various families of cytokines in myocarditis. The class of IFNs have generally been found to be very protective, especially during the acute stages of the disease. However, both the ILs and TNF families have been found to be harmful as promoters of inflammation during later chronic phase of myocarditis. However, they may be protective during the very acute phase immediately following viral inoculation.

Therefore, to maintain the most optimal biological homeostasis, it will be important in the future in terms of therapeutic strategy to maintain the acute protective properties of the cytokines, but have the ability to turn the system off once the initial conditions have been controlled, to avoid chronic disease induced by excessive cytokine production.

Acknowledgements. Supported in part by grants from the Heart & Stroke Foundation and Medical Research Council of Canada.

References

Aitken K, Penninger J, Mak T, Chow L, Dawood F, Wen WH et al (1994) Increased susceptibility to coxsackieviral myocarditis in IRF-1 transgenic knockout mice. Circulation 90: 1139

Buetler B, Cerami A (1987) Cachectin: more than a tumor necrosis factor. N Engl J Med 316: 379–385

DeBelder AJ, Radomski MW, Why HJF, Richardson PJ, Bucknall CA, Salas E et al (1993) Nitric oxide synthase activities in human myocardium. Lancet 341: 84–85

DeBelder AJ, Radomski MW, Why HJF, Richardson PJ, Martin JF (1995) Myocardial calcium-independent nitric oxide synthase activity is present in dilated cardiomyopathy, myocarditis and postpartum cardiomyopathy but not in ischaemic or valvar heart disease. Br Heart J 74: 426–430

Dressler KA, Mathias S, Kolesnick RN (1992) Tumor necrosis factor-alpha activates the sphingomyelin signal transduction pathway in cell-free system. Science 255: 1715–1718

Ferrari R, Bachetti T, Confortini R, Opasich C, Febo O, Corti A et al (1995) Tumor necrosis factor soluble receptors in patients with various degrees of advanced congestive heart failure. Circulation 1995: 1479–1486

Figulla HR, Stille-Siegener M, Mall G, Heim A, Kreuzer H (1995) Myocardial enterovirus infection with left ventricular dysfunction: a benign disease compared with idiopathic dilated cardiomyopathy. J Am Coll Cardiol 25: 1170–1175

Finkel MS, Oddis CV, Jacob TD, Watkins SC, Hattler BG, Simmons RL (1992) Negative inotropic effects of cytokines on the heart mediated by nitric oxide. Science 257: 387–389

Gulick T, Chung MK, Pieper SJ, Lange LG, Schreiner GF (1989) Interleukin 1 and tumor necrosis factor inhibit cardiac myocyte beta-adrenergic responsiveness. Proc Natl Acad Sci USA 86: 6753–6757

Han RO, Ray PE, Baughman KL, Feldman AM (1991) Detection of interleukin and interleukin-receptor mRNA in human heart by polymerase chain reaction. Biochem Biophys Res Commun 181: 520–523

Haywood GA, Tsao PS, Von der Leyen HE, Mann MJ, Keeling PJ, Trindada PT et al (1996) Expression of inducible nitric oxide synthase in human heart failure. Circulation 93: 1087–1094

Higuchi M, Aggarwal BB (1993) P80 form of the human tumor necrosis factor receptor is involved in DNA fragmentation. FEBS Lett 331: 252–255

Hoshino E, Pichard C, Greenwood CE, Kuo GC, Cameron RG, Kurian R et al (1991) Body composition and metabolic rate in rat during a continuous infusion of cachectin. Am J Physiol 260: E27–36

Huber SA, Polgar J, Schultheiss P, Schwimmbeck P (1994) Augmentation of pathogenesis of coxsackievirus B3 infections in mice by exogenous administration of interleukin-1 and interleukin-2. J Virol 68: 195–206

Kanda T, Yokoyama T, Iama S, Suzuki T, Murata K, Kobayashi I (1995) Effect of combination therapy with OK432 and recombinant human interferon-alpha A/D on atrial natriuretic peptide gene expression in mice with viral myocarditis. J Ph Exp Th 274: 494–498

Kishimoto C, Crumpacker CS, Abelmann WH (1988) Prevention of murine coxsackie B3 viral myocarditis and associated lymphoid organ atrophy with recombinant human leucocyte interferon alpha A/D. Cardiovasc Res 22: 732–738

Kishimoto C, Kuroki Y, Hiraoka Y, Ochiai H, Kurokawa M, Sasayama S (1994) Cytokine and murine coxsackievirus B3 myocarditis. Interleukin-2 suppressed myocarditis in the acute stage but enhanced the condition in the subsequent stage. Circulation 89: 2836–2842

Lane JR, Neumann DA, Lafond-Walker A, Herskowitz A, Rose NR (1992) Interleukin 1 or tumor necrosis factor can promote Coxsackie B3-induced myocarditis in resistant B10.A mice. J Exp Med 175: 1123–1129

Lange LG, Schreiner GF (1994) Immune mechanisms of cardiac disease. N Engl J Med 330: 1129–1135

Levine B, Kalman J, Mayer L, Fillit HM, Packer M (1990) Elevated circulating levels of tumor necrosis factor in severe chronic heart failure. N Engl J Med 323: 236–241

Lowenstein CJ, Snyder SH (1992) Nitric oxide, a novel biologic messenger. Cell 70: 705–707

Lutton CW, Gauntt CJ (1985) Ameliorating effect of IFN-beta and anti-IFN-beta on coxsackievirus B3-induced myocarditis in mice. J interferon Res 5: 137–146

Martino T, Liu P, Sole MJ (1994) Viral infection and the pathogenesis of myocarditis and dilated cardiomyopathy. Circ Res 74: 182–188

Matsui J, Cameron RG, Kurian R, Kuo GC, Jeejeebhoy KN (1993) Nutritional, hepatic and metabolic effects of cachectin/tumor necrosis factor in rats receiving total parenteral nutrition. Gastroenterology 104: 235–243

Matsumori A, Crumpacker CS, Abelmann WH (1987) Prevention of viral myocarditis with recombinant human leukocyte interferon alpha A/D in a murine model. J Am Coll Cardiol 9: 1320–1325

Matsumori A, Tomioka N, Kawai C (1988) Protective effect of recombinant alpha interferon on coxsackievirus B3 myocarditis in mice. Am Heart J 115: 1229–1232

Matsumori A, Yamada T, Suzuki H, Matoba Y, Sasayama S (1994) Increased circulating cytokines in patients with myocarditis and cardiomyopathy. Br Heart J 72: 561–566

McMurray J, Abdullah I, Dargie HJ, Shapiro D (1991) Increased concentrations of tumour necrosis factor in "cachectic" patients with severe chronic heart failure. Br Heart J 66: 356–358

Neumann DA, Lane JR, Allen GS, Herskowitz A, Rose NR (1993) Viral myocarditis leading to cardiomyopathy: do cytokines contribute to pathogenesis? Clin Immunol Immunopathol 68: 181–190

Schulz R, Nava E, Moncada S (1992) Induction and potential biological relevance of Ca2+-independent nitric oxide synthase in the myocardium. Br J Pharmacol 105: 3629–3632

Schutze S, Potthoff K, Machleidt T, Berkovic D, Wiegmann K, Kronke M (1992) TNF activates NF-kappa B by phosphatidylcholine-specific phospholipase C-induced "acidic" sphingomyelin breakdown. Cell 71: 765–776

Schwimmbeck PL, Badorff C, Schultheiss HP, Strauer BE (1994) Transfer of human myocarditis into severe combined immunodeficiency mice. Circ Res 75: 156–164

Seko Y, Matsuda H, Kato K, Hashimoto Y, Yagita H, Okumura K, et al (1993) Expression of intercellular adhesion molecule-1 in murine hearts with acute myocarditis caused by coxsackievirus B3. J Clin Invest 91: 1327–1336

Smith JC, Allen PM (1992) Neutralisation of endogenous tumor necrosis factor ameliorates the severity of myosin-induced myocarditis. Circ Res 70: 856–863

Sobotka PA, McMannis J, Fisher RI, Stein DG, Thomas JX (1990) Effects of interleukin 2 on cardiac function in isolated rat heart. J Clin Invest 86: 845–850

Sole MJ, Liu P (1993) Viral myocarditis: developing a paradigm for pathogenesis and treatment of dilated cardiomyopathy. J Am Coll Cardiol 22(4A): 99–105

Tartaglia LA, Pennica D, Goeddel DV (1993) Ligand passing: the 75kDa tumor necrosis factor receptor recruits TNF for signaling by the 55kDa TNF receptor. J Biol Chem 268: 18542–18548

Torre-Amione G, Kapadia S, Lee J, Bies RD, Lebovitz R, Mann DL (1995) Expression and functional significance of tumor necrosis factor receptors in human myocardium. Circulation 92: 1487–1493

Yamada T, Matsumori A, Sasayama S (1994) Therapeutic effect of anti-tumor necrosis factor-alpha on the murine model of viral myocarditis induced by encephalomyocarditis virus. Circulation 89: 846–851

Yokoyama T, Vaca L, Rossen RD, Durante W, Hazarika P, Mann DL (1993) Cellular basis for the negative inotropic effects of tumor necrosis factor-alpha in the adult mammalian heart. J Clin Invest 92: 2303–2312

The Role of Heart Infiltrating Cells in Myocyte Injury

W.H. Barry and L. Zhao

Introduction

There remains considerable uncertainity regarding the mechanisms of myocyte injury that is caused during myocarditis, or cardiac allograft rejection. Many investigators have proposed that immune mediated cardiac injury is due to an effect of CD8+ cytotoxic T lymphocytes (CTL). CTL may directly injure cardiac myocytes in an allospecific manner, by reacting with major histocompatibility complex (MHC) class 1 antigens expressed on the surface of the myocyte in the case of transplant rejection, or by reacting against viral antigens expressed on the surface of the myocyte in the case of myocarditis (for review see Barry 1994). Indeed there is considerable evidence that CD8+ CTLs can cause injury or lysis of cardiac myocytes in a variety of experimental situations. The work of Felzen et al. (1994) has demonstrated that Con A-activated CTL can induce lysis of cardiac myocytes. Hassin et al. (1987) showed that lymphocytes isolated from the spleen of Mingo virus infected rats can lyse Mingo virus infected cultured cardiac myocytes, and Huber et al. (1984) have demonstrated CTL-mediated lysis of Coxsackie virus infected myocytes by sensitized CTL. Work from our group (Woodley et al. 1991; Ensley et al. 1994) has demonstrated that CD8+ CTL obtained from a mixed lymphocyte reaction (MLR) in a murine heterotopic transplant model can induce contractile abnormalities and lysis of cultured fetal murine cardiac ventricular myocytes in an allospecific manner.

These studies clearly demonstrate the ability of CTL to injure cardiac myocytes. However, although CTL are present during cardiac rejection, (Frisman et al., 1991; Sell et al. 1992) little work has been done to demonstrate that in the in vivo setting, CTL are involved in direct myocyte injury. Indeed, a number of investigators have suggested that CD4+ cells may be the principal mediators of allograft rejection, possibly by recruitment and activation of macrophages resulting in a delayed type hypersensitivity (DTH) response (Hall 1991; Bishop et al. 1992, 1993; Bradley et al. 1992).

We have investigated these issues in a murine heterotopic cardiac transplant system, by determining the nature of inflammatory cells infiltrating a rejecting cardiac allograft, and assaying for cytotoxicity caused by various cell types in

Cardiology Division, University of Utah Medical Center, 50 North Medical Drive, Salt Lake City, UT 84132, USA

an in vitro cultured adult myocyte system. Our results indicate that CD8 + CTL cells do participate in direct myocardial injury during allograft rejection, but that other cell types, possibly macrophages, also contribute significantly to the injury observed.

Methods

Animals

BALB/c, C3H/heN and C57 BL/6 mice were obtained from the National Cancer Institute in Frederick, Maryland, Cancer Research and Development Center. Heterotopic cardiac transplantation was performed as described by Shelby and Corry (1982). After anesthesia, the abdomen of the recipient animal was opened and the donor heart was transplanted by anastamosing the donor to the recipient aorta and the donor pulmonary artery to the inferior vena cava in an end-to-side fashion. The transplanted heart is thus arterially perfused via the coronary arteries and contracts spontaneously but does perform work. In these experiments, the recipient animal was C57 BL/6 and the donor animal BALB/c.

Production of MLR

As described previously (Woodley et al. 1991) spleens were obtained from recipient animals 6–9 days after transplantation processed into single cell suspensions. They were cultured with irradiated donor strain lymphocytes for 6 to 8 days. This process thus includes in vitro and in vivo allostimulation of lymphocytes, and produces a culture in which effector cells causing myocyte lysis are primary CD8+ CTL (Woodley et al. 1991). Non-sensitized control lymphocytes (NSL) were obtained from non transplanted recipient animals and cultured without exposure to irradiated donor strain lymphocytes.

Culture of Activated Peritoneal Macrophages

The method of Higuchi et al. (1990) was used to prepare activated peritoneal macrophages. Briefly, C57B6 mice were injected intraabdominally with 3% thioglycollate broth, 2 ml per mouse. After 3 days, the peritoneal fluid was harvested, and cells were cultured for 24 h in the presence of 100 ng/ml lipopolysaccharide (LPS) and 25 units/ml of interferon-γ, to further activate macrophages present.

Isolation of HIC

Donor hearts were removed 6–8 days after transplantation and five to eight hearts were pooled and minced. The tissue was digested with collagenase. After red blood cells were lysed with sterile water, the inflammatory heart infiltrating cells (HIC) were washed and resuspended in myocyte culture medium.

Dissociation and Culture of Adult Mouse Ventricular Myocytes

Adult mouse myocyte isolation was performed by aortic cannulation and collagenase retrograde perfusion of individual hearts as described (Wagoner et al. 1996). After mincing of the tissue to separate the myocytes, they were suspended in gradually increasing calcium containing medium and finally in myocyte culture medium.

Measurement of Lysis of Adult Ventricular Myocytes

Suspensions of MLR cells, HIC, NSL, or macrophages were added to 300 µl cultured adult myocytes in 2-ml tubes. The concentration of rod shaped adult myocytes was adjusted to give a desired effector–to–target cell ratio. Myocytes and effector cells were allowed to settle to the bottom of the tube by gravity, and they were incubated in a 5% CO_2 and 95% air environment at 37 °C for a predetermined time. Subsequently, trypan blue was added to the co-culture and the number of viable myocytes was determined by counting the non-trypan blue stained rod-shaped cells with clear cross striations in a modified hemocytometer. The relative survival of myocytes incubated with the various effector cells was determined by comparing the survival of myocytes to that of myocytes in tubes containing medium alone. Measurements were performed in quadruplicate, and the average of four values was determined.

Results

Comparison of the cell types present in HIC and MLR populations revealed that the MLR population contained a higher percentage of lymphocytes (81%) as compared to the HIC population (44% lymphocytes). The HIC population also contained numerous macrophages (30%) and a significant number of polymorphonuclear leukocytes (PMN) (20%). Limiting dilution analysis (Orosz et al. 1989) was carried out to determine the relative number of alloantigen reactive CTL present in these populations. The total population of allo-responsive CTL was 1 in 93 and the HIC population versus 1 in 72 and the MLR population. These differences were not statistically significant. Thus both HIC and MLR populations contained a similar number of allo-reactive cytotoxic T lymphocytes.

Results of the examination of the relative cytotoxicity of MLR and HIC cells against cultured adult ventricular myocytes is shown in Fig. 1. As can be seen in Fig. 1A, the cytotoxicity produced by HIC was much less marked than that produced by MLR cells. As shown in Fig. 1B, the cytotoxicity also developed somewhat more slowly. The results in Fig. 1A suggested that the CTL present

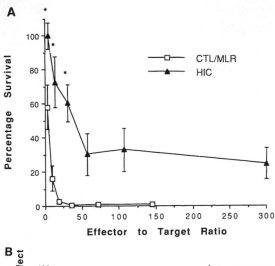

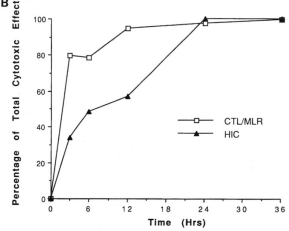

Fig. 1A,B. Injury produced by HICs against donor-strain myocytes. **A** Plot shows percentage survival of donor-strain myocytes incubated with varying dilutions of HICs and MLR cells for 36 h at 37 °C. MLR cells have significantly greater cytotoxic effects than HICs at E/T ratios up to 125:1. $n=4$ separate experiments; *$p < .05$. **B** Cumulative cytotoxicity of HICs and MLR cells over time. Plotting the cumulative cytotoxicity of HICs and MLR cells against donor-strain adult ventricular myocytes over time demonstrates that most of the cytotoxic effect of MLR cells occurs in the first 6 h, whereas the cytotoxic effect of HICs is more gradual and continuous, with a greater amount of cytotoxicity occuring between 12 and 24 h from HICs compared with MLR cells. This time course is derived from data from a representative experiment. Modified from Wagoner et al. (1996) with permission of authors and publisher

within the HIC population were not as effective killers as the CTL present in an MLR; and the findings shown in Fig. 1B also indicated that the mechanism of injury being caused might differ between these two cell populations.

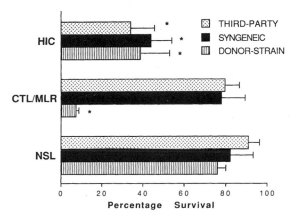

Fig. 2. Alloantigen-specificity of HIC vs MLR cytotoxicity. Bar graph represents experiments performed simultaneously on myocytes isolated from donor-strain (BALB/c), syngeneic (C57BL/6), and third-party (C3H) adult mice. The survival of myocytes from all three strains coincubated with HICs, MLR cells, or medium alone at 37 °C was determined; cytotoxicity was assessed at 12 h. The average E/T ratio for each strain varied between 137:1 for the target strain and 325:1 for the syngeneic strain. Whereas MLR cells were cytotoxic against only the donor-strain, HICs killed donor-strain, syngeneic, and third-party adult ventricular myocytes. $n=8$ separate experiments; $*p < .05$ by ANOVA Intragroup analysis comparing survival of cell type between strains. From Wagoner et al. Circ 93: 111–119, 1996, with permission of authors and publisher

To investigate the latter possibility, we compared the extent of myocyte lysis caused by HIC and MLR cells directed against donor strain, syngeneic or self strain, and third party unrelated strain myocytes. The results are shown in Fig. 2. MLR cells caused lysis that was allospecific, that is donor strain myocytes were lysed but not syngeneic or third party cells. The injury caused by HIC was much less allospecific, and syngeneic and third party myocytes were lysed equally well by HIC as were the donor strain cells. These results clearly indicated that the type of injury being produced by the HIC cells was distinct from that produced by the MLR cells. Since the injury produced by MLR cells has been shown to be due primarily to the CD8+ CTL component of the MLR (Woodley et al. 1991), this finding clearly suggested that CTL were not accounting for the majority of cell injury produced by the HIC.

To investigate this issue more directly, we examined the effects of depletion of the CTL by exposing these cell populations to anti-CD8 antibody (hybridoma 2.43) plus complement. These experiments showed that although anti-CD8 antibody plus complement significantly decreased HIC induced cytotoxicity (9.23% ± 1.89% increase in survival), this was markedly less than the effect of anti-CD8 antibody treatment on MLR cytotoxicity (59.4% ± 3.71% increase in survival, $p < 0.0001$).

As mentioned previously, a major difference in the composition of the HIC and MLR populations was the presence of a large number of macrophages in the HIC cell population. We therefore examined the effects of activated mouse peritoneal macrophages on myocytes in vitro. The results are shown in Fig. 3.

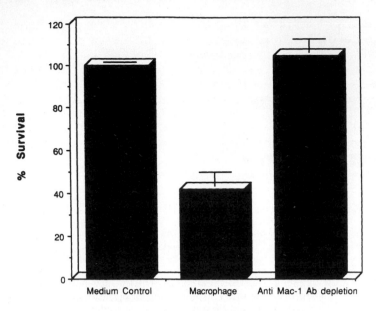

REACTION MIXTURE

Fig. 3. Effects of activated macrophages on myocyte survival. The column on the *left* shows survival of myocytes in culture medium (control). The column in the *middle* shows survival of myocytes in the co-cultured with activated macrophages for 12 h (100:1 E–T ratio). On the *right*, the effects on myocyte lysis of removal of activated macrophages by means of anti-MAC-1 antibody treatment are shown. Macrophages caused significant lysis ($p < 0.01$) of myocytes, (means ± SEM, $n=6$)

In these experiments, cultured activated macrophages were shown to induce significant myocyte lysis. This lysis could be inhibited by removing macrophages from the cultures by treatment with an anti-MAC-1 antibody, followed by exposure to magnetic beads coated with a secondary antibody, and placing the cells in a strong magnetic field. This indicates that macrophages in the peritoneal exudate fluid culture were causing the injury to myocytes.

Discussion

Our results demonstrate that while the HIC population contains a significant number of alloreactive cytotoxic T lymphocytes, only a small portion of the injury produced in our in vitro assay utilizing cultured adult ventricular myocytes can be ascribed to the CTL component of the HIC population. Myocyte lysis produced by the HIC was less intense than that caused by CTL in an MLR, developed more slowly, and was less allospecific. Furthermore, only a relative small proportion of the HIC-induced myocyte injury could be inhibited by monoclonal antibody-mediated CTL lysis. These findings taken together provide strong evidence that cell types other than allosensitized CTL in the HIC population are causing direct myocyte injury during cardiac allograft rejection.

Our experiments with activated macrophages demonstrate that the macrophage component of the infiltrating cell population could be causing myocyte injury. This would be consistent with the recent results of Bishop et al. (1993). This group showed that in vivo depletion of CD8+ cells from the recipient animal did not inhibit allograft rejection in the murine heterotopic transplant model. However, depletion of CD4+ cells did prevent rejection. These results are consistent with the hypothesis that CD4+ cells are mediating allograft rejection. Since previous work from our laboratory have shown that CD4+ cells have no direct cytoxic effect on myocytes (Woodley et al. 1991), these findings strongly suggest that CD4 cells are mediating allograft injury indirectly possibly by production of cytokines, which promote the infiltration of the graft by macrophages (Barry 1994), and contribute to the activation of macrophages.

It is not clear by what mechanism activated macrophages may cause myocyte injury. Activated macrophages can promote acute inflammation through mediators such as platelet activating factor, prostaglandins, leucotrienes, and free radicals (Cramer 1987; Marboe et al. 1990; Balbiar 1984). Cytokines such as tumor necrosis factor and nitric oxide secreted by macrophages may also have direct effects on myocytes (Higuchi et al. 1990). Other inflammatory cells present in the HIC population that could injure myocytes include neutrophils (Entman et al. 1992) and eosinophils (Chan et al. 1995). Further studies will be necessary to define the mechanisms by which HIC mediated myocyte injury is occuring during allograft rejection and myocarditis, and the cell types involved.

Acknowledgement. Supported in part by NIH Grant RO1 HL42535.

References

Babiar BM (1984) The respiratory burst of macrophages. J Clin Invest 73: 599–601

Barry WH (1994) Mechanisms of immune-mediated myocyte injury. Circulation 89: 2421–2432

Bishop DK, Shelby J, Eichwald EJ (1992) Mobilization of T lymphocytes following cardiac transplantation: Evidence that CD4-positive cells are required for cytotoxic T lymphocyte activation, inflammatory endothelial development, graft infiltration, and acute allograft rejection. Transplantation 53: 849–857

Bishop DK, Chan S, Li W, Ensley RD, Xu S, Eichwald EJ (1993) CD4-positive helper T lymphocytes mediate mouse cardiac allograft rejection independent of donor alloantigen specific cytotoxic T lymphocytes. Transplantation 56: 892–897

Bradley JA, Sarawar SR, Porteous C, Wood PJ, Card S, Ager A, Bolton EM, Bell EB (1992) Allograft rejection in CD4+ T cell-reconstituted athymic nude rat: the nonessential role of host-derived CD8+ cells. Transplantation 53: 477–482

Chan SY, DeBruyns LA, Goodman RE, Eichwald EJ, Bishop DK (1995) In vivo depletion of CD8+ T cells results in Th2 cytokines production and alternate mechanisms of allograft rejection. Transplantation 59: 1155–1161

Cramer DV (1987) Cardiac transplantation: immune mechanisms and alloantigens involved in graft rejection. CRC Crit Rev Immunol 7: 1–30

Ensley RD, Ives M, Zhao L, McMillen M, Shelby J, Barry WH (1994) Effects of alloimmune injury on contraction and relaxation in cultured myocytes and intact cardiac allografts. J Am Coll Cardiol 24: 1769–1778

Entman ML, Youker K, Shappel SB, Siegel C, Rothlein R, Dreyer WJ, Schmalstieg FC, Smith

CW (1990) Neutrophil adherence to isolated adult canine myocytes. J Clin Invest 85: 1497–1506

Felzen B, Bers G, Rosen D, Binah O (1994) Mechanisms whereby cytotoxic T lymphocytes damage guinea-pig ventricular myocytes in vitro. Eur J Physiol 427: 422–431

Frisman DM, Fallon JT, Hurwitz AA, Dec WG, Kurnick JT (1991) Cytotoxic activity of graft-infiltrating lymphocytes correlated with cellular rejection in cardiac transplant patients. Hum Immunol 32: 241–245

Hall B (1991) Cells mediating allograft rejection. Transplantation 51: 1141–1151

Hassin D, Fixler R, Shimoni Y, Rubinstein E, Raz S, Gotsman MS, Hasin Y (1987) Physiological changes induced in cardiac myocytes by cytotoxic T lymphocytes. Am J Physiol 252: C10–C16

Higuchi M, Higashi N, Taki H, Osawa T (1990) Cytolytic mechanisms of activated macrophages. J Immunol 144: 1425–1431

Huber SA, Job LP, Woodruff JF (1980) Lysis of infected myofibers by coxsackievirus B-3 immune T lymphocytes. Am J Pathol 115: 1326–1332

Marboe CC, Buffaloe A, Fenoglio JJ (1990) Immunologic aspects of rejection: Prog Cardiovasc Dis 32: 419–432

Orosz CG, Horstemeyer B, Zinn NE, Bishop DK (1989) Development and evaluation of an LDA technique that can discriminate in vivo alloactivated CTL from their naive CTL precursors. Transplantation 43: 189–194

Sell KW, Kanter K, Rodey GE, Wang YC, Ansari AA (1992) Characterization of human heart-infiltrating cells after transplantation. V. Suppression of donor-specific allogeneic responses by cloned T-cell lines isolated from heart biopsy specimens of patients after transplantation. J Heart Lung Transplant 11: 500–510

Shelby J, Corry RJ (1982) The primarily vascularized mouse heart transplant as a model for the study of immune response. J Heart Transplant 2: 32–36

Wagoner LE, Zhao L, Bishop DK, Chan S, Xu S, Barry WH (1996) Lysis of adult ventricular myocytes by cells infiltrating rejecting murine cardiac allografts. Circulation 93: 111–119

Woodley SL, McMillen M, Shelby J, Lynch DH, Roberts LK, Ensley RD, Barry WH (1991) Myocyte injury and contraction abnormalities produced by cytotoxic T lymphocytes. Circulation 83: 1410–1418

The Significance of T Cell Responses in Human Myocarditis

P. Schwimmbeck, C. Badorff, K. Schulze, and H.-P. Schultheiss

Introduction

The pathogenesis of myocarditis (MC) and dilated cardiomyopathy (DCM) is still poorly understood. It is assumed that an enteroviral infection, for example, by coxsackie B (CB) viruses is initiating the inflammatory process in human MC. This is supported by epidemiological studies showing an increased in cidence of viral MC following endemics of CB virus infections (Helin et al. 1968). In addition, the recent demonstration of enteroviral RNA in endomyocardial tissue of patients, suggested a pathophysiological significance of the infection. Using molecular biological methods such as dot-blot analysis, insitu hybridization or polymerase chain reaction (PCR), enteroviral RNA could be demonstrated in up to 50% of patients with MC and in an almost equally high percentage of cases with DCM (Bowles et al. 1986). However, the percentage of positive samples differs widely between the different studies, possibly due to different probes used for hybridization, differences in the primers utilized for amplification, or contamination with viral RNA, especially in the PCR, thus giving false-positive results.

The viral etiology of MC could also be demonstrated in animal models. Using CB3 virus, strain Nancy, it was possible to induce inflammatory heart disease, very much resembling human MC, in susceptible mice like Balb/c (Huber et al. 1984). By the infection of mice with different major histocompatibility complex (MHC) (H2) backgrounds, the genetic basis for susceptibility or resistance to the infection could be determined. In these experiments an acute viremic state of the disease could be differentiated from a more chronic stage that was characterized by the clearance of the virus and an autoimmune response against uninfected host tissue by sensitized T cells. However, the antigen of the T cell response is not known so far.

In human MC and DCM, an autoimmune response is also suspected. This is supported by the demonstration of autoantibodies against different autoantigens such as cardiac myosin (De Scheerder et al. 1991), the β-adrenergic receptor (Limas and Limas 1991), or the adenine nucleotide translocator (ANT) (Schultheiss et al. 1983) in the sera of patients with MC and DCM. Auto-

Department of Internal Medicine/Cardiology, Benjamin Franklin Hospital, Free University of Berlin, Hindenburgdamm 30, 12200 Berlin, Germany

antibodies against the ANT have in particular been shown to cause an impairment of the energy metabolism both in vitro and in vivo in the animal model (Schulze et al. 1989, 1990). Here it was possible to induce autoantibodies in guinea pigs after immunization with the isolated ANT that caused a shortage of energy rich nucleotides in the cytosol of myocytes and led to a decrease in the left ventricular function in a working heart model.

Another characteristic finding in human MC are infiltrating lymphocytes in the myocardium. These can be found both in the acute and in the chronic stages of the disease that often present clinically as DCM. Especially when immunohistological methods with monoclonal antibodies against lymphocyte surface markers were used, an inflammatory response in DCM could also often be found where the routine histological examination was not able to detect a relevant cellular infiltration (Kuehl et al. 1992). In addition, using monoclonal antibodies against human leukocyte antigens (HLA) class I and II and against adhesion molecules, an upregulation of these proteins could be shown that proves the presence of an immune reaction in these hearts. Such an immune reaction is independent of the presence of enteroviral sequences in the hearts and can be found in the myocardium of patients with DCM as well as with MC. Thus, also these results suggest a common origin and pathogenesis of MC and DCM, whereby DCM may represent a later stage of the initial MC.

However, many questions regarding the function and significance of sensitized T cells in MC and DCM remain unanswered. Among these is the identification of epitopes recognized by lymphocytes in MC, the specificity and phenotype of infiltrating cells in the myocardium of patients with MC and DCM, and the pathogenetic significance of the T cell response in human MC and DCM. In our experiments, we tried to address at least some of these questions.

T Cell Epitopes of CB3

Infection of mice with CB3, strain Nancy, is a well-studied animal model of MC. After infection of susceptible mice such as Balb/c, an inflammation in the hearts of the animals is seen that is characterized by myocyte necrosis and massive cellular infiltrates. Previous experiments have shown that at least in the initial state of the disease these infiltrating lymphocytes are directed against the virus used for the infection (Wolfgram et al. 1986). Since it had been shown that it is possible to map T cell epitopes using synthetic peptides (Schrier et al. 1988), we wanted to study which epitopes of CB3 are recognized by the sensitized T cells in the mice.

Previously, experiments using Western blot methodology had identified the viral coat protein VP1 of CB3 as harboring main B cell epitopes (Mertens et al. 1983). We, therefore, synthesized overlapping peptides of 15 amino acids (AA) each, representing the entire sequence of VP1 of CB3. All together, 31 peptides were prepared using the simultaneous multiple peptide synthesis method. When these peptides were tested in an enzyme-linked immunosorbent assay (ELISA) system for reactivity with sera from CB3 infected mice, the AA1–15,

AA 21–35, and AA 229–243 could be identified as antigenic determinants recognized by the anti-CB3 antibodies (Haarmann et al. 1994). In additional studies with type-specific antisera against the serotypes 1–6 of CB viruses it was possible to differentiate between serotype-specific (AA 1–15), semi-specific (AA 21–35), and nonserotype-specific epitopes (AA 229–243). This is of major interest for the development of a serological test system for CB viruses. It is highly conceivable to design both nonserotype-specific antibody screening tests and serotype-specific assays for the further differentiation of the infection using the appropriate peptides.

The epitopes represented by the peptides are accessible on the native virus, since sera raised against the peptides can be used for the immunohistological demonstration of the virus in myocardial sections of infected mice. In addition, the antipeptide antibodies bound the isolated virus in a Western blot.

To identify the T cell epitopes on VP1 of CB3, we used the overlapping peptides and tested them in a proliferation assay with [^{3}H] thymidine incorporation for reactivity with lymph node cells from CB3 infected mice. At least six different peptides induced significant proliferation of the lymphocytes, thus identifying them as T cell epitopes of CB3 virus. These contained the AA 1–15, AA 21–35, AA 79–93, AA 119–133, AA 129–143, and AA 199–213. The proliferating cells were shown to be T lymphocytes, since the treatment of the animals with monoclonal antibodies against pan T lymphocytes resulted in complete loss of reactivity of the lymph node cells.

In subsequent studies done in collaboration with S. Huber from the University of Vermont, USA, the pathogenetic significance of the T cell epitopes was investigated (Huber et al. 1993). Mice were immunized with the peptides and subsequently infected with CB3 virus 2 weeks later. After preimmunization with a peptide representing the AA 1–15 of CB3 a significant reduction of the virus titer in the heart and decreased inflammation was observed. In contrast, after immunization with the AA 21–35, the viral titers in the myocardium after infection were unchanged when compared with those in animals without preimmunization. However, both the degree of inflammation in the heart and mortality of the animals, which is normally rather low in this model of infection, were significantly increased. Thus, these experiments showed that an immune response against different T cell epitopes of CB3 virus can either have a protective or a detrimental effect in the pathogenesis of MC. Therefore, experiments testing possible vaccines such as peptides or viral proteins or parts thereof should be tested carefully in order to avoid the induction of an immune response causing additional damage in the pathogenesis of MC.

Human T-Cell Responses Against CB Viruses

After infection with CB viruses, a T-cell response is induced in humans. However, so far the epitopes recognized by the T lymphocytes are not known. In order to identify the T cell antigens recognized by the T cells and especially in order to see if they are identical to the epitopes reactive in murine myocarditis, we tested the peripheral blood leukocytes (PBL) of patients with immunohistologically proven myocarditis for reactivity with the overlapping peptides representing the viral coat protein VP1 of CB3 in a proliferation assay with thymidine incorporation. In tests of more than 30 patients, we found different reactivity patterns: about half of the patients showed reactivity with peptides representing the AA 41–55, 139–153, 239–253 and 269–283. The epitopes recognized by the T cells from patients with MC also differed between the individual patients and were different from the epitopes recognized by the T cells in murine MC after the infection of Balb/c mice with CB3. This is most likely due to the differences in the antigen presenting cells (MHC) between mice and humans, where only restricted peptides are presented to the immune systems and can thus be recognized by the effector cells. This may also be one of the reasons for a different reactivity pattern between the various patients. However, our population of patients studied so far is not yet large enough to allocate a certain reactivity pattern to an individual MHC type. It is highly conceivable that the reported HLA class II correlations in DCM are due to the restricted presentation of pathogenetically important antigens (Bjorkmann et al. 1987). Another reason for the differences in the reactivity pattern to CB viruses between mice and humans is certainly that in humans it is mostly impossible to determine what serotype of virus caused the infection, since there is a high rate of immunity against enteroviruses in the adult population and there is a considerable cross reactivity between the single types of coxsackie viruses (Mertens et al. 1983).

Lymphocyte Cultures Established from Endomyocardial Biopsies of Patients with MC and DCM

A characteristic finding in human MC is the presence of activated, infiltrating leukocytes in the myocardium. However, neither the phenotype nor the specificity of the infiltrating cells is known. We, therefore, studied whether it is possible to culture the infiltrating mononuclear cells present in endomyocardial, right ventricular biopsies of patients with clinically suspected MC or DCM. Using cocultivation with irradiated autologous PBL in the presence of recombinant interleukin-2 and restimulation with myocardial tissue, we were able to establish primary lymphocyte cultures in about 50% of the biopsies from MC and DCM patients (see Table 1) within 30 days. There was no major difference in the percentage of positive biopsies between both diseases. As controls, we cultured myocardial biopsies from patients with arterial hypertension and hypertrophic cardiomyopathy. In none of these cases it was possible to establish positive cell cultures.

For phenotyping of the cells, we used fluorescence-activated cell sorter (FACS) analysis with double labeling of the cells. The majority of cells were CD3-positive, identifying them as T lymphocytes. Most of these cells were also either CD4 (helper/inducer) or CD8 (suppressor/cytotoxic)-positive (see Table 2). The CD8-positive cultures had a tendency to be present more frequently in patients with healing myocarditis; however, this did not reach statistical significance. Only in a very low percentage macrophages or natural

Table 1. Lymphocytes cultured from myocardial biopsies of patients with myocarditis (MC) or dilated cardiomyopathy (DCM)

Patients	Positive culture		Negative culture	
	n	%	n	%
MC (n=71)	38	54	33	46
DCM (n=47)	25	53	22	47
Controls (n=8)	0	0	8	100

Cultures were considered to be positive if more than 1×10^6 cells could be grown within 30 days. Biopsies from patients with arterial hypertension or hypertrophic cardiomyopathy were used as controls.

Table 2. Immune phenotype of cells cultured from myocardial biopsies

Marker	Percentage	Range (%)
CD3-positive (pan T) cells	95	84–99
CD4-positive (helper/inducer) cells	42	18–89
CD8-positive (suppressor/cytotoxic) cells	51	13–95
MA100-positive cells (macrophages)	0	0
CD57-positive (natural killer) cells	3	0–10

The average number of positive cells are given for the different markers and the range of positive cells. Cells were evaluated by FACS analysis after staining with monoclonal antibodies.

killer cells were observed. Despite the fact that our culture conditions may have influenced the phenotype and number of cells that grew, it was possible to demonstrate that there are infiltrating, activated leukocytes in the myocardium of patients with MC as well as patients with DCM.

The cultured cells were tested for proliferation after stimulation with CB3 virus, the isolated ANT and peptides derived from these proteins. In five patients, we found significant proliferation with a stimulation index of more than 3 against the ANT or peptides derived from it. These experiments demonstrate that the ANT is a myocardial autoantigen in MC and DCM and is recognized by infiltrating cells in the myocardium of patients. When we tested for proliferation against CB3 or peptides derived thereof, we found proliferation in nine cultures. Here we again found proliferation against different epitopes; however, most of the cultures reacted with the AA 51–65 and 139–153 of VP1 of CB3 virus. Of course, the question remains as to why not more or even all of the cultures reacted with CB3 virus or the ANT. One explanation is certainly that different enteroviruses are thought to be involved in the pathogenesis of MC and DCM, and that those may not share T cell epitopes with the CB3 virus used here as an antigen. In addition, microbes other than enteroviruses may also cause MC, since enteroviral sequences can be found in only about 50% of biopsies of patients with MC and in an even lower percentage of biopsies with DCM. The same is also true for the identification of autoantigens in MC and DCM. Several other autoantigens besides the ANT were identified and characterized in patients with MC and DCM. Therefore, testing with different viruses or autoantigens would have probably yielded a larger number of positive cultures. In addition, the cells cultured from the myocardial biopsies may have an impaired capacity of proliferation due to the long culture times, thus giving a lower degree of proliferation or even none. Another problem in these proliferation assays is the quality of the antigen presenting cells. A high proliferation rate could perhaps be achieved by using irradiated Epstein-Barr virus (EBV)-transformed, immortal autologous leukocytes as antigen presenting cells, since the quality of antigen presenting cells is a crucial factor for proliferation. However, in our experiments we used only irradiated PBL as antigen presenting cells since we wanted to avoid a possible unspecific proliferation due to EBV.

Significance of T Cell Responses: Transfer of Human MC into SCID Mice

Despite the demonstration of autoimmune phenomena in patients with MC and DCM, there is no proof of the autoimmune pathogenesis of these diseases. This is due to the lack of a transfer model for the human diseases. In the animal experiment it is possible to transfer MC from CB3 infected mice after the clearance of the virus to uninfected mice by lymphocyte transfer. Similarly, autoimmune MC can be induced by the infusion with sensitized T cells from animals immunized with cardiac myosin (Smith and Alan 1991). However, in the human disease, transfer experiments were so far unsuccessful, since human mononuclear cells will be rejected and eliminated when transfered into xenogenic, immunocompetent animals.

Severe combined immunodeficient (SCID) mice lack functional T and B lymphocytes in the peripheral blood due to a genetic defect (Bosma et al. 1983). Therefore, these animals can be used in transfer experiments to receive allogenic or even xenogenic transplants (Phillips and Spaner 1991). In previous experiments it had been possible to transfer normal human leukocytes and also PBL from patients with lupus erythematodes (Duchusal et al. 1990), primary biliary cirrhosis (Krams et al. 1989), rheumatoid arthritis (Tighe et al. 1990), or Grave's disease into SCID mice (Macht et al. 1991).

Following these lines we wanted to investigate the possibility of transferring PBL from patients with chronic MC into SCID mice to examine the animals for the presence of autoimmune phenomena normally seen in the human disease and to measure the left ventricular function in the animals after transfer. As donors we isolated the PBL from 13 patients with immunohistologically proven myocarditis that had persisted for more than 6 months. Viral persistence in the myocardial biopsies of these patients was excluded by in-situ hybridization and PCR using enteroviral-specific probes. Only patients with a negative serology for EBV were included, since EBV-positive donors can induce lymphomas in the animals after transfer (Rowe et al. 1991). All the patients included had positive titers of autoantibodies against the ANT, and the left ventricular function of the heart was impaired. As controls we isolated PBL from seven healthy blood donors also with negative EBV serology. For the transfer 50×10^6 PBL were injected intraperitoneally into 8–10 week old male CB17 SCID mice. For each experiment, at least three animals per patient were used and kept under specific pathogen-free conditions in the animal quarters. After 60 days, the animals were evaluated for the presence of immunoglobulins and autoantibodies in the peripheral blood, human mononuclear cells in the peripheral blood and different tissues and the left ventricular function was determined by measuring the slope of the left ventricular pressure pulse after direct puncture of the left ventricle of the heart under ether anesthesia.

At 60 days after transfer, human immunoglobulin (Ig) levels of up to 4 mg/ml of human IgG and IgM could be found in the sera of the SCID mice. There was no difference in the human Ig levels in the peripheral blood of the animals receiving PBL from either controls or patients with MC. These Ig were due to a polyclonal immune response as shown by the distribution of the human IgG subclasses in the SCID mouse sera. Quite similar to the IgG subclass distribution in the donor sera with the usual predominance of IgG1, the SCID mouse sera in the reconstituted animals showed all four IgG subclasses. Due to the exclusion of EBV-positive donors, no monoclonal Ig in the transfused SCID mice was observed. When we tested for the presence of autoantibodies against the ANT in the SCID mice, no relevant autoantibody titers were observed in the animals which received PBL from controls. In contrast, more than 90% of animals which received PBL from MC patients had significant levels of autoantibodies against the isolated ANT, both IgG and IgM (Schwimmbeck et al. 1994). Thus, these experiments suggest an ongoing human immune response against the ANT in the animals after transfer of PBL.

When we tested for the presence of human PBL in the peripheral blood of the SCID mice by FACS analysis, human mononuclear cells, representing up to 10% of the total leukocytes in the peripheral blood of the SCID mice could be demonstrated. These cells consisted in about equal parts of human B and T lymphocytes. The T lymphocytes could be further differentiated into CD4-positive helper/inducer cells and CD8-positive suppressor/cytotoxic cells (see Fig. 1). There was no difference in the levels of human leukocytes between the animals receiving cells from patients with MC or healthy controls. The human leukocytes in the peripheral blood of the SCID mice were activated, since the sera of animals receiving PBL from patients with MC contained elevated levels of the human soluble interleukin-2 receptor, which is released during the activation of T cells. In comparison, mice receiving cells from controls had normal levels of the soluble interleukin-2 receptor.

Staining of the myocardium of the SCID mice showed no relevant infiltrating human cells in the animals receiving PBL from controls. However, animals receiving leukocytes from patients with MC had in the average upto 6.1 infiltrating CD3-positive human T cells in their myocardium per ten high-power light microscopic fields. These cells formed focal infiltrations in the heart, a finding seen quite similarly in myocardial biopsies of patients with

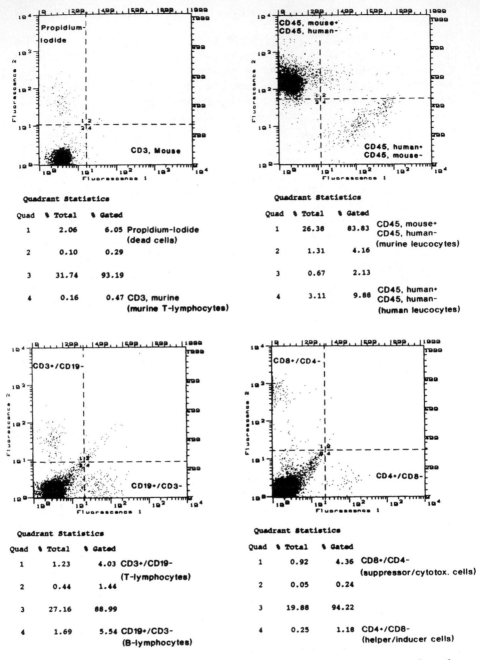

Quadrant Statistics

Quad	% Total	% Gated	
1	2.06	6.05	Propidium-Iodide (dead cells)
2	0.10	0.29	
3	31.74	93.19	
4	0.16	0.47	CD3, murine (murine T-lymphocytes)

Quadrant Statistics

Quad	% Total	% Gated	
1	26.38	83.83	CD45, mouse+ CD45, human- (murine leucocytes)
2	1.31	4.16	
3	0.67	2.13	
4	3.11	9.88	CD45, human+ CD45, human- (human leucocytes)

Quadrant Statistics

Quad	% Total	% Gated	
1	1.23	4.03	CD3+/CD19- (T-lymphocytes)
2	0.44	1.44	
3	27.16	88.99	
4	1.69	5.54	CD19+/CD3- (B-lymphocytes)

Quadrant Statistics

Quad	% Total	% Gated	
1	0.92	4.36	CD8+/CD4- (suppressor/cytotox. cells)
2	0.05	0.24	
3	19.88	94.22	
4	0.25	1.18	CD4+/CD8- (helper/inducer cells)

Fig. 1a,b. FACS analysis of peripheral blood mononuclear cells in SCID mice at 60 days after transfer of 50×10^6 PBL from a patient with immunohistologically proven MC. Double labeling was used in all experiments. **a** On the *left panel,* labeling of dead cells with propidium-iodide and a monoclonal antibody against murine CD3, a murine pan T cell marker. The *right panel* shows staining of the cells with a monoclonal antibody against murine respectively human leukocytes. **b** On the *left panel,* the results of staining with a human B and T cell marker and *on the right panel*, the further differentiation of the cells into suppressor/cytotoxic and helper/inducer cells. The number of positive cells is given below each panel

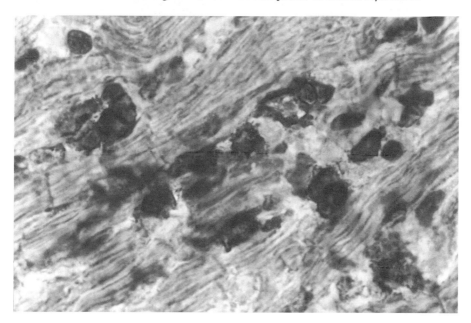

Fig. 2. Infiltrating human lymphocytes in the myocardial tissue of a SCID mouse transfused with PBL from a patient with myocarditis. Immune peroxidase staining with a murine monoclonal antibody against human CD3. ×400

MC (see Fig. 2). The peripheral skeletal muscle of the animals transfused with either PBL from MC patients or from controls were free of infiltrating human leukocytes. Additional sections were obtained from the liver of the reconstituted animals. Also here, no relevant levels of infiltrating human leukocytes were observed, thus excluding clinically apparent graft-versus-host disease. Another indicator for the absence of relevant graft-versus-host disease was the survival of all animals after transfer and the obviously healthy look of the animals without runting, necrosis of the tips of the toes, or diarrhoea (Murphy et al. 1992).

The antigen recognized by the infiltrating human leukocytes in the SCID mouse hearts is not known. However, since obviously an ongoing B-cell response against the ANT is present in the SCID mice, it can be speculated that the T cell response is also directed, at least in part, against the ANT (Schwimmbeck et al. 1991). In order to investigate the antigen specificity of the human infiltrating cells in the myocardium of the SCID mice, we are now attempting to culture these cells in order to determine their antigen specificity.

In additional experiments, SCID mice were transfused with either only CD4-positive cells or with CD4-depleted PBL from patients with MC. Hereby only low levels of human Ig or infiltrating cells in the myocardium could be achieved. These results demonstrated the necessity of an ongoing human immune response besides the transfer of sensitized T cells for the full development of MC.

The mechanisms by which the obviously sensitized human T cells are directed to the heart and recognize their antigen are not known so far. However, adhesion molecules could play an important role for the T cell trafficking as also shown for other diseases (Bankert et al. 1989).

When we tested the myocardial function of the SCID mouse hearts after transfer of PBL, normal left ventricular function was observed in the animals receiving PBL from healthy controls. Their slope of the left ventricular pressure pulse (dp/dt) was on an average 2450 mmHg/s and thus not significantly different from the values measured in untreated animals (2570 mmHg/s). However, animals receiving PBLs from patients with MC showed a decreased left ventricular pressure pulse of about 1750 mmHg/s (see Fig. 3). The exact mechanism leading to the impairment of the left ventricular function is not known. Regarding the relative low number of infiltrating human leukocytes, it is obviously not due to direct damage of the infiltrating cells but rather due to either the release of cytokines from the infiltrating cells or to another humoral factor. In order to address this question it is necessary to determine the levels of human cytokines in the myocardium of the SCID mice by, for example, determining their mRNA levels.

In summary, the transfer of MC from patients with MC into SCID mice with PBLs gives proof to the hypothesis of an autoimmune pathogenesis for MC and DCM.

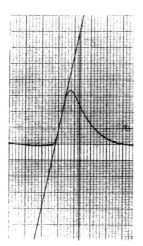 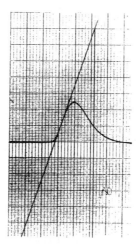

Fig. 3. Measurement of the left ventricular pressure in SCID mice after direct puncture of the left ventricle. A tangent was added to the curve in order to determine the slope of the left ventricular pressure pulse (dt/dp). The *left panel* gives a representative example of the measurement in a SCID mouse after transfer of PBLs from a healthy control, showing a dp/dt of 2360 mmHg/s. The *right panel* gives an example of a SCID mouse heart after transfer of PBLs from a patient with MC with a dp/dt of 1480 mmHg/s. The heart rates in the animals were comparable

Conclusions

Sensitized T cells can be demonstrated both in the murine models of MC as well as in human MC and DCM. These lymphocytes are antigen-specific for coxsackie viruses and/or myocardial autoantigens such as the ANT. Using isolated proteins and peptides derived from their sequences, it is possible to identify the epitopes recognized by the immune cells. The sensitized T cells play an important role in the pathogenesis of MC and DCM since it is possible to transfer the immune phenomena and the impairment of the function of the heart into SCID mice with the PBL isolated from patients with MC. With this model it seems to be feasible to test the significance (or insignificance) of the immune response against single (auto-)antigens in MC and DCM by the transfer of cells specific for the (auto-)antigen.

Acknowledgements. This work was supported by a grant from the Deutsche Forschungsgemeinschaft. PLS was the recipient of a grant from the NATO for international collaboration.

References

Bankert RB, Umemoto T, Sugiyama Y, Chen FA, Repasky E, Yokota S (1989) Human lung tumors, patients' peripheral blood lymphocytes and tumor infiltrating lymphocytes propagated in SCID mice. Curr Top Microbiol Immunol 154: 201–210

Bjorkmann PJ, Saper MA, Samraouni B, Bennett WS, Strominger JL, Wiley DC (1987) Structure of the human class I histocompatibility antigen HLA-A2. Nature 329: 506–512

Bosma GC, Custer RP, Bosma MJ (1983) A severe combined immunodeficiency mutation in the mouse. Nature 301: 527–530

Bowles NE, Richardson PJ, Olsen EGJ, Archard LC (1986) Detection of Coxsackie-B-virus-specific RNA sequences in myocardial biopsy samples from patients with myocarditis and dilated cardiomyopathy. Lancet 1: 1120–1123

De Scheerder IK, De Buyzere M, Delanghe J, Maas A, Clement DL, Wieme R (1991) Humoral immune response against contractile proteins (actin and myosin) during cardiovascular disease. Eur Heart J 12 [suppl D]: 88–94

Duchusal MA, McConahey PJ, Robinson CA, Dixon FJ (1990) Transfer of human lupus erythmatodes in severe combined immunodeficient (SCID) mice. J Exp Med 172: 985–988

Haarmann CM, Schwimmbeck PL, Mertens T, Schultheiss HP, Strauer B (1994) Identification of serotype-specific and nonserotype-specific B-cell epitopes of Coxsackie B viruses using synthetic peptides. Virology 200: 381–389

Helin M, Savola J, Lapinleimu K (1968) Cardiac manifestations during a coxsackie B5 epidemic. Br Med J 3: 97–99

Huber SA, Lodge PA (1984) Coxsackie B3 myocarditis in Balb/c mice: evidence for autoimmunity to myocyte antigens. Am J Physiol 116: 21–27

Huber SA, Polgar J, Moraska A, Cunningham M, Schwimmbeck P, Schultheiss HP (1993) T lymphocyte responses in CVB3-induced murine myocarditis. Scand J Infect Diseases 88: 67–78

Krams SM, Dorshkind K, Gershwin ME (1989) Generation of biliary lesions after transfer of human lymphocytes into severe combined immunodeficient (SCID) mice. J Exp Med 170: 1919–1930

Kuehl U, Daun B, Seeberg B, Schultheiss HP, Strauer BE (1992) Dilated cardiomyopathy – a chronic myocarditis? Herz 17(2): 97–106

Limas CJ, Limas C (1991) Beta-adrenoreceptor antibodies and genetics in dilated cardio-myopathy: an overview and review. Eur Heart J 12[suppl D]: 175–177

Macht L, Kukuma N, Leader K, Sarsero D, Pegg CAS, Phillips DIW, Yates P, McLachlan SM, Elson C, Smith BR (1991) Severe combined immunodeficient (SCID) mice: A model for investigating human thyroid autoantibody synthesis. Clin Exp Immunol 84: 34–42

Mertens T, Pika U, Eggers HJ (1983) Cross antigenicity among enteroviruses as revealed by immunoblot technique. Virology 129: 431–442

Murphy WJ, Bennett M, Anver MR, Baseler M, Longo DL (1992) Human-mouse lymphoid chimeras: Host-vs.-graft and graft-vs.-host reactions. Eur J Immunol 22: 1421–1427

Phillips RA, Spaner DE (1991) The SCID mouse: Mutation in a DNA repair gene creates recipients useful for studies on stem cells, lymphocyte development and graft-versus-host disease. Immunol Rev 124: 63–73

Rowe M, Young LS, Crocker J, Stokes H, Henderson S, Rickinson AB (1991) Epstein-Barr virus (EBV) -associated lymphoproliferative disease in the SCID mouse model: Implications for the pathogenesis of EBV-positive lymphomas in man. J Exp Med 173: 147–158

Rubin LA, Nelson DL (1990) The soluble interleukin-2 receptor: biology, function and clinical application. Ann Intern Med 113: 619–627

Schrier RD, Gnann JW, Langlois AJ, Shriver K, Nelson JA, Oldstone MBA (1988) B- and T-lymphocyte responses to an immunodominant epitope of human immunodeficiency virus. J Virology 62: 2531–2536

Schultheiss HP, Bolte HD, Schwimmbeck P, Klingenberg M (1983) The antigenic character-istics and the significance of the adenine nucleotide translocator (ANT) as a major auto-antigen for antimitochondrial antibodies in myocarditis and congestive cardiomyopathy. J Mol Cell Cardiol 15: 85–93

Schulze K, Becker BF, Schultheiss HP (1989) Antibodies to the ADP–ATP carrier – an auto-antigen in myocarditis and dilated cardiomyopathy – penetrate into myocardial cells and disturb energy metabolism in vivo. Circ Res 64: 179–192

Schulze K, Becker BF, Schauer R, Schultheiss HP (1990) Antibodies to ADP–ATP carrier – an autoantigen in myocarditis and dilated cardiomyopathy – impair cardiac function. Circ 81: 959–969

Schwimmbeck PL, Schultheiss HP, Strauer BE (1991) Demonstration of antigen-specific lymphocytes cultured from myocardial tissue of patients with viral heart disease. Circ 84[suppl II]: II–440 (abstract)

Schwimmbeck PL, Badorff C, Schultheiss HP, Strauer BE (1994) Transfer of human myo-carditis into severe combined immunodeficiency mice. Circ Res 75: 156–164

Smith SC, Allen PM (1991) Myosin-induced acute myocarditis is a T cell-mediated disease. J Immunol 147: 2141–2147

Tighe H, Silverman GJ, Kozin F, Tucker R, Gulizia R, Peebles C, Lotz M, Rhodes G, Machold K, Mosier DE, Carson DA (1990) Autoantibody production by severe combined im-munodeficient mice reconstituted with synovial cells from rheumatoid arthritis patients. Eur J Immunol 20: 1843–1848

Wolfgram LJ, Beisel KW, Herskowitz A, Rose NR (1986) Variations in the susceptibility to coxsackie B3 virus induced myocarditis among different strains of mice. J Immunol 136: 1846–1852

The Possible Pathogenic Role of Autoantibodies in Myocarditis and Dilated Cardiomyopathy

G. Wallukat[1], H.-P. Luther[1], J. Müller[2], and A. Wollenberger[1]

Introduction

A chronic β-adrenergic overdrive in patients with dilated cardiomyopathy (DCM) has been postulated to be one of the pathogenic features of this disease (Thomas and Marks 1978; Swedberg et al. 1979; Cohn et al. 1984). The marked elevation of the plasma norepinephrine level in patients with heart failure may have a number of consequences such as (a) a catecholamine-triggered alteration of the β-adrenergic reaction cascade represented by a desensitization of the β_1-adrenoceptor (Bristow, 1982, 1984; Brodde 1991; Steinfahrt et al. 1991; Ungerer et al. 1993), (b) an inhibition of the adenylate cyclase by overexpression of the Giα protein (Böhm et al. 1990), and (c) a reduction in the inotropic responsiveness of the heart (Bristow 1993). These changes, induced specifically by β_1-adrenergic agonism, might play a role in the pathogenesis of DCM. This idea is supported by the finding that the use of β_1-adrenergic antagonists may be helpful in the treatment of DCM (Waagstein et al. 1975, 1993). Treatment of a weakened heart using β-blocking agents, a seemingly paradoxical therapy, leads to an improvement in the function of the heart and to a reduction in mortality of the patients (Swedberg et al. 1979).

Another characteristic of DCM is the presence of functional autoantibodies in the serum of patients with this disease. One such antibody is directed against the ADP/ATP translocator of the inner mitochondrial membrane and is responsible for a reduction in the cytosolic ATP concentration (Schulze et al. 1989; Schultheiss 1993; Schultheiss et al. 1995). It can crossreact with the sarcolemmal L-type Ca^{++}-channel, increasing the sarcolemmal Ca^{++} current into cardiac myocytes (Morad et al. 1988). Another functional autoantibody present in the serum of DCM patients recognizes parts of the extracellular structures of the muscarinic cholinergic M_2 receptor (Fu et al. 1993) and/or the β_1-adrenoceptor (Wallukat and Wollenberger 1987; Wallukat et al. 1995). Autoantibodies directed against the M_2 receptor were found in the sera of 38% of the DCM patients investigated (Fu et al. 1994). Antibodies recognizing the β_1-adrenoceptor were present in 80% of the serum probes of the investigated DCM patients. The sensitive bioassay system, cultured neonatal rat cardiac

---

[1]Max Delbrück Centre for Molecular Medicine, Robert-Rössle-Str. 10, 13125 Berlin, Germany
[2]German Heart Centre, Augustenburger Platz 1, 13353 Berlin, Germany

myocytes, including not only the second (Magnusson et al. 1990) but also the first extracellular loop of the β_1-adrenoceptor was used in our experiments. Because this antibody acts like a β-adrenergic agonist, it is very likely that it plays an important part in the adrenergic overdrive characteristic of many patients with DCM. It may also play an additional role in the development of this disease.

Characterization of the Anti-β_1-Adrenoceptor Autoantibody

Autoantibodies recognizing β-adrenoceptors were first described by Venter et al. (1980), who found anti-β_2-adrenoceptor antibodies in the serum of patients with asthma and allergic rhinitis. This antibody acted like a β-adrenergic antagonist (Wallukat and Wollenberger 1991; Turki and Liggett 1995) and recognized the third extracellular loop of the β_2-adrenoceptor (Wallukat and Wollenberger 1991). In Chagas' heart disease, which is endemic in South and Central America, Goin and coworkers (1991) detected autoantibodies that recognized both the β_1- and the β_2-adrenoceptor subtypes. These antibodies acted like a β-adrenergic agonist (Borda et al. 1984) and exerted a positive chronotropic effect in cultured neonatal rat cardiomyocytes (Ferrari et al. 1995). Similar autoantibodies were also found in the serum of patients with DCM, a disease that resembles Chagas' heart disease.

In serum samples of DCM patients, autoantibodies directed against the β_1-adrenoceptor subtype were detected (Wallukat and Wollenberger 1987; Limas et al. 1989; Magnusson et al. 1994). These antibodies, which were of the IgG isotype, were able to influence the function of cardiomyocytes. Their targets were epitopes on the first or the second extracellular loop of the rat β_1-adrenoceptor (Wallukat et al. 1995) with which they cross-reacted (both loops are identical in humans and rats). In spontaneously beating cultured neonatal rat cardiomyocytes, they induced a positive chronotropic effect that was blocked by the β_1-subtype selective adrenergic antagonist bisoprolol, but not by β_2-selective adrenoceptor antagonists ICI 118.551 (Wallukat et al. 1991a). Moreover, it was possible to neutralize the anti-β_1-adrenoceptor autoantibodies using synthetic peptides corresponding to the amino acid sequence of the first and the second extracellular loops of the β_1-adrenoceptor (Wallukat et al. 1995). From this finding it can be concluded that the anti-β_1-adrenoceptor antibodies recognize epitopes on both of these extracellular loops. Using these amino acid sequences we succeeded in purifying the antibodies by affinity chromatography. As shown in Fig. 1 the purified anti-β_1-adrenoceptor antibodies recognized the β_1-adrenoceptor with high affinity. Their maximal effect was attained at a concentration of 1 nM; the EC_{50} was 0.14 nM.

As mentioned above, these antibodies acted in cultured neonatal rat ventricular cardiomyocytes like a β-adrenergic agonist by increasing the rate of beating. This effect occurred via the β-adrenoceptor–adenylate cyclase–protein kinase A cascade. Involvement of this cascade is evidenced by the fact that the antibodies displaced the radioligand [^{3}H]dihydroalprenolol from the β-receptor. Furthermore the addition of the antibodies to the cultured cardio-

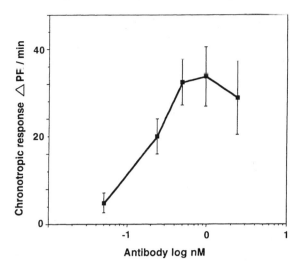

Fig. 1. Effect of an affinity purified anti-β_1-adrenoceptor autoantibody on the beating rate of spontaneously beating cultured cardiomyocytes. *PR*, pulsation rate

myocytes led to a significant accumulation of the second messenger cyclic AMP and to an activation of the protein kinase A. The latter effect was measured directly by estimating the activity ratio of the enzyme or indirectly by using RP-cAMP S a specific inhibitor of this enzyme.

Possible Pathogenic Role of the Anti-β_1-Adrenoceptor Autoantibodies and New Therapeutic Approaches

As mentioned above, the anti-β_1-adrenoceptor antibodies exerted their effect, at least to a major extent, via the β-adrenoceptor-mediated effector system. But in contrast to a classic β-adrenergic agonist, the action of which is subject to desensitization, the anti-$\beta_1$adrenoceptor autoantibody was unable to desensitize the β-adrenergic reaction cascade. In cultured cardiomyocytes, a prolonged treatment (2 h) of the cells with the β-adrenergic agonist isoprenaline led to a diminishment of the β-adrenergic responsiveness. This was accompanied by a reduction in the number of β-adrenoceptors. Treatment of cultured cardiomyocytes for the same length of time with the agonist-like anti-β_1-adrenoceptor autoantibody led to neither a reduction in the antibody-induced positive chronotropic response (Wallukat et al., 1991a) nor to a significant loss of the number of β-adrenergic binding sites (Wallukat et al. 1996). This lack of tachyphylaxis could be of pathogenic relevance in DCM, contributing to chronic adrenergic overdrive which is considered to be a feature of DCM (Bristow 1993) and a factor in ventricular tachyarrhythmias which in a substantial percentage of DCM patients are the cause of sudden death (Tamburo and Wilber, 1992). On these grounds the repeatedly reported beneficial effect of β-blockers in DCM is readily understood.

That the anti-β_1-adrenoceptor autoantibodies may play a role in the pathogenesis of DCM was indicated by findings in patients with myocarditis. Patients with this disease, a possible precursor of DCM (Abelmann 1988), do not differ from those with DCM with respect to the presence and the level of circulating autoantibodies that recognize the β_1-adrenoceptor (Wallukat et al. 1991b). It is therefore also of interest that in a patient with acute myocarditis, the healing process (as reflected by a normalization of the ejection fraction and the heart rate) was correlated with a disappearance of the anti-β_1-adrenoceptor autoantibodies from the blood (Fig. 2a,b).

Related data were obtained using immunoadsorption on Ig-Therasorb columns (Baxter, Munich, Germany) to remove the antibodies from the serum of DCM patients. If autoantibodies play either a primary or secondary role in the

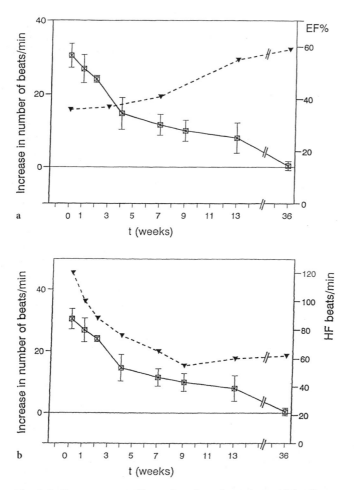

Fig. 2a,b. Improvement of heart function of a patient with healing myocarditis. **a** The ejection fraction (EF; ▼) of the heart in comparison to the anti-β_1-adrenoceptor autoantibody value (□). **b** The heart frequency (HF; ▼) of the patient during healing

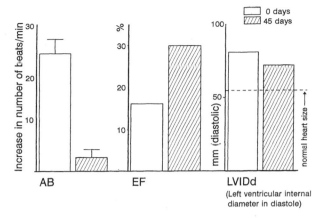

Fig. 3. Effect of immunoadsorption on the amount of anti-β_1-adrenoceptor autoantibody (*AB*), the ejection fraction (*EF*), and the left ventricular internal diameter in diastole (*LVIDd*) in a patient with DCM. The parameters were measured before and 45 days after immunoadsorption

pathogenesis of DCM, removal of the antibodies can be expected to lead to an improvement of cardiac function. The effect of immunoadsorption on the function of the heart of a patient with DCM whose serum contained autoantibodies against the β_1-adrenoceptor is shown in Fig. 3. The β-adrenergic agonist-like action of the anti-β_1-adrenoceptor antibody was used to monitor the efficiency of the immunoadsorption. After the treatment (four immunoadsorptions per week) and a subsequent substitution with a human immunoglobulin preparation, the antibody level was markedly reduced. In parallel to the reduction of the anti-β_1-adrenoceptor autoantibody level, an improvement of the function of the heart was observed. Figure 3 shows the antibody level, the ejection fraction, and the left ventricular internal diameter in diastole (LVIDd) both before and 45 days after the immunoadsorption. After this time the level of antibodies was reduced to 11.5% of the original value and the ejection fraction increased from 16% to 30%. In parallel a reduction in the left ventricular internal diameter in diastole from 81 mm to 72 mm was observed. From this finding it can be inferred that autoimmune processes could play a role in the development and maintenance of this disease and that the elimination of the autoantibodies from the patient's sera can have a beneficial effect.

An improvement of the function of the heart and a normalization of the heart size was also observed in 18 patients with end-stage dilated cardiomyopathy (ejection fraction <15%), implanted with a left ventricular cardiac assist device for bridging the period until transplantation. Under the influence of this cardiac support system the left ventricular ejection fraction of the hearts increased on average to 40% and the heart size was reduced to normal (Müller et al. 1995). In parallel to the improvement of cardiac function, a disappearance of circulating anti-β_1-adrenoceptor autoantibodies was observed (Table 1). Explantation of the assist device in four patients either 160, 200, 243, or 348

Table 1. Effect of an implanted cardiac assist device on the heart function and anti-β_1-adrenoceptor autoantibody value

Weeks after implantation	LVEF (%)	HR (beat/min)	LVIDd (mm)	Auto AB (relative unit)
0	15	129	72	6.0
2	21	115	60	5.0
5	33	85	52	2.6
10	55	75	48	0.6
22	50	82	52	0.0

LVEF, left ventricular ejection fraction; HR, heart rate; LVIDd, left ventricular internal diameter in diastole; AutoAB, autoantibody.

days after the implantation, was not followed by a deterioration in the performance of the heart. Measurements of hemodynamic parameters in these patients indicate that the normalization of cardiac performance has up to now been maintained for as long as 237, 153, 145, and 33 days, respectively, after explantation of the cardiac support system. Four other patients with heart failure who lacked the autoantibodies to the β_1-adrenoceptor in the sera, failed to respond to implantation of this support system. This points to a hitherto unrecognized aspect of the function of these antibodies. The anti-β_1-adrenoceptor antibodies can in any case usefully serve as a sensitive tool for monitoring the autoimmunological activity in patients with DCM.

The remarkable correlation between the reduction in the circulating autoantibodies against the β_1-adrenoceptor and the improvement of the function of the heart may imply that the anti-β_1-adrenoceptor antibodies, possibly in concert with other autoantibodies detected in the serum of DCM patients (Schultheiss et al. 1995), may play a part in the pathophysiology of myocarditis and DCM.

Acknowledgements. The authors are grateful to Mrs. M. Wegener, Mrs. H. Schmidt and Mrs. K. Karczewski for skillful technical assistance.

References

Abelman WH (1988) Myocarditis as a cause of dilated cardiomyopathy. In: Engelmeier BS, O'Connel JB (eds) Drug therapy in dilated cardiomyopathy and myocarditis. Marcel Dekker, New York, pp 221–231

Böhm M, Gierschik P, Jacobs KH, Pieske B, Schnabel P, Ungerer M, Erdmann E (1990) Increase of Giα in human hearts with dilated but not ischemic cardiomyopathy. Circulation 82: 1249–1265

Borda ES, Pascual J, Cossio PM, Vega M, Arana RM, Sterin-Borda L (1984) A circulating IgG in Chagas' disease which binds to beta adrenoceptor of myocardium and modulates its activity. Clin Exp Immunol 57: 679–686

Bristow MR (1984) The adrenergic nervous system in heart failure. N Engl J Med 311: 850–851

Bristow MR (1993) Pathophysiologic and pharmacologic rationales for clinical management of chronic heart failure with beta-blocking agents. Am J Cardiol 71: 12C–22C

Bristow MR, Ginsburg R, Monobe W, Cubiciotti RS, Sageman WS, Lurie K, Billingham ME, Harrison DE, Stinson EB (1982) Decreased catecholamine sensitivity and beta-adrenergic receptor density in failing human hearts. N Engl J Med 307: 205–211

Brodde, OE (1991) β_1 and β_2 adrenoceptors in the human heart: Properties, function, and alterations in chronic heart failure. Pharmacol Rev 43: 203–242

Cohn JN, Levine TB, Olivari MT, Garberg V, Lura D, Francis GS, Simon AB, Rector T (1984) Plasma norepinephrine as a guide to prognosis in patients with chronic congestive heart failure. N Engl J Med 311: 819–823

Ferrari I, Levin MJ, Wallukat G, Elies R, Lebesgue D, Chiale P, Elizari M, Rosenbaum M, Hoebeke J (1995) Molecular mimicry between the immunodominant ribosomal protein PO of Trypanosoma cruzi and a functional epitope on the human β_1-adrenergic receptor. J Exp Med 182: 59–65

Fu LX, Magnusson Y, Bergh CH, Liljeqvist JÅ, Waagstein F, Hjalmarson Å, Hoebeke J (1993) Localization of a functional epitope on the second extracellular loop of the human muscarinic receptor in patients with idiopathic dilated cardiomyopathy. J Clin Invest 91: 1964–1968

Fu MLX, Hoebeke J, Matsui S, Matoba M, Magnusson Y, Hedner T, Herlitz H, Hjalmarson Å (1994) Autoantibodies against cardiac G-protein-coupled receptors define different populations with cardiomyopathies but not with hypertension. Clin Immunol Immunopathol 72: 15–20

Goin JC, Borda E, Segovia A, Sterin-Borda L (1991) Distribution of antibodies against β-adrenoceptors in the course of human Trypanosoma cruzi infection. Proc Soc Exp Biol Med 197: 186–192

Limas CJ, Goldenberg IF, Limas C (1989) Autoantibodies against β-adrenoceptors in human idiopathic dilated cardiomyopathy. Circ Res 64: 97–103

Magnusson Y, Marullo S, Höyer S, Waagstein F, Andersson B, Vahlne A, Guillet JG, Strosberg AD, Hjalmarson Å, Hoebeke J (1990) Mapping of a functional autoimmune epitope on the β_1-adrenergic receptor in patients with idiopathic dilated cardiomyopathy. J Clin Invest 86: 1658–1666

Magnusson Y, Wallukat G, Waagstein F, Hjalmarson Å, Hoebeke J (1994) Autoimmunity in idiopathic dilated cardiomyopathy. Characterization of antibodies against the β_1-adrenoceptor with positive chronotropic effect. Circulation 89: 2760–2767

Morad M, Davies NW, Ulrich G, Schultheiss HP (1988) Antibodies against ADP-ATP carrier enhance Ca^{2+}-current in isolated cardiac myocytes. Am J Physiol 255: H960–H964

Müller J, Wallukat G, Weng Y, Siniawski H, Hummel M, Hetzer R (1995) Abfall der β-Rezeptoren-Autoantikörper in Patienten mit idiopathischer dilatativer Kardiomyopathie (DKMP) während mechanischer Linksherzunterstützung. Z Kardiol 84(Suppl): 132

Schultheiss HP (1993) Disturbances of the myocardial energy metabolism in dilated cardiomyopathy due to autoimmunological mechanisms. Circulation 87(Suppl IV): 48

Schultheiss HP, Schulze K, Schauer R, Witzenbichler B, Strauer BE (1995) Antibody-mediated imbalance of myocardial energy metabolism. A causal factor of cardiac failure? Circ Res 76: 64–72

Schulze K, Becker BF, Schultheiss HP (1989) Antibodies to the ADP/ATP carrier - an autoantigen in myocarditis and dilated cardiomyopathy - penetrate into myocardial cells and disturb energy metabolism in vivo. Circ Res 64: 179–192

Steinfahrt M, Geertz B, Schmitz W, Scholz H, Haverich A, Breil I, Hanrath P, Reupcke C, Sigmund M, Lo HB (1991) Distinct down-regulation of cardiac β_1- and β_2- adrenoceptors in different human heart diseases. Naunyn Schmiedebergs Arch Pharmacol 343: 217–220

Swedberg K, Hjalmarson Å, Waagstein F, Wallentin I (1979) Prolongation of survival in congestive cardiomyopathy by β-receptor blockade. Lancet i: 1374–1376

Swedberg M, Eneroth P, Kjekshus J, Wilhelmsen L (1990) Hormones regulating cardiovascular function in patients with severe congestive heart failure and their relation to mortality. Circulation 82: 1730–1736

Tamburo P, Wilber D (1992) Sudden death in idiopathic dilated cardiomyopathy. Am Heart J 124: 1035–10452

Thomas JA, Marks BH (1978) Plasma norepinephrine in congestive heart failure. Am J Cardiol 41: 233–243

Turki J, Liggett SB (1995) Receptor-specific properties of β_2-adrenergic receptor autoantibodies in asthma. Am J Respir Cell Mol Biol 12: 531–539

Ungerer M, Böhm M, Elce JS, Erdmann E, Lohse MJ (1993) Altered expression of β-adrenergic receptor kinase and β_1-adrenergic receptors in the failing human heart. Circulation 87: 454–463

Venter JC, Fraser LM, Harrison LC (1980) Autoantibodies to β_2-adrenergic receptors: a possible cause of adrenergic hyporesponsiveness in asthma and allergic rhinitis. Science 207: 1361–1363

Waagstein F, Hjalmarson Å, Varnauskas E, Wallentin I (1975) Effect of chronic beta-adrenergic receptor blockade in congestive cardiomyopathy. Br Heart J 37: 1022–1036

Waagstein F, Bristow MR, Swedberg K, Camerini F, Fowler MB, Silver MA, Gilbert EM, Johnson MR, Goos FG, Hjalmarson Å (1993) Beneficial effects of metoprolol in idiopathic dilated cardiomyopathy. Lancet 342: 1441–1446

Wallukat G, Wollenberger A (1987) Effects of the gamma globulin fraction of patients with allergic asthma and dilated cardiomyopathy on chronotropic β-adrenoceptor function in cultured neonatal rat heart myocytes. Biomed Biochim Acta 78: S634–S639

Wallukat G, Wollenberger A (1991) Autoantibodies to β_2-adrenergic receptors with anti-adrenergic activity from patients with allergic asthma. J Allergy Clin Immunol 88: 581–587

Wallukat G, Boewer V, Förster A, Wollenberger A (1991a) Anti-β-adrenoceptor autoantibodies with β-adrenergic activity from patients with myocarditis and dilated cardiomyopathy. In: Lewis BS, Kimchi A (eds) Heart Failure – Mechanisms and Management. Springer, Berlin Heidelberg New York, pp 21–29

Wallukat G, Morwinski R, Kowal K, Förster A, Boewer V, Wollenberger A (1991b) Autoantibodies against the β-adrenergic receptor in human myocarditis and dilated cardiomyopathy: β-adrenergic agonism without desensitization. Eur Heart J 12(Suppl D): 178–181

Wallukat G, Wollenberger A, Morwinski R, Pitschner H-F (1995) Anti-β_1-adrenoceptor autoantibodies with chronotropic activity from the serum of patients with dilated cardiomyopathy: Mapping of epitopes in the first and second extracellular loops. J Mol Cell Cardiol 27: 397–406

Wallukat G, Fu MLX, Magnusson Y, Hjalmarson Å, Hoebeke J, Wollenberger A (1996) Agonistic effect of anti-peptide antibodies and autoantibodies directed against adrenergic and cholinergic receptors: Absence of desensitization. Blood Press (in press)

The Adenine Nucleotide Translocator: A Major Autoantigen in Myocarditis and Dilated Cardiomyopathy

H.-P. Schultheiss, K. Schulze, P. Schwimmbeck, and A. Dörner

Introduction

Current concepts of autoimmunity emphasize the significance of antibodies in the development and maintenance of autoimmune disorders. However, it is difficult to show that a given autoantibody is an essential component of a pathological mechanism which leads to tissue damage and organ dysfunction. Beside contributing to an understanding of the pathogenesis, a precise characterization of the antibodies involved in the autoimmunological process may have diagnostic and prognostic value.

In this study we investigated the relevance of autoantibodies against the adenine nucleotide translocator (ANT) in the pathogenesis of myocarditis and dilated cardiomyopathy (DCM). The autoantibodies found in the sera of these patients are highly heart-specific and inhibit the nucleotide transport in vitro [1–5].

ANT is an integral protein of the inner mitochondrial membrane that allows the exchange of extramitochondrial and intramitochondrial ADP and ATP [6–8]. The ANT protein complex consists of two identical 32-kDa subunits whose single nucleotide binding site alternatively faces the matrix (m conformation) and the cytosolic (c conformation) side of the membrane. Depending on the conformational change of the carrier, mitochondrial ATP is exchanged for cytosolic ADP in a ratio of 1:1.

Since ANT is the only transport system for ADP and ATP, it is the most important link of energy-producing and energy-consuming processes. If a pathogenetic role of the antibodies against ANT is suggested, restricted nucleotide transport across the inner mitochondrial membrane would be expected not only in vitro but also in vivo. This would lead to an imbalance between energy production and energy consumption in failing hearts. Infact, there is substantial evidence that failing hearts of patients with DCM are in an energy-depleted state. We were able to show a significant increase in lactate dehydrogenase isoform 5 (LDH 5) associated with a decrease in LDH 1 in myocardial biopsies from patients with severe chronic heart failure resulting from DCM. A decrease in myocardial ATP was found, accompanied by the shift in the LDH isoform pattern [9]. These data are in accordance with the results of

Department of Internal Medicine/Cardiology, Benjamin Franklin Hospital, Free University of Berlin, Hindenburgdamm 32, 12200 Berlin, Germany

^{31}P magnetic resonance spectroscopy demonstrating a creatine phosphate/ATP ratio which is significantly reduced in patients with advanced heart failure due to DCM compared to controls [10, 11]. In light of the finding of ANT-reacting autoantibodies in viral heart disease and altered energy metabolism, we investigated the function and expression of ANT in order to examine the influence of the autoantibodies on their target protein. In addition, we immunized guinea pigs with purified ANT protein and infected A/J mice with Coxsackie B3 virus, which is known to induce myocarditis. Both treatments resulted in autoimmunological reactions producing antibodies against ANT. Using these animal models, it was possible to elucidate the connection between the energy metabolism and the heart work.

Methods and Results

Characterization of the Autoantibodies

Sera of patients with proven DCM and patients with clinically suspected myocarditis were tested. The diagnosis of DCM was established according to the criteria of the WHO/ISFC task force as a chronic disorder of heart muscle of unknown cause or association. Cases of specific heart muscle disease or secondary cardiomyopathy were excluded. The diagnosis of myocarditis was established on the basis of the patient's history, especially with regard to a common cold infection, an accompanying change in viral neutralization titer on follow-up, clinical features, and morphological evidence of myocarditis in myocardial biopsy samples. The biopsies were classified into three major groups: active myocarditis, healing myocarditis, and healed myocarditis. Sera from patients with proven coronary heart disease (CHD; $n=30$) and from healthy blood donors (controls; $n=40$) were used for comparison.

When sera of patients with clinically suspected myocarditis were tested in the enzyme-linked immunosorbent assay (ELISA) against the ANT from heart, a significant antibody titer was seen in 20 of 22 patients with acute or healing myocarditis and in 26 to 44 patients with a histological diagnosis of healed myocarditis (Fig. 1). In 57% of patients with DCM the antibody titer against the ANT was significantly elevated. Unlike sera from the controls, the sera from patients with CHD did not contain autoantibodies against the ANT protein. When positive sera from patients with suspected myocarditis reacting to the ANT protein from heart were tested, binding to kidney or liver protein was significantly lower than binding to heart protein [12, 13], indicating organ specificity of the antibodies.

Altered ANT Function and Expression in Hearts of Patients with DCM and Myocarditis

If a pathogenetic role of these antibodies is suggested, it must be asked whether these immune-inactivating antibodies can act as antagonists not only in vitro but also in vivo, resulting in decreased nucleotide transport across the inner

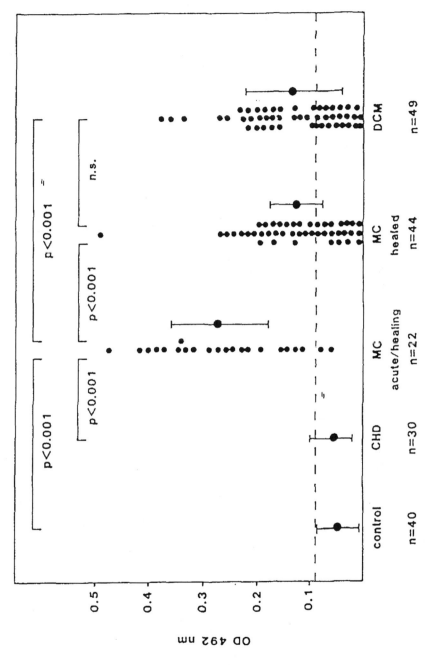

Fig. 1. The binding of autoantibodies to the ANT from heart in enzyme-linked immunosorbent assay from patients with myocarditis (MC) (acute/healing, healed), dilated cardiomyopathy (DCM), coronary heart disease (CHD), and healthy blood donors (control)

mitochondrial membrane. Therefore, we isolated mitochondria from explanted hearts of patients with DCM undergoing heart transplantation and measured the nucleotide exchange rate of the ANT.

We observed a markedly diminished maximum transport rate of ANT in mitochondria of DCM patients who underwent heart transplantation. The maximum myocardial transport capacity of the translocator was reduced by 37% in 16 of 25 DCM patients (Fig. 2). There was no alteration of ANT exchange capacity in myocardial mitochondria of patients with ischemic or valvular heart disease compared to controls. The reduced nucleotide exchange rate of ANT obviously reflects a disease-specific process in DCM.

To check the hypothesis that the diminished transport rate might be caused by a lowered ANT protein density in mitochondria of DCM patients, we determined total mitochondrial ANT protein by immunoblotting using a specific antibody. In comparison to controls, total ANT protein content was significantly increased in the cardiac mitochondria of DCM patients. In contrast, none of the patients with heart disease of other etiologies demonstrated an elevation of total ANT in their myocardial tissue (Fig. 3). These findings underline the disease-specificity of ANT in DCM. However, a reduction in mitochondrial ANT protein content cannot be responsible for the diminished transport rate of ADP and ATP.

Immunological studies pointed for the first time to the existence of ANT isoforms [14, 15]. These data were confirmed by molecular biological investigations showing the presence of at least three different human genes for ANT, designated ANT1, ANT2, and ANT3 [16, 17]. Since the three ANT isoforms are thought to have different kinetic properties, as demonstrated for the

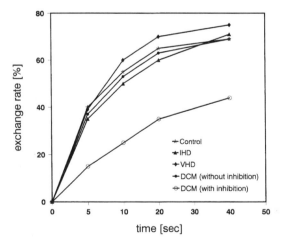

Fig. 2. Nucleotide exchange rate in mitochondria from explanted hearts from patients with coronary ($n=17$) or valvular ($n=5$) heart disease, from DCM patients ($n=16$) with exchange rates outside the normal range found for controls ($n=12$), and from DCM patients ($n=9$) with transport rates equivalent to those of controls. Isolated mitochondria were preloaded with ^{14}C-ADP and the exchange rate was determined by the inhibitor stop method combined with the back exchange [14]. Exchange times were 5 s, 10 s, 20 s, and 40 s

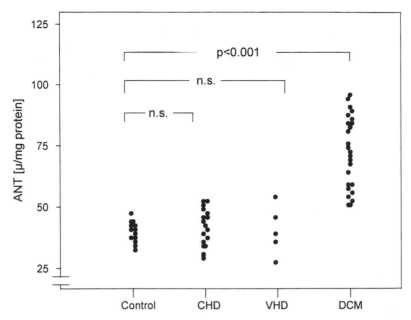

Fig. 3. Quantification of the ANT protein content in human mitochondria isolated from explanted hearts from controls ($n-13$) and patients suffering from ischemic (CHD, $n=17$) valvular (VHD, $n=5$) heart disease or DCM ($n=25$) and undergoing heart transplantation. Quantification of the carrier protein was done by an immunobinding assay on nitrocellulose membranes using antibodies raised against total myocardial ANT protein. The specific binding of antibodies to the ANT protein was detected by ^{35}S-protein A. The radioactivity was subsequently assayed in a β-counter

three adenine nucleotide translocase isoforms in yeast [18], we determined the ANT isoform transcription pattern in endomyocardial biopsies of patients suffering from myocarditis or DCM in comparison to controls and in patients with ischemic or valvular heart disease.

The ANT mRNA isoform patterns of the control population ($n=29$) showed a predominant expression of ANT1 with an average of $68.1 \pm 4.5\%$, with $24.9 \pm 5.0\%$ for ANT2 and $7.0 \pm 2.7\%$ for ANT3. None of the patients suffering from ischemic or valvular heart disease ($n=25$) exhibited any differences in their isoform pattern compared to the control values (Fig. 4c). In contrast, 37% (14 of 39) of the myocarditis patients with a disease history of less than 1 year (group A) demonstrated an alteration in the ANT mRNA pattern with percentages outside the range of distribution found for controls. Here, the relative amount of ANT1 mRNA was markedly elevated to an average of $85.2 \pm 3.9\%$, while ANT2 was decreased to $8.8 \pm 2.8\%$. ANT3 remained constant. Sixty-one percent of the patients with chronic myocarditis (14/23, group B) had a modified ANT isoform distribution. However, the highest percentage of patients with an altered isoform pattern was found in the group of DCM patients (82%). The percentage of patients with a modified isoform distribution increased obviously with the duration of the disease.

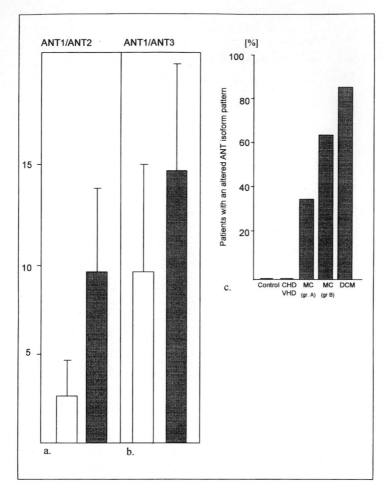

Fig. 4. Ratios ANT1/ANT2 (**a**) and ANT1/ANT3 (**b**) show non-equivalent increases indicating that the elevation in ANT1 isoform mRNA is associated with a decrease in ANT2 mRNA, ANT 3 remaining constant. *Open bars,* Controls; *filled bars,* patients with an altered isoform pattern. **c** Percentages of patients with an altered isoform distribution. MC group A are myocarditis patients with a disease history of less than 1 year; MC group B are patients with chronic myocarditis chronic myocarditis

The unequal increase in the proportions ANT1/ANT2 (2.7 ± 1.1 to 9.7 ± 3.6) and ANT1/ANT3 (9.7 ± 6.3 to 14.2 ± 9.7; Fig. 4a,b) clearly shows the isoform shift, characterized by a rise in the amount of ANT1 mRNA associated with a decrease in the amount of ANT2 mRNA, whereas the amount of ANT3 mRNA remains constant.

Long-term investigations in 37 myocarditis patients have shown that the alteration in isoform pattern occurs at the beginning of the disease and does not return to a normal isoform distribution during therapy. Additionally, patients with a normal isoform pattern at the beginning of myocarditis did not show any change in isoform distribution at a later date. Thus, the isoform shift is not a progressive process but an event during early period of the disease. If a modification occurs, it is permanent. Furthermore, patients with an enteroviral myocardial infection have about four times as high a risk of isoform pattern alteration as those without any enteroviral RNA in their heart muscle tissue. However, viral persistence is not required to maintain the ANT isoform pattern shift.

Determining the amount of ANT1 and total ANT protein in myocardial tissue of patients with an altered isoform pattern by immunodot blotting using specific antibodies showed that the proportion of ANT1 mRNA is equivalent to the proportion of ANT1 protein. Thus, the alteration in mRNA level affects the distribution of the ANT isoform proteins in myocardial mitochondria of patients suffering from DCM or myocarditis.

Subcellular Distribution of Adenine Nucleotides and Hemodynamic Function in the hearts of Guinea Pigs Immunized with ANT Protein

The ability of antibodies against the ANT to inhibit nucleotide exchange activity from heart mitochondria was demonstrated in vitro. If a pathophysiological role for these antibodies is postulated, it has to be shown that they are an essential component in the pathological mechanism leading to organ dysfunction. Therefore, we immunized guinea pigs with purified carrier protein, leading to autoimmune reactions, and measured the subcellular distribution of the adenine nucleotides and the hemodynamic parameters of the immunized animals in comparison to control animals. Analysis of subcellular distribution of ATP and ADP provides a sensitive marker for defining the transport activity of the ANT protein. Dependent on the membrane potential, the nucleotide exchange is greatly disproportionate in energized mitochondria. Therefore, ATP and ADP are highly asymmetrically disturbed across the mitochondrial membrane; the concentration ratio ATP/ADP is significantly higher in the extra- than in the intramitochondrial space. In regard to these characteristics, it was shown by Klingenberg and Heldt [7] that the force for the regulation of the adenine nucleotide exchange is derived from the potential difference between the cytosolic and mitochondrial ATP. As energization of the inner mitochondrial membrane, which is expressed by the cytosolic-mitochondrial phosphorylation potential difference for ATP ($\Delta G_{(cyt-mit)}$), modulates ANT activity, a decrease in $\Delta G_{(cyt-mit)}$ can be taken as an indicator of reduced transport capacity of the translocator.

Hearts of control animals exhibited a normal intracellular distribution of ATP (Table 1). In hearts of guinea pigs showing immunoinactivating antibodies against ANT, the concentration of ATP was slightly lower in the cytosol but markedly increased in mitochondria. Consequently, both the ADP/ATP ratio and the phosphorylation state – expressed as the ratio $[ATP]/[ADP] \times P_i]$ – were significantly lower in the cytosol, whereas a substantial increase was observed in the mitochondria. $\Delta G_{(cyt-mit)}$was only 0.7 kJ/mol in the hearts of

Table 1. Subcellular distribution of myocardiac high-energy phosphates in isolated perfused guinea pig hearts. Ratios for free cytosolic ATP/ADP were calculated from the mass action ratio of the creatine kinase reaction

	Control ($n=5$)		After immunization ($n=6$)	
	Cytosol	Mitochondria	Cytosol	Mitochondria
ATP (mmol/l)	13.2 ± 2.0	8.1 ± 2.3	11.3 ± 2.9	$18.3 \pm 5.9^{**}$
ADP (mmol/l)	1.9 ± 0.4	1.6 ± 0.3	$2.5 \pm 0.5^{*}$	$1.1 \pm 0.2^{*}$
ATP/ADP (overall)	6.7 ± 0.4	5.1 ± 0.5	$4.5 \pm 1.1^{**}$	$17.1 \pm 4.9^{**}$
ATP/ADP (free)	61.8 ± 7.9	–	$50.2 \pm 8.8^{*}$	–
(ATP)/ADP) × (P_i)	5487 ± 644	926 ± 215	$4105 \pm 624^{**}$	$3349 \pm 1445^{**}$
$\Delta G_{(cyt-mit)}$[a]	4.6 ± 0.5		$0.7 \pm 1.2^{**}$	

[a] $\Delta G_{(cyt-mit)}$: difference in phosphorylation potential between cytosol and mitochondria
$^{*}f<0.01$, $^{**}f<0.001$ vs control

immunized animals, while $\Delta G_{(cyt-mit)}$ was significantly higher (4.6 kJ/mol, $p<0.001$) in myocardial tissue of control animals. As discussed previously, under physiological conditions, the asymmetric transport of ATP creates a high cytosolic and a low mitochondrial ATP/ADP ratio. A decrease in the cytosolic-mitochondrial phosphorylation potential difference for ATP indicates an imbalance between energy delivery and demand in the cell. Thus, the data demonstrate that the total transport capacity for ATP of the ANT is diminished in immunized animals, leading to inadequate delivery of high-energy phosphates to the cytosol.

This result raised the question of whether myocardial function is altered by the disturbance of cellular energy balance caused by reducing the ATP efflux from mitochondria into cytosol. To evaluate this hypothesis we measured the hemodynamic data from immunized guinea pig hearts which were stimulated by high calcium concentration and maximum elevation of the afterload. The hearts were isolated and perfused as working heart preparations, as described previously. The preload of 12 cm H_2O and the mean developed determined the pressure-volume work of the left ventricle. External heart work was calculated as the sum of pressure-volume work and acceleration work [½ × ejection volume × (mean velocity of flow)^2] during ejection.

Beating heart preparations from guinea pigs immunized with ANT protein showed a marked decrease in cardiac function compared to control animals. (Table 2). Mean aortic pressure, stroke volume, stroke work, and external heart work of the left ventricle were 40%–80% lower. External heart work was reduced from 344 to 132 mJ/g per minute. Similarly, myocardial oxygen extraction was found to be reduced while myocardial lactate production was significantly increased.

These functional data support the hypothesis that the antibodies reacting against ANT alter myocardial function by means of an antibody-mediated restriction of the translocator protein, leading to an imbalance between energy demand and energy supply, resulting in heart dysfunction. This is confirmed by recent data demonstrating a direct relation between the impairment of

Table 2. Hemodynamic data from isolated perfused hearts of guinea pigs immunized with ANT protein

	Controls	Immunized animals	p
Heart rate (bpm)	224 ± 30	219 ± 15	NS
Mean aortic pressure (mmHg)	87 ± 8	61 ± 1	<0.005
Coronary flow (ml/min)	30 ± 4	19 ± 11	<0.005
Stroke volume (μl/g)	132 ± 15	89 ± 40	<0.005
External heart work (mJ/g min)	344 ± 67	132 ± 24	<0.005
Myocardial O_2 consumption (μmol/g min)	18 ± 4	11 ± 5	<0.005
O_2 extraction (%)	70 ± 8	69 ± 12	NS
Coronary lactate release (μmol/g min)	1.4 ± 0.6	3.0 ± 1.6	<0.01

energy metabolism and myocardial function. It was shown that the magnitude of the reduction in $\Delta G_{(cyt\text{-}mit)}$ correlates directly with the maximum heart work of guinea pigs performed after being immunized with ANT protein.

Characterization of Myocardial Energy Metabolism in Coxsackie-B3-Infected Mice

In view of a possible link between viral infection and induction of auto-immunity, we investigated whether an immunological reaction against the ANT could be incited by viral infection (Fig. 5). Circulating heart-reactive

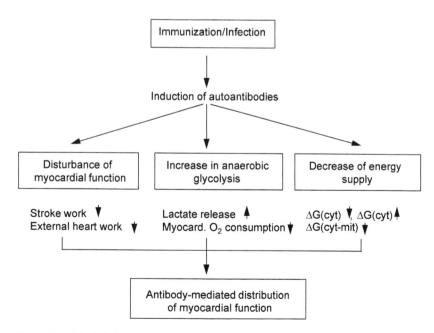

Fig. 5. Possible link between viral infection and induction of autoimmunity

Table 3. Subcellular distribution of myocardiac high-energy phosphates in perfused hearts of mice infected with Coxsackie B3 virus

	Controls	Immunized animals	p
ATP (mM)			
Cytosolic	7.6 ± 1.6	4.7 ± 1.8	<0.01
Mitochondrial	5.1 ± 1.2	11.4 ± 1.8	<0.005
ADP (mM)			
Cytosolic	3.3 ± 0.8	5.4 ± 1.8	<0.05
Mitochondrial	4.4 ± 1.1	2.8 ± 0.6	<0.005
Phosphocreatine (mM)			
Cytosolic	20.4 ± 2.2	11.8 ± 1.8	<0.005
ATP/ADP ratio			
Cytosolic	64.5 ± 22.8	33.5 ± 10.9	< 0.005
Mitochondrial	1.2 ± 0.3	4.2 ± 1.0	<0.005
G (kJ/mol ATP)			
Cytosolic	17.6 ± 0.8	17.4 ± 1.2	NS
Mitochondrial	8.3 ± 0.7	12.3 ± 1.1	<0.005
$\Delta G_{(cyt\text{-}mit)}$ (kJ/mol ATP)	9.3 ± 0.3	5.1 ± 1.2	<0.005

G, Phosphorylation potential

antibodies were found after infection of H-2 congenic mice (A.SW/Sn-J) with Coxsackie B3 virus (CB3). Further characterization of the antibodies by western blotting showed that they stained a 30-kDa protein in mitochondrial protein extract which was identified as the ANT.

To evaluate the ANT function in hearts of virus-infected mice, we measured the intracellular distribution of high-energy phosphates as described above by nonaqueous fractionation and calculated $\Delta G_{(cyt\text{-}mit)}$. Determination of subcellular concentrations of high-energy phosphates revealed significant differences between the infected animals showing autoantibodies and the control group. Mitochondrial ATP increased from 5.1 ± 1.2 mM to 11.4 ± 1.8 (Table 3). The ATP/ADP ratio diminished from 64.5 ± 22.8 to 33.5 ± 10.9 in the cytosol. In contrast, the mitochondrial ATP/ADP ratio is seen to be markedly elevated from 1.2 ± 3.3 to 4.2 ± 1.0. A significant reduction of the cytosolic-mitochondrial phosphorylation potential difference could be observed, indicating dysfunction of the ANT.

Molecular Mimicry: A Possible Cause of Developing Autoimmunity

A relationship between infectious agents (viruses) and the development of autoimmune disease has been shown. Several theories have been proposed to explain the connection. One of the mechanisms by which a virus could trigger an autoimmune response is by molecular mimicry, defined as the sharing of antigenic determinants by the virus and host cell [19]. Structural similarities have frequently been noted between a number of RNA and DNA viruses and "self" proteins. Since CB3 has been shown to induce myocarditis, we searched for homologous determinants between the sequence of CB3 and that of ANT. A region of homology was found between the ANT (amino acid 27-36) and CB3 (amino acid 1218-1228) [20]. Further experiments demonstrated that this homology translated into immunological cross-reactivity [21]. These results show that the sharing of cross-reacting antigenic determinants between ANT and CB3 may play a role in induction of an autoimmune process following viral myocarditis. This assumption is confirmed by the fact that more than 60% of sera from patients with DCM or myocarditis bind to the viral sequence, while only 5% of the control sera showed a positive binding on ELISA [22]. Thus molecular mimicry may account for the enigma of persistent immunity in the absence of continued exposure to the virus.

Discussion

A number of investigations have suggested that immunopathological mechanisms, both humoral and cellular, may contribute, at least in part, to the pathogenesis of myocarditis and dilated cardiomyopathy [23,24]. Recent data demonstrating persistence of viral RNA in the myocardium of patients with myocarditis and DCM make a persistent viral infection in the latter quite likely [25-27]. The interest is now focused on the link between viral infection, the induction of autoimmunity, and the alteration of differentiated functions of the heart in myocarditis and DCM. A possible explanation for virus-induced autoimmunity is that antigenic determinants of a virus can induce the formation of antibodies during an infection which may cross-react with homologous but not identical epitopes on a host protein. Depending on the biological function of the host protein that is recognized by viral antibodies, the result of the interaction may lead to a physiological disorder in which persistence of the virus in the tissue is not imperative. The virus infection may lead to tissue injury that in turn releases more self-antigens normally not present in the immune system, resulting in an elevated production of auto-antibodies (Fig. 6).

We were able to identify autoantibodies against the adenine nucleotide translocator (ANT) in the sera of patients suffering from myocarditis and DCM, which were highly heart-specific and capable of inhibiting nucleotide exchange activity in vitro. These antibodies show cross-reactivity to the VP protein of Coxsackie B3 virus [21,28] known to induce myocarditis in humans and animals. These antibodies seem to be involved in a process leading to a dysfunction of the ANT in the heart muscle tissue of DCM patients. The lowered ANT nucleotide transport is accompanied by an elevation in total ANT protein. Thus, reduced carrier density in myocardial mitochondria cannot be responsible for the restricted ANT transport capacity. Moreover, a shift in normal ANT isoform expression was found to be characterized by an increase in ANT1 and a decrease in ANT2 mRNA. ANT3 remains unaffected. The mRNA pattern was found to be equivalent to the ANT isoform protein distribution in mitochondria. This isoform shift was induced during the early period of myocarditis and did not return to a normal expression, although inflammatory cells disappeared and no persistence of virus could be detected

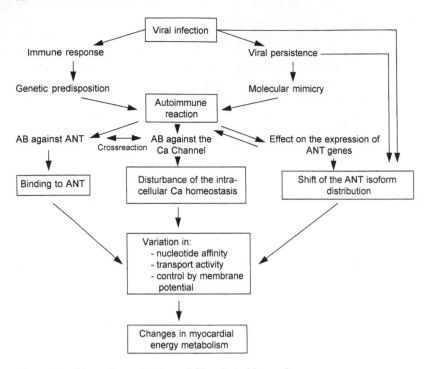

Fig. 6. Possible pathomechanism of dilated viral heart disease

in the hearts of patients. The importance of the virus in this process is shown by the fact that patients harboring the virus have about four times as high a risk of isoform pattern alteration as those without enterovirus infection. However, the virus infection only seems to be an inducing factor, since persistence of the virus is not necessary for maintenance of the isoform shift. Additionally, the alteration in ANT function and expression is seen to be highly disease-specific, since no modifications according to the ANT were observed in the heart muscle tissue of patients with ischemic valvular heart disease. Finding several alterations in myocardial gene expression in various heart diseases led to the assumption that there is a common tendency towards a "fetal gene program" in severe heart failure [29,30]. Since ANT2 is predominantly transcribed in myoblasts still undergoing proliferation, whereas a high level of ANT1 mRNA is observed in finally differentiated muscle cells [31], we would have expected that the isoform shift is characterized by an accumulation of ANT2 and a decrease in ANT1. However, a reciprocal behavior to the fetal program was found in the heart muscle tissue of DCM and rc patients. Thus, the unusual isoform shift emphasizes that there is an activation of an individual gene program in patients with DCM and myocarditis. Nevertheless, it is still unknown whether the ANT isoform shift is the reason for the lowered ANT transport capacity, or whether it is a compensating effect for the ANT dysfunction caused by other mechanisms. Here, the autoantibodies may be mediators of the alterations at the molecular level [32–34].

The disease-specific restriction of ANT function in DCM is additionally supported by experimental studies using guinea pigs immunized with ANT protein and A/J mice infected with Coxsackie B3 virus, both leading to auto-immune reactions against the ANT. We found a significant alteration in the myocardial cytosolic-mitochondrial distribution of high-energy phosphates in both animal models, showing a decrease in cytosolic-mitochondrial phosphorylation potential difference $\Delta G_{mit\text{-}cyt}$. Since the phosphorylation potential difference is a suitable measure of the energy state or the balance between mitochondrial phosphorylation and cytosolic ATP consumption, our findings indicate an inhibition of the nucleotide transport in the hearts of infected and immunized animals. In parallel with the disturbed energy metabolism, the functional data of the isolated perfused hearts from immunized guinea pigs performing maximum pressure-volume work showed significantly altered myocardial function. Stroke volume, stroke work, and external heart work, calculated as the sum of pressure-volume work and acceleration work during ejections, were greatly reduced. Thus, the biochemical and functional data clearly support the hypothesis that the antibodies against the ANT cause a dysfunction of the heart via an antibody-mediated distribution of cellular energy metabolism.

Nevertheless, the mechanism by which the antibodies are enable to exert their deleterious effect on energy metabolism and myocardial function needs to be elucidated. Using immunofluorescence techniques and peroxidase-an-tiperoxidase staining, we found immunoglobulin deposits in mitochondrial membranes in cryosections of the myocardium of immunized animals [35]. In isolated cardiac myocytes, the formation and cytosolic internalization of immunoglobulin-containing membrane-coated vesicles could be shown. These results might support the hypothesis of a direct binding of the cyto-solically internalized antibodies to ANT. Cytosolic uptake of the plasma membrane-bound antibodies could be a result of receptor-mediated en-docytosis [36].

A second possibility of antibody effect is that antibody binding to the cell surface indirectly influences ANT function by activating a messenger system. This is supported by the observation of cross-reactivity between the ANT protein and the calcium channel [37,38]. By electrophysiological and functional studies, it was demonstrated that ANT antibodies bind specifically at the calcium channel of the cell surface and change calcium influx into the cell. A raised intracellular calcium concentration could cause an intramitochondrial calcium overload and lower the mitochondrial transmembrane potential, which seems to be dependent on the intramitochondrial calcium concentration and on calcium fluxes through the mitochondrial membrane. Any lowered mitochondrial transmembrane potential would downregulate the activity of the electrogenic nucleotide exchange via the ANT, finally decreasing the cytosolic-mitochondrial phosphorylation potential difference for ATP. Thus, an anti-body-mediated change in cellular calcium homeostasis would initiate cellular metabolic impairment via calcium. Indeed, there is intense discussion about the possibility that abnormalities in calcium metabolism of the myocardium are involved in the pathogenesis of cardiomyopathies.

According to these hypotheses, the alteration in ANT isoform expression would try to offset the insufficient transport capacity of the translocator, leading to a deficit of cytosolic ATP.

On the other hand, disturbed calcium homeostasis – calcium is an important component in signal transduction – could lead to changes in gene expression. The imbalance in the ANT isoform distribution could result in a lowered ANT transport rate. Klingenberg found that the capacity of bovine ANT is lower in heart than in liver mitochondria. Our recent studies indicate a predominant expression of ANT2 in liver tissue ($63 \pm 11\%$), assuming that ANT2 has a tendentially higher nucleotide transport rate than ANT1. Thus, the imbalance in isoform expression characterized by an increase in ANT1 and a decrease in ANT2 could indeed be a potential reason for the lowered transport capacity of the carrier found in the myocardial tissue of DCM patients.

Regardless of the mechanism of antibody interaction – whether directly through antibody-mediated inhibition of the ANT function or indirectly through antibody-mediated disturbance of intracellular calcium homeostasis – our data indicate that an antibody-mediated dysfunction of the ANT is of relevance in myocarditis and DCM.

References

1. Schultheiss H-P, Schwimmbeck P (1986) Autoantibodies to the adenine nucleotide translocator (ANT) in myocarditis (MC): prevalence, clinical correlates and diagnostic value. Circulation 74 [Suppl 2]: 142
2. Schultheiss H-P (1986) The significance of autoantibodies against the ADP/ATP carrier for the pathogenesis of myocarditis and dilated cardiomyopathy: clinical and experimental data. Springer Semin Immunopathol 11: 15–30.
3. Schultheiss H-P, Schulze K, Kühl U, Ulrich G, Klingenberg M (1987) The ADP/ATP carrier as an mitochondrial autoantigen: facts and perspectives. Ann NY Acad Sci 488: 44–64
4. Schultheiss HP, Kühl U, Schauer R, Schulze K, Kemkes B, Becker BF (1988) Antibodies against the ADP/ATP carrier alter myocardial function by disturbing cellular energy metabolism. In: Schultheiss HP (ed) New concepts in viral heart disease. Springer, Berlin Heidelberg New York, pp 243–258
5. Schulze K, Becker BF, Schauer R, Schultheiss HP (1990) Antibodies to ADP-ATP carrier – an autoantigen in myocarditis and dilated cardiomyopathy – impair cardiac function. Circulation 81: 959–969
6. Klingenberg M (1985) The ADP/ATP carrier in mitochondrial membranes. In: Martonosi AN (ed) The enzymes of biological membranes, vol 4. Plenum, New York, pp 511–533
7. Klingenberg M, Heldt HW (1982) The ADP/ATP translocation in mitochondria and its role in intracellular compartmentation. In: Sies H (ed) Metabolic compartmentation. Academic, London, pp 101–122
8. Klingenberg M (1980) The ADP/ATP carrier translocation in mitochondria: a membrane potential controlled transport. J Membr Biol 56: 97
9. Schultheiss HP (1990) Effect on the myocardial energy metabolism of angiotensin-converting enzyme inhibition in chronic heart failure. Am J Cardiol 65: 74G–81G
10. Hardy CJ, Weiss RG, Bottomley PA, Gerstenblith G (1991) Altered myocardial high-energy phosphate metabolites in patients with dilated cardiomyopathy: Am Heart J 122: 795–801
11. Neubauer S, Krahe T, Schindler R, Horn M, Hillenbrand H, Entzeroth C, Mader H, Kromer EP, Riegger GAJ, Lackner K, Ertl G (1992) 31P magnetic resonance spectroscopy in dilated cardiomyopathy and coronary artery disease: altered cardiac high-energy phosphate metabolism in heart failure. Circulation 86: 1810–1818

12. Schultheiss HP (1987) The mitochondrium as an autoantigen in inflammatory heart disease. Eur Heart J 8[Suppl]: 203–210
13. Schultheiss HP, Bolte HD (1985) Immunological analysis of autoantibodies against the adenine nucleotide translocator in dialted cardiomyopathy. J Mol Cell Cardiol 17: 603–617
14. Schultheiss HP, Klingenberg M (1984) Immunochemical characterization of the adenine nucleotide translocator: organ- and conformation-specifity. Eur J Biochem 143: 599–605
15. Schultheiss HP, Klingenberg M (1985) Immunoelectrophoretic characterization of the ADP/ATP carrier from heart, kidney and liver. Arch Biochem Biophys 239: 273–279
16. Ku DF, Kagan J, Chen ST, Chang CD, Basergo R, Wurzel J (1990) The human fibroblast adenine nucleotide translocator gene. J Biol Chem 265: 16060–16063
17. Cozens AL, Runswick MJ, Walker JE (1989) DNA sequences of two expressed nuclear genes for human mitochondrial ADP/ATP translocase. J Mol Biol 206: 261–280
18. Gawaz M, Douglas MG, Klingenberg M (1990) Structure-function studies of adenine nucleotide transport in mitochondria. II. Biochemical analysis of distinct AACI and AAC2 in yeast. J Biol Chem 265: 14202–14208
19. Oldstone MBA, Dyrberg TI, Fujinami R (1986) Mimicry by virus of host molecules: implications for autoimmune disease. Prog Immunol 6: 787–795
20. Schwimmbeck PL, Schultheiss H-P, Strauer BE (1989) Identification of a main auto-immunogenic epitope of the adenine nucleotide translocator which cross-reacts with Coxsackie B3 virus: use in the diagnosis of myocarditis and dilative cardiomyopathy. Circulation 80 [Suppl II]: 665
21. Schwimmbeck PL, Schultheiss H-P, Strauer BE, Oldstone MBA (1989) Sharing of antigenic determinants between Coxsackie B3 virus and autoantigens in viral myocarditis and dilative cardiomyopathy. J Am Coll Cardiol 13: 253–A
22. Schwimmbeck PL, Schultheiss HP, Strauer BE (1990) Isolation of myocardial auto-antibodies using immunoadsorption with synthetic peptides as antigens. Eur Heart J 11 [Suppl]: 280
23. Zanetti M (1986) New concepts in autoimmunity. Immunol Invest 15: 287
24. Rose NR, Herskowitz A, Neumann DA, Neu N (1988) Autoimmune myocarditis: a paradigm of post-infection autoimmune disease. Immunol Today 9: 117–119
25. Archard LC, Freeke AC, Richardson PJ, Meany B, Olson EGJ, Morgan-Capner P, Rose ML, Taylor P, Banner NR, Yacoub MH, Bowles NE (1988) Persistence of enterovirus RNA in dilated cardiomyopathy: a progression from myocarditis. In: Schultheiss H-P (cd) New concepts in viral heart disease. Springer, Berlin Heidelberg New York, pp 349–362
26. Kandolf A, Kirschner P, Ameis D, Canu A, Erdmann E, Schultheiss H-P, Kemkes B, Hofschneider P (1989) Enteroviral heart disease: diagnosis by in-situ hybridization. In: Schultheiss HP (ed) New concepts in viral heart disease. Springer, Berlin Heidelberg New York, pp 337–348
27. Editorial (1990) Dilated cardiomyopathy and enteroviruses. Lancet 336: 971–973
28. Oldstone MBA, Dyrberg TI, Fujinami R (1986) Mimicry by virus of host molecules: implications for autoimmune disease. Prog Immunol 6: 787–795
29. Izumo S, Nadal-Ginard B, Mahdavi V (1988) Protooncogene induction and reprogramming of cardiac gene expression produced by pressure overload. Proc Natl Acad Sci USA 85: 339–343
30. Komuro I, Yazaki Y (1993) Control of cardiac gene expression by mechanical stress. Annu Rev Physiol 55: 55–75
31. Stepien G, Torroni A, Chung AB, Hodge JA, Wallace DC (1992) Differential expression of the adenine nucleotide translocator isoforms in mammalian tissues and during muscle cell differentiation. J Biol Chem 267: 14592–14597
32. Schultheiss HP, Bolte HD (1985) Immunological analysis of autoantibodies against the adenine translocator in dilated cardiomyopathy. J Mol Cell Cardiol 17: 603–617
33. Schultheiss HP (1987) The mitochondrion as antigen in inflammatory heart disease. Eur Heart J 8: 23–210
34. Schultheiss HP, Kühl U, Schauer R, Schulze K, Kemkes B, Becker BF (1988) Antibodies against adenosine di-triphosphate carrier alter myocardial function by disturbing cellular energy metabolism. In: Schultheiss HP (ed) New concepts in viral heart disease. Springer, Berlin Heidelberg New York, pp 243–258

35. Schulze K, Becker BF, Schultheiss H-P (1989) Antibodies to the ADP/ATP carrier – an autoantigen in myocarditis and dilated cardiomyopathy – penetrate into myocardial cells and disturb energy metabolism in vivo. Circ Res 64: 179–192
36. Janda I, Herzog V, Kühl U, Schultheiss H-P (1990) Biochemical and immunocytochemical evidence for endocytosis of antibodies against the ADP/ATP carrier – an autoantigen in dilated cardiomyopathy. Circulation 82[Suppl III]: 268
37. Schultheiss H-P, Kühl U, Janda I, Melzner B, Ulrich G, Morad M (1988): Antibody-mediated enhancement of calcium permeability in cardiac myocytes. J Exp Med 168: 2105–2116
38. Morad M, Davies NW, Ulrich G, Schultheiss H-P (1988) Antibodies against ADP-ATP carrier enhance Ca^{2+} current in isolated cardiac myocytes. Am J Physiol 255: H960–H964

Immunohistochemical Analysis of Inflammatory Heart Disease

U. Kühl, M. Noutsias, and H.-P. Schultheiss

Introduction

Cardiomyopathies are diseases of the heart characterized by ventricular dysfunction that is not due to secondary causes such as hypertension, congenital, valvular, coronary, arterial, or pericardial abnormalities. They are described as primary cardiomyopathies if the origin of cardiac dysfunction is unknown, and as secondary or specific cardiomyopathies if the heart is involved by specific infectious, metabolic, neuromuscular or toxic diseases. According to the new definition of the WHO, primary cardiomyopathies are classified as dilated cardiomyopathy, hypertrophic cardiomyopathy, restrictive cardiomyopathy, and arrhythmogenic right ventricular cardiomyopathy [1].

Idiopathic dilated cardiomyopathy is the most common cause of chronic heart failure. The disease is clinically characterized by chamber dilatation and impaired diastolic and systolic ventricular function of a variable degree, ranging from mild or moderate, well-compensated heart failure to poorly contracting left ventricle. It may be idiopathic, familial/genetic or, as shown for a number of cases, of specific origin due to viral and/or immune involvement of the heart, the latter of which means post-myocarditic. Although the term "myocarditis" is commonly used in conjunction with acute infectious or hypersensitive inflammation of the heart, recent experimental and clinical data have provided evidence for a causal relationship between dilated cardiomyopathy and myocarditis, suggesting that an "inflammatory cardiomyopathy" exists [1–6]. The pathogenetic mechanisms involved and the incidence and exact time course of the disease, especially for the transition of acute myocarditis into chronic heart failure, are still a matter of discussion, mainly for diagnostic reasons.

Except in the very early state, the clinical symptoms of myocarditis vary and bear no relation to the localization and extension of the inflammatory process. In addition, a history of a systemic viral infection does not necessarily mean that the heart itself is affected. The viral origin of myocarditis can only be proven if the virus is detected within the injured myocardium. Viral myocarditis, however, can cause heart failure by at least two different mechanisms.

Department of Internal Medicine/Cardiology, Benjamin Franklin Hospital, Free University of Berlin, Hindenbargdamm 32, 12200 Berlin, Germany

In early stages of the disease, the infected myocardium is injured by the direct cytotoxic effect of the virus. In this case, the extent of tissue damage and depression of cardiac function depends on the pathogenicity of the infectious agent. Replicating virus, however, will be cleared from the myocardium within 10 or 12 days. This initial phase is followed by a humoral and cellular immune process which might limit further expansion of the destructive process or, by itself, cause an ongoing, immune-mediated injury to the myocardium. These secondary immune responses may then be responsible for the progression of myocardial impairment. In the first case, a viral infection of the heart or its persistence is required for the development of myocarditis and developing heart failure, while in the second case a direct attack on the heart by a virus is not necessary, and progression of the disease is mediated by the persisting immune process.

The fact that clinical parameters are missing for a diagnosis of chronic myocarditis has led to histological analysis of endomyocardial biopsies being considered the "gold standard" for diagnosing cardiomyopathies and especially myocarditis. This is true for acute myocarditis, but the interpretation of chronic myocarditis can be exceedingly difficult using light microscopy, as is shown by the great variation in the diagnosis of myocarditis when this is only based on histological analysis [7]. The reason is that, at the morphological level, lymphocytes may mimick other cellular elements of the interstitium, and electron-microscopic examination might be necessary in order to evaluate the cell type accurately [8, 9]. The lymphocytic infiltrates are often focally distributed and, therefore, are easily missed by sampling error [10]. Furthermore, it is well-established that some lymphocytes can occur in absolutely normal cardiac tissue and, therefore, the mere presence of lymphocytes in the myocardium, especially if not activated, does not necessarily constitute myocarditis. Other possible causes for the great variation include patient selection and time point of the biopsy after onset of clinical symptoms, because histological interpretation of endomyocardial biopsies is markedly influenced by the time, the biopsy is taken. Problems in histological diagnosis can be summarized as follows:

1. High interobserver variability
   a. Identification of inflammatory cells
   b. Differentiation from interstitial cells
   c. Quantification of lymphocytes
2. Missing of morphologic criteria
3. Sampling error
   a. Size of biopsies
   b. Number of biopsies
   c. Location of biopsies

Immunohistological methods have now been successfully introduced into the diagnosis of an inflammatory myocardial process [11–14]. Due to the sensitivity of monoclonal antibodies used against specific epitopes of inflammatory cells, this method allows the identification, characterization, and quantification of different cell types infiltrating the myocardial tissue. Thus, in contrast to routine histology with the difficulties explained above in the detection of lymphocytes, cardiac inflammation can be easily identified immuno-histo-chemically. The immune process is characterized immuno-histochemically not only by infiltrating lymphocytes but also by the expression of additional immune markers of cell activation and different markers of tissue inflammation. This allows a reproducible diagnosis of cardiac inflammation especially in those cases where the involvement of a chronic immune process with focal type of cell infiltration is assumed [14–17].

In this chapter, we introduce different immunohistological markers and discuss their meaning for the diagnosis of myocarditis and their role for the developing immune process. We compare the results of the histological and immunohistological analysis of endomyocardial biopsies and provide evidence that immunohistochemistry is an indispensable tool for an accurate diagnosis of chronic myocardial inflammation.

Methods

Characterization of Patients

In all, 658 patients were enrolled in this study. All patients underwent full non-invasive and invasive analysis including physical examination, routine laboratory tests, electrocardiography (ECG), exercise ECG, echocardiography, coronary angiography, and left ventriculography. After exclusion of specific causes of cardiac dysfunction (e.g., hypertension or congenital, valvular, coronary, arterial, or pericardial abnormalities), right-sided heart endomyocardial biopsies were performed to further elucidate the origin of cardiac dysfunction.

Clinical Classification

Myocarditis. The clinical diagnosis of myocarditis is based on the acute onset of chest pain, laboratory changes (e.g., increased levels of creatine kinase (CK) or CK-MB, blood sedimentation rate, BSR), conspicuous electrocardiographic disturbances with ST segment or T deviations, arrhythmias, echocardiographically or angiographically documented segmental wall motion abnormalities, or pericardial effusions in previously healthy people after exclusion of other specific causes of heart diseases. These patients report a sudden onset of faintness, development of reduced working capacity and dyspnoe at exertion in association with a recent history of viral infection. Global ventricular contractility in most cases is only slightly impaired, although severe cardiac dysfunction may also be present at early stages of the disease occasionally.

Dilated Cardiomyopathy. The clinical presentation of dilated cardiomyopathy patients is similar to and often indistinguishable from that of the myocarditis group, although symptoms might be more pronounced. In contrast to the patients with myocarditis, dilated cardiomyopathy is clinically suggested when the history of cardiac symptoms is prolonged and dates back months or even years without any evidence of a viral infection in association with onset of symptoms. Cardiac dysfunction ranges from mild or moderate impairment of cardiac contractility, but is normally characterized by a more severe depressed systolic and/or diastolic ventricular dysfunction with a reduction in ejection fraction, stroke volume, and cardiac index resulting in clinical symptoms of congestive heart failure. After exclusion of specific causes of ventricular contractility these patients are clinically classified as cardiomyopathies of unknown origin (dilated cardiomyopathy).

Histological Classification

Myocarditis is histologically defined as an "inflammatory cell infiltrate of the myocardium in association with myocyte necrosis and/or degeneration of adjacent myocytes, not typical of ischaemic damage associated with coronary arterial disease" (Dallas Classification, [18, 19]). If lymphocytic infiltrates are not accompanied by myocytolysis in the first biopsy ("borderline myocarditis"), a definitive histologic diagnosis of myocarditis cannot be made at this moment. The histological definition of chronic myocarditis according to the Dallas Classification (histologically "ongoing myocarditis") demands the persistence of an unchanged lymphocytic infiltrate in a follow-up biopsy. If the inflammatory process resolves in comparison with the initial biopsy, a "healing myocarditis" has to be suggested. Fibrosis might be present at all time points except in the acute phase of myocarditis. If neither inflammation nor fibrosis nor any other cardiomyocyte abnormalities are present, patients cannot be classified according to histological criteria and the diagnosis according to the Dallas classification will be "no myocarditis". Unspecific morphological changes without any signs of inflammation may be consistent with dilated cardiomyopathy, especially if ventricular contractility is impaired and volumes are enlarged. Normal ventricular function and diameters may point to a postmyocarditic state.

Immunohistological Classification

The detection of cell necrosis needs an optimal preservation of tissue morphology, which cannot be achieved in cryostat sections, but demands paraffin-embedded material. Acute myocarditis according to the Dallas Criteria, therefore, is a histological diagnosis which cannot be obtained from frozen sections. Chronic/ongoing myocarditis is immunohistochemically characterized by a lymphocytic infiltration with more than 2.0 cells per high power field (HPF, magnification $\times$ 400) equivalent to more the 7.0 cells/mm^2 and the enhanced expression of additional markers of cell activation or immune cell regulation (Table 1). In myocarditis, the most frequently encountered cellular infiltrate is lymphocytic, but inflammatory infiltrates may also contain a mixture of different types of activated immunocompetent cells, for example

Table 1. Immunohistological diagnosis of inflammatory heart disease

Cells/antigens	CD	Definition of pathologically/positive
Infiltrating cells		
Lymphocytes	CD3	> 2.0 cells/HPF (> 7.0 cells/mm^2)
		> 1.5 cells/HPF if focal
and/or		
Macrophages	27E10	> 1.5 cells/HPF
Markers of cell activation		
HLA-antigens	HLA-I/II	enhanced expression
and/or		
Adhesion molecules	CD18, VCAM	enhanced expression
	CD54	

HPF; high power field (magnification × 400, equivalent to 0.28 mm^2)

macrophages, neutrophils, eosinophils, giant cells, or granulomas (Fig 1). An immunologically active immune process with activated interstitial and endothelial cells is characterized not only by activated inflammatory cells, but also by the enhanced expression of numerous adhesion molecules on both cell compartments. The most important of these immunologic markers belonging to the selectin, β2-integrin, and immunoglobulin superfamilies are shown in Table 2. Biopsy sections were screened semiquantitatively for relative levels of expression of major histocompatibility complex (MHC) class I and II antigens and adhesion molecules on both the vascular endothelium and interstitial cells, and the immunoperoxidase techniques mentioned below were performed. Immunoperoxidase staining of HLA antigens and adhesion molecules were graded as follows:

1. Grade 0–1+: No immunoreactivity or weak staining similar to that seen in negative control samples, with endothelial cells faintly stained; few interstitial cells are marked.

Table 2. Immunohistological cell markers

Reactive cell compartment	Antigen
T-lymphocytes	CD3
Helper/inducer lymphocytes	CD4
Cytotoxic/suppressor lymphocytes	CD8
B-lymphocytes	CD19–22
Natural Killer (NK) cells	CD57
Macrophages	CD14
Activated lymphocytes	HLA-I/II, ILR2, CD25, CD18, CD54, CD45RO, CD71
Activated macrophages	27E10, 25F9, RM 3/1, HLA-DR
Activated endothelial cells	HLA-DR, HLA-I, CD54, CD62E, VCAM-1

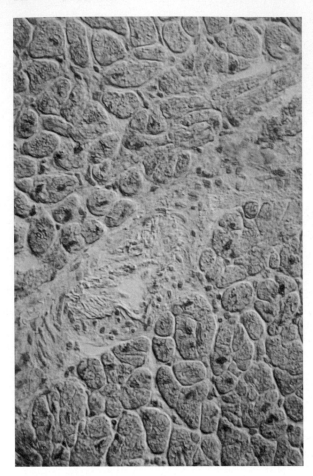

Fig. 1a–d. Normal cardiac myocardium (a) lymphocytic infiltration in a diffuse (b) and focal (c) distribution; activated macrophages (d) ×400

2. Grade 2+: Enhanced expression on endothelial cells and increased number of positively stained interstitial cells.
3. Grade 3+: Endothelial cells are strongly immunoreactive. There are more positive interstitial cells and the intensity of staining on each cell is increased (Fig. 2).

Sample Preparation

At least ten endomyocardial biopsy specimens were obtained from each patient. The average dimension of each specimen was 1.0–2.0 mm^3. For histology, two biopsies were fixed in formalin. For immunohistology, five biopsy specimens were snap-frozen in a slurry of dry ice and methylbutane at −70° C and covered with Tissue Tec (O.C.T. Compound, Miles Inc., USA) as an embedding medium. For routine immunohistological analysis, only one biopsy specimen was serially cut into sections of 5 μm thickness; six to nine serial sections were

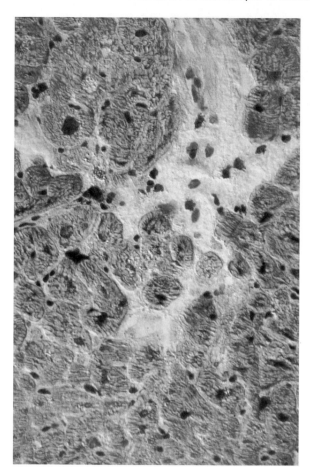

Fig. 1b

analyzed from this first biopsy for each antibody (see below). Biopsies were examined by two independent observers in a blinded fashion. If additional sections had to be made from a second or third biopsy specimen, staining with some of the routine markers (CD3, HLA I and II, CD54) was repeated on every biopsy to rule out sampling error. Results obtained for additional immune markers (e.g., adhesion molecules or cytokines) were only taken into consideration if routine marker analysis was identical in all analyzed biopsies.

Immunohistological Staining

Cryotome sections (5 μm) were preincubated with fetal calf serum (FCS) to saturate nonspecific immunoglobulin binding sites. Specific monoclonal-mouse anti-human antibodies in pretested dilutions were then incubated on the sections for 45 min at room temperature in a humidified chamber. Unbound antibodies were removed by three washes with phosphate-buffered saline

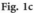

Fig. 1c

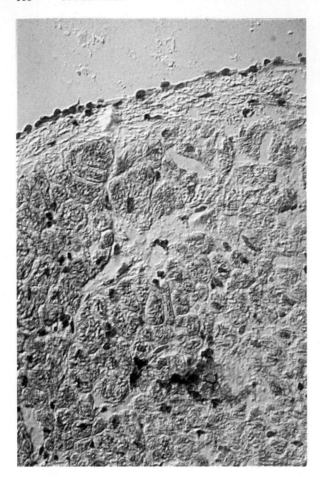

(PBS), each of 3 min duration. Peroxidase labeled rabbit-anti-mouse immuno-globulin (Dianova), diluted at 1:200 in PBS containing 10% FCS (30 min, room temperature) was used to detect specifically bound primary antibodies. Staining was performed with 3-amino-9-ethylcarbazole as a chromogene against a hematoxylin counterstain. Sections were coverslipped with Kaiser's gelatin (Merck, Darmstadt, FRG).

Results

Histology

Endomyocardial biopsies of 359 patients with clinically suspected myocarditis (group 1) and 299 patients with clinically suspected dilated cardiomyopathy (group 2) were analyzed according to histological and immunohistological criteria of cardiac inflammation. Histologically, cardiac inflammation was seen

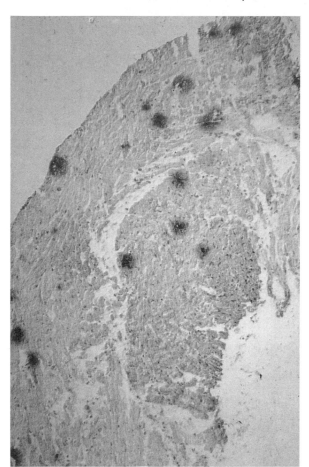

Fig. 1d

in 3.3% of the myocarditis group (12 patients) and 1.3% biopsies (four patients) with dilated cardiomyopathy (Table 3). The biopsies were consistent
with the diagnosis of borderline myocarditis in 6.7% of patients in group 1 and
4.3% of patients in group 2. No myocarditis was diagnosed in 90.0% of samples
of group 1, and 94.4% of biopsies were consistent with the diagnosis of dilated
cardiomyopathy in group 2.

Immunohistology

Immunohistochemical analysis revealed an active immune process with pathologically increased lymphocytic infiltrates and enhanced expression of adhesion molecules in 198 biopsies (55%) of patients with myocarditis and 129
biopsies (43%) of patients with dilated cardiomyopathy (Table 3). Mean cell
counts (per HPF) of lymphocytes and percentages of enhanced expression of

Table 3. Histological and immunohistological analysis of endomyocardial biopsies

	Myocarditis (n=359)		Dilated cardiomyopathy (n=299)	
	%	n	%	n
Histology				
Myocarditis	3.3	12	1.3	4
Borderline myocarditis	6.7	24	4.3	13
No myocarditis	90.0	323	94.4	282
Immunohistology				
Positive	55	198	43	129
Negative	45	161	57	170

histocompatibility antigens or adhesion molecules in immunohistologically
positive and negative biopsies are given in Table 4. In immunohistologically
negative tissues as well as control tissues, only few lymphocytes are detected
[14]. Mean lymphocyte numbers of these biopsies were 0.6 ± 0.4 cells/HPF.

Analyzing the data in more detail, it becomes evident that even low numbers
of infiltrating lymphocytes characterize an activated immune process with
interstitial and endothelial cell activation. Endomyocardial biopsies with more
than 2.0 lymphocytes per HPF show a pathologically enhanced expression of
different immune markers, for example histocompatibility antigens (Tables 4
and 5). While a slightly enhanced expression of HLA classes I and II is seen in
less then 30% of normal cardiac tissues, expression of these molecules is clearly
up-regulated in over 90% of biopsies with more than 2 lymphocytes per HPF.
Similar results are obtained for other adhesion molecules. Integrins (CD11a/
LFA-1, CD11b/Mac-1, CD11c/p150,95 CD49d/VLA-4, and CD29/VLA-β-chain)
can be demonstrated in 55%–89% of interstitial cells. Similarly, members of the
immunoglobulin (CD54/ICAM-1, VCAM-1 and LFA-3) and selectin families
(CD62E/ELAM-1, CD62P/GMP140) are pathologically enhanced in 36%–88%
[14] (Tables 4 and 5).

Endothelial cell activation, as analyzed by adhesion molecule expression,
(Fig. 2, Table 5) is seen in the majority of lymphocyte-positive biopsies (ICAM-

Table 4. Expression of immune markers on interstitial cells

	n	CD3	CD4	CD8	CD45RO	mac	CD54	CD18	CD11a	CD11b
Myocarditis	359									
Positive (> 2.0 cells/HPF)	198	3.6	2.2	1.9	2.7		1.7	17.8	7.3	6.2	6.1
Negative (< 2.0 cells/HPF)	161	0.6	0.3	0.3	0.4		0.8	7.9	1.3	1.0	1.4
Dilated cardiomyopathy	299									
Positive (> 2.0 cells/HPF)	129	2.8	1.4	1.4	1.2		1.6	17.8	3.5	3.7	3.0
Negative (< 2.0 cells/HPF)	170	0.6	0.3	0.3	0.4		0.8	10.4	2.1	1.9	2.0

HPF, high-power field

1, 88%, VCAM-1, LFA-3, 60%). Analysis of inflammatory cell adhesion molecules and their endothelial cell counter receptors reveals that both molecules, ligands and receptors, are coexpressed in a similar fashion in positive biopsies, indicating a costimulation of both interacting molecules (Fig 3). In CD3-lymphocyte negative tissues, expression of these molecules is only slightly enhanced (ICAM-1, 23%, VCAM-1, 20%, LFA-3, 13%). The reason for the up-regulation of HLA and adhesion molecules in tissues without cellular infiltration is not known. It is possible that focal lymphocytic infiltrates in these biopsies have been missed due to sampling error.

For the immunohistologic diagnosis of cardiac inflammation, it is important that the expression pattern of HLA antigens and adhesion molecules is independent of a diffuse or focal type of cellular infiltration. Activated endothelial cells are found equally distributed over the entire cardiac tissue (Figure 2). This independence of the focal type of cellular infiltration reduces sampling error and indicates that the immunologic process, which is postu-

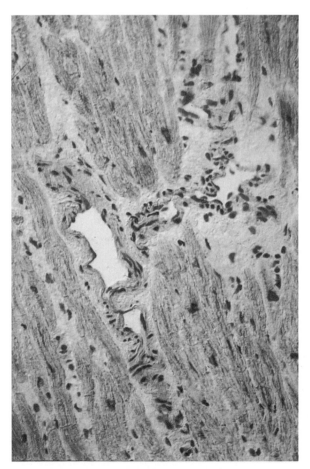

Fig. 2a–e. Activated vascular endothelium. Staining for VCAM-1 in normal, noninflamed (a) and inflamed (b) cardiac tissue. Enhanced expression of CD54 (ICAM-1) (c) and HLA-DR (d) in a biopsy with increased CD3-positive lymphocytes. Cytokine release (interferon-γ) from activated macrophage (e) a–c, e, ×400; d, ×40

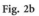

Fig. 2b

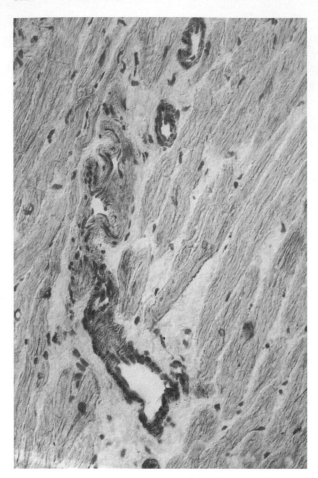

Table 5. Activated vascular endothelium: percentage of enhanced expression of adhesion molecules in lymphocyte positive and negative biopsies

Antigen	Positive (> 2.0 T-lymphocytes/ HPF) %	Negative (< 2.0 T-lymphocytes/ HPF) %
HLA-I/II	93	31
HLA-I	58	10
HLA-DR	67	20
CD54	88	23
VCAM-1	85	20
LFA-3	60	13

HPF, high-power field

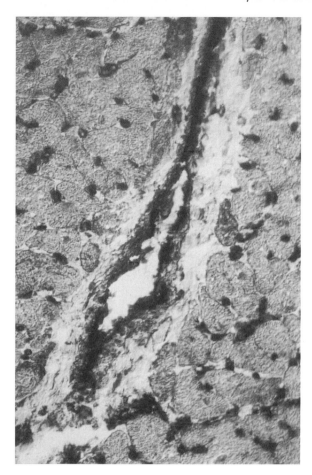

Fig. 2c

lated to be responsible for cardiac impairment and progression of the disease is activated within the entire myocardium.

Activated macrophages are detected in more than 80% of tissues with pathologically increased inflammatory lymphocytes. In addition to lymphocytes and endothelial cells, these macrophages are suggested to be the main source of different cytokines. This can be shown by our immunohistologic data which demonstrate that different cytokines are preferentially found to be released in immunohistologically positive biopsy specimens from activated inflammatory cells (Fig 2E; Table 6).

Discussion

The term "myocarditis" is commonly used in connection with acute infectious or hypersensitive inflammation of the heart, although the existence of a

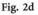

Fig. 2d

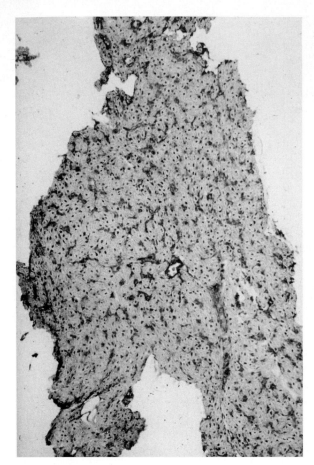

chronic form of cardiac inflammation has been demonstrated by clinical and experimental data. In the majority of patients, myocarditis is considered to be a benign condition which recovers completely within several weeks. Those patients who suffer from residual myocardial abnormalities and progress to a chronic cardiac dysfunction are of poor predictive outcome. The responsible pathogenetic mechanisms involved, the incidence and exact time course are yet unknown.

Myocarditis can be caused by a multitude of viruses but, in Western countries, enteroviral infections – especially Coxsackie B1-6 serotypes – are the most frequent viral pathogens that attack the heart, and viral infections have been suggested as one possible precursor of myocarditis and dilated cardio-myopathy. On the other hand, viral infection has been discussed controversially for a long time, mostly because virological methods had failed to detect the virus in the myocardium. This situation changed completely since molecular biological methods have been developed as diagnostic tools for heart diseases. By using in-situ hybridization or polymerase chain reaction (PCR),

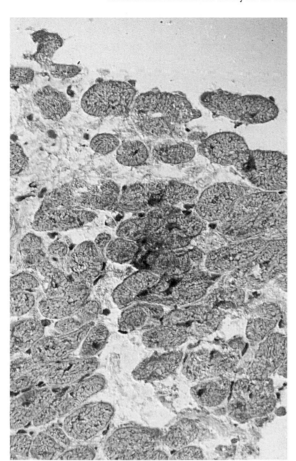

Fig. 2e

persisting viral RNA could be demonstrated in the myocardium of patients with clinically suspected myocarditis and chronic heart failure (dilated cardiomyopathy). These data, demonstrating enteroviral mRNA in the myocardium over months or even years, corroborate the concept of a possible viral persistence in the myocardium and suggest that the infection may cause the development of myocarditis that further progresses towards chronic heart failure in an unknown percentage of patients [20–24].

In the acute phase of viral invasion and replication, tissue destruction is caused by a direct cytotoxic effect of the responsible virus. This initial phase is followed by a humoral and cellular immune process which might limit further expansion of the destructive process or, by itself, cause an ongoing injury to the myocardium [25–30]. The developing immune process is characterized by the appearance of organ-specific autoantibodies, immunoglobulin deposits at the cardiac myocyte cell surface, a humoral and/or cellular cytotoxic reactivity directed against cardiac myocytes, and cellular infiltration of the myocardium. Until now, however, it is still a matter of discussion whether viral persistence,

Table 6. Percentage of cytokine-expressing inflammatory cells in immunohistological positive and negative biopsies

	Immunohistology(%)	
	Positive	Negative
Cytokines		
IL-1α	35	6
IL-2	29	8
IL-8	30	13
TNF-α	44	16
TNF-β	40	11
Cytokine receptors		
TNF-R	45	18
Receptor antogonists		
IL-2RA	48	2

IL, interleukin; TNF, tumor necrosis factor

the virally induced secondary immune process, or both are responsible for development and progression of the disease.

No specific clinical parameters to identify viral heart disease or other forms of cardiomyopathies exist. This restriction is also true for left-sided heart catheterization, by which only secondary causes of myocardial dysfunction can be shown or excluded. An indubitable diagnosis for specific heart muscle diseases can only be obtained from histological analysis of cardiac tissue. Therefore, endomyocardial biopsies should be performed in all cases of un-explained heart failure after exclusion of other secondary causes of cardiac diseases.

Histological analysis has been considered as the "gold standard" for diagnosing inflammatory heart disease. This is true for acute myocarditis with biopsy-proven myocyte necrosis adjacent to infiltrating lymphocytes, but the histological diagnosis of chronic myocarditis causes difficulties and the results

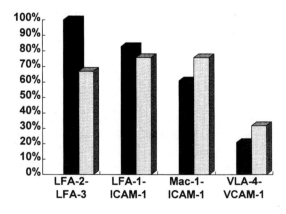

Fig. 3. Coexpression of lymphocyte adhesion molecules (LFA-2, LFA-1, Mac-1, VLA-1) and their endothelial cell counter receptors (LFA-3, ICAM-1, VCAM-1) in immunohistologically positive biopsies

obtained are contradictory. The histological definition of chronic myocarditis according to the Dallas Classification (histologically borderline or ongoing myocarditis) demands the presence of infiltrating lymphocytes without further histomorphological signs of myocyte injury or immunohistologic features of a persisting, activated inflammatory process. The cellular infiltrates in chronic heart failure, however, are often sparse or focal and therefore might be missed by sampling error. Moreover, it is difficult to differentiate noninflammatory interstitial cells from infiltrating lymphocytes. Misinterpretation of interstitial cells as inflammatory lymphocytes thus leads to an over- or underestimation of the degree of the inflammatory process. Ultimately, one has to keep in mind that infiltrating lymphocytes, especially if they are not activated, are not necessarily representative of an ongoing immune process that affects the entire myocardium. These two mechanisms (i.e.) misinterpretation of interstitial cells and sampling error) are responsible for a low diagnostic yield in the histological analysis and might explain the often reported high interobserver variability [7]. The difficulties of the histological diagnosis of inflammatory heart disease are demonstrated by the results of our histological analysis of endomyocardial biopsies in which cardiac inflammation could only be demonstrated in only 16 out of 658 analyzed tissues (2.5%).

Immunohistological methods have now been successfully introduced into the diagnosis of an inflammatory myocardial process. As shown by our data, cardiac inflammation is immunohistochemically easily identified and can be demonstrated in 55% of biopsy specimens of patients with clinically suspected myocarditis and 43% of cardiac tissues from patients with suggested dilated cardiomyopathy. The observed picture of infiltration depends on the pathogenicity of the infectious agent and the time the biopsy is taken. Immunohistological analysis of mild cardiac inflammation reveals that activated macrophages might be the very first and only indication of the beginning immune process. After a short and variable time lymphocytic infiltrates arise which often primarily consist of CD4-positive helper-inducer cells. A focal infiltration is more commonly seen than a diffuse distribution (Fig 1). A persisting immune process in chronic myocarditis is characterized by mixed diffuse or focal cellular infiltrates containing activated leukocytes, CD4- and CD8-positive lymphocytes and macrophages (Table 4). Activation of interstitial cells is characterized by an enhanced expression of activation markers or histocompatibility antigen classes I and II and numerous other adhesion molecules (Tables 4 and 5).

Lymphocyte numbers in chronic myocarditis are relatively low when compared with acute myocarditis, where hundreds of infiltrating cells per high power microscopic field might be present. An ongoing active immune process, however, is immunohistologically not only characterized by lymphocytic infiltrates, but also by the enhanced expression of different additional immune markers of interstitial and endothelial cell activation [31–34]. In biopsies with increased lymphocytic infiltrates exceeding 2 cells per high power field, expression of histocompatibility antigen classes I and II and other adhesion molecules is pathologically enhanced in more than 90% of cases. Up-regulation of these immune markers is not restricted to the neighbourhood of lymphocytic infiltrates, but seen in the entire biopsy specimen. Due to this pattern of distribution, the diagnosis of cardiac inflammation is markedly improved in comparison with the routine histological analysis of endomyocardial biopsies, and sampling error is reduced considerably because the distribution pattern of these markers is independent of the diffuse or focal type of cellular infiltration. In addition to the improvement in the diagnosis of inflammatory heart disease, these immune markers corroborate the concept of a generalized activated immune process in the entire cardiac tissue with pathologically increased lymphocytic infiltrates.

For immune cell activation and infiltration of blood- borne inflammatory cells into inflamed tissues, stimulatory and regulatory immune events have to be induced. Inflammatory processes are supported by interactions between activated immunocompetent and endothelial cells and signal transducing plasma- and cell-derived humoral factors. Immune-modulating cytokines directly modify leukocytes and endothelial cells both structurally and functionally, and the enhanced expression of adhesion molecules, induced by pro-inflammatory cytokines such as interleukin (IL)-1α, tumor necrosis factor (TNF)-α and interferon (IFN)-γ is a crucial prerequisite for the commencement of the immunologic cascade [35–38]. These cell adhesion molecules provide position-specific information, enabling immunocompetent cells to selectively adhere and traffic through vascular endothelium adjacent to an inflamed area and then to migrate into and infiltrate the impaired tissue [35, 36].

Most adhesion molecules are induced by cytokines which are locally released by activated immunocompetent cells, e.g., macrophages, lymphocytes, or endothelial cells. Immunohistological staining for different cytokines demonstrates a release of IL-1, IL-2, IL-8, TNF-α and TNF-β, or IFN-γ from areas of focally distributed inflammatory cells, mostly macrophages (Table 6; Fig 2). It, therefore, has to be assumed that the enhanced expression of HLA antigens and other adhesion molecules as well as the endothelial cell activation within the entire myocardium of positive biopsies is caused by a local cytokine release from activated immune cells. Moreover, the cytokine-rich microenvironment and its developing tissue gradient may contribute to the inflammatory traffic of immune cells into the inflamed areas (Fig. 4). In an animal model of virally induced heart disease, it has been shown recently that the use of cytokines may contribute to the lymphocytic infiltration into heart tissue [39].

Conclusion

In summary, immunohistological techniques can successfully be used to identify, characterize and quantify mononuclear cell infiltrates in myocardial biopsies, especially in cases of sparse or focal tissue distribution, as often seen in patients with dilated cardiomyopathy. The whole cascade of immune events known to be involved in immune cell activation and lymphocyte or macrophage infiltration is activated in biopsies with more than 2 lymphocytes per HPF (Table 7). This supports the hypothesis of a chronically smoldering inflammatory process even in biopsies with low numbers of infiltrating lym-

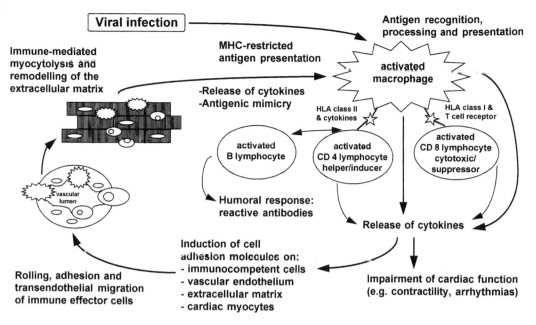

Fig. 4. Activation of immune processes in inflammatory heart disease

phocytes. In addition to the diagnostic advantages, immunohistochemical analysis of endomyocardial biopsies has become helpful in selecting patients for an anti-inflammatory treatment of patients, because an immuno-suppressive therapy can only be successful if an ongoing immune process is still active at the time of introduction of therapy. Furthermore, the possibility of analyzing different key steps of immune regulation enables a follow up of patients during treatment. This will improve future diagnostic and therapeutic strategies in future [40] (see also Kühl et al., this volume).

References

1. WHO (1996) Report of the 1995 World Health Organization/International Society and Federation of Cardiology Task Force on the definition and classification of cardiomyopathies. Circulation 93: 841–842
2. Zee-Cheng CS, Tsai CC, Palmer DC, Codd JE, Pennington DG, Williams GA (1984) High incidence of myocarditis by endomyocardial biopsy in patients with idiopathic congestive cardiomyopathy. J Am Coll Cardiol 3: 63–70
3. Steenbergen C, Kolbeck PC, Wolfe JA, Anthony RM, Sanfilippo FP, Jennings RB (1986) Detection of lymphocytes in endomyocardium using immunohistochemical techniques. Relevance to evaluation of endomyocardial biopsies in suspected cases of lymphocytic myocarditis. J Appl Cardiol 1: 63–73
4. MacArthur CGC, Tarin D, Goodwin JF, Hallidie-Smith KA, (1984) The relationship of myocarditis to dilated cardiomyopathy. Eur Heart J 5: 1023–1035
5. Kawai C, Matsumori A, Fujiwara H (1987) Myocarditis and dilated cardiomyopathy. Ann Rev Med 38: 221–239

6. Dec GW Jr, Palacios IF, Fallon JT, Aretz HT, Mills J, Mills DCS, Johnson RA (1985) Active myocarditis in the spectrum of acute dilated cardiomyopathies. N Engl J Med 312: 885–890
7. Shanes JG, Ghali J, Billingham ME, Ferrans VJ, Fenoglio JJ, Edwards WD, Tsai CC, Saffitz JE, Isner J, Furner S, Subramanian R (1987) Interobserver variability in the pathologic interpretation of endomyocardial biopsy results. Circulation 75: 401–405
8. Billingham MB (1987) Acute myocarditis: a diagnostic dilemma. Br Heart J 58: 6–8
9. Ohlsen EGJ (1985) The problem of viral heart disease: how often do we miss it? Postgrad Med J 61: 479–480
10. Hauck AJ, Kearney DL, Edwards WD (1989) Evaluation of postmortem endomyocardial biopsy specimens from 38 patients with lymphocytic myocarditis: Implication for role of sampling error. Mayo Clin Proc 64: 1235–1245
11. Edwards WD, Holmes DR, Reeder GS (1982) Diagnosis of active lymphocytic myocarditis by endomyocardial biopsy. Quantitative criteria for light microscopy. Mayo Clin Proc 57: 419–425
12. Fenoglio JJ, Ursell PC, Kellogg CF, Drusin RE, Weiss MB (1983) Diagnosis and classification of myocarditis by endomyocardial biopsy. N Engl J Med 308: 12–18
13. Mason JW, Billingham ME (1982) Acute inflammatory myocarditis In: Fenoglio JJ (ed) Endomyocardial biopsy: technique and applications. Boca CRC Press, Boca Raton
14 Kühl U, Seeberg B, Noutsias M, Schultheiß H-P (1995) Immunohistochemical analysis of the chronic inflammatory process in dilated cardiomyopathy. Br Heart J 75: 295–300
15. Linder J, Cassling RSM, Rogler WC, Wilson JE, Markin RS, Sears TD, McManus BM (1985) Immunohistological characterization of lymphocytes in uninflamed ventricular myocardium. Arch Pathol Lab Med 109: 917–920
16. Kühl U, Noutsias M, Seeberg B, Schannwell M, Welp LB, Schultheiß H-P, Strauer BE (1994) Chronic inflammation in dilated cardiomyopathy. J Cardiac Failure 1: 13–25
17. Kühl U, Noutsias M, Seeberg B, Schannwell M, Welp LB, Schultheiß H-P, Strauer BE (1994) Chronic inflammation in the myocardium of patients with clinically suspected dilated cardiomyopathy. J Heart Failure (January): 231–245
18. Aretz HT (1987) Myocarditis, the Dallas Criteria. Hum Pathol 18: 619–624
19. Aretz HT, Billingham ME, Edwards WD (1986) Myocarditis: a histopathological definition and classification. J Cardiovasc Pathol 1: 3–14
20. Anonymous (1990) Dilated cardiomyopathy and enteroviruses (Editorials) Lancet 336: 971–973
21. Bowles NE, Ohlsen EGJ, Richardson PJ, Archard LC (1986) Detection of Cocksackie B-virus-specific RNA sequences in myocardial biopsy samples from patients with myocarditis and dilated cardiomyopathy. Lancet 1: 1120–1122
22. Grasso M, Arbusti E, Silini E, Diegoli M, Percivalle E, Ratti G, Bramerio M, Gavazzi A, Vigano M, Milanesi G (1992) Search for coxsackie B3 RNA in idiopathic dilated cardiomyopathy using gene amplification by polymerase chain reaction. Am J Cardiol 69: 658–664
23. Kandolf R, Ameis D, Kirschner P, Canu A, Hofschneider PH (1985) In situ detection of enteroviral genomes in myocardial cells by nucleic acid hybridization: An approach to the diagnosis of viral heart disease. Proc Natl Acad Sci 82: 4818–4822
24. Archard LC, Bowles NE, Cunningham l, Freeke CA, Olsen EG, Rose ML, Meany B, Why HJF, Richardson FJ (1991) Molecular probes for detection of persisting enterovirus infection of human heart and their prognostic value. Eur Heart J 12[Suppl D]: 56–59
25. Neu N, Beisel KW, Traysman MD, Rose NR, Craig SW (1987) Autoantibodies specific for cardiac myosin isoform are found in mice susceptible to Coxsackie B3-induced myocarditis. J Immunol 138: 2488–2492
26. Limas CJ, Goldenberg JF, Limas C (1989) Autoantibodies against β-adrenoceptors in human idiopathic dilated cardiomyopathy. Circ Res 64: 97–103
27. Schultheiss HP, Ulrich G, Janda I, Kühl U, Morad M (1988) Antibody-mediated enhancement of calcium permeability in cardiac myocytes. J Exp Med 168: 2105–2119
28. Wolff P, Kühl U, Schultheiss HP (1989) Laminin distribution and autoantibodies to laminin in dilated cardiomyopathy and myocarditis. Am Heart J 117: 1303–1309

29. Schulze K, Becker BF, Schauer R, Schultheiss HP (1990) Antibodies to the ADP/ATP carrier – and autoantigen in myocarditis and dilated cardiomyopathy – impair cardiac function. Circulation 81: 959–969
30. Schulze K, Becker BF, Schultheiß HP (1989) Antibodies to the ADP/ATP carrier, an autoantigen in myocarditis and dilated cardiomyopathy, penetrate into myocardial cells and disturb energy metabolism in vivo. Circ Res 64: 179–192
31. Duijvestijn A, Hamann A (1990) Mechanisms and regulation of lymphocyte migration. Immunology Today 10: 23–28
32. van Seventer GA, Shimizu Y, Horgan KJ, Shaw S (1990) The LFA-1 ligand ICAM-1 provides an important costimulatory signal for T-cell receptor-mediated activation of resting T cells. J Immunol 144: 4579–4586
33. Hughes CCW, Savage COS, Pober JS (1990) The endothelial cell as regulator of T-cell function. Immunol Rev 117: 85–102
34. Cotran RS, Pober JS (1988) Endothelial activation: its role in inflammatory and immune reactions. Endothel Cell Biol: 335–347
35. Pober JS (1987) Effects of tumor necrosis factor and related cytokines on vascular endothelial cells. Ciba Foundation Symposium
36. Dustin ML, Rothlein R, Bhan AK, Dinarello CA, Springer TA (1986) Induction by Il-I and interferon-gamma: tissue distribution, biochemistry and function of a natural adherence molecule (ICAM-1). J Immunol 137(1): 245–254
37. Springer TA (1990) Adhesion receptors of the immune system. Review article. Nature 346: 425–434
38. Yong K, Khwaja A (1990) Leukocyte cellular adhesion molecules. Blood Rev 4: 211–225
39. Neumann DA, Lane JR, Allen GS, Herskowitz A, Rose NR (1993) Viral myocarditis leading to cardiomyopathy: do cytokines contribute to pathogenesis? Clin Immunol Immunpathol 68: 181–190
40. Kühl U, Schultheiß HP, Strauer BE (1994) Methylprednisolone in chronic myocarditis. Postgrad Med J 70: S35–S42

Immunological Mediators in Inflammation of the Heart

Adhesion Molecule Induction and Expression in Neutrophil-Induced Myocardial Injury

K.A. Youker[1], N. Frangogiannis[1], M. Lindsey[1], C.W. Smith[2], and M.L. Entman[1]

Introduction

Reperfusion of a previously ischemic myocardium has become a standard therapeutic approach to acute myocardial infarction. The efficacy of this approach in reducing mortality and morbidity has been well established. However, there is also substantial evidence that the reperfusion process is accompanied by cardiac injury. In theory, attenuating this reperfusion-dependent injury would further improve the results of thrombolytic or angioplastic interventions of acute myocardial infarction.

One of the proposed mechanisms by which reperfusion might induce myocardial injury relates to the observation that reperfusion is associated with an intense acute inflammatory reaction that is not seen in myocardial infarction in the absence of reperfusion until much later [1]. This intense inflammatory reaction is extremely rapid in onset; it has also been proposed that it may occur so rapidly that it might overwhelm normal defense mechanisms and may result in an acute inflammatory injury of viable myocardium. Intervention in this inflammatory response, however, must be carefully considered; substantial evidence associates the inflammation accompanying myocardial infarction and reperfusion with healing [2]. Reperfusion of the myocardium has been shown to reduce noxious myocardial remodeling, an event which is associated with the rapid influx of leukocytes [3]. In the 1970s, evidence that anti-inflammatory agents might reduce myocardial infarct size led to a clinical trial of large doses of methylprednisolone in patients with acute myocardial infarction; the short-lived study is a tragedy [4]. Subsequent studies in animals demonstrated that such an approach to inflammatory reactions in the infarcted myocardium markedly impaired the normal healing process [5].

Our approach to inflammation in the ischemic and reperfused myocardium reveals a dilemma. Therapeutic strategies must be aimed at reducing the acute inflammatory injury occurring early after reperfusion. These strategies must avoid impairing the positive effects of inflammation on healing of the myocardial infarction. Our laboratory has approached this problem by attempting

[1]Section of Cardiovascular Sciences, Department of Medicine, The Methodist Hospital and, The DeBakey Heart Center, Houston, TX 77030, USA
[2]Speros P. Martel Section of Leukocyte Biology, Department of Pediatrics and Texas Children's Hospital, Baylor College of Medicine, Houston, TX 77030, USA

to dissect the cellular and molecular processes which orchestrate the inflammatory process in the previously ischemic myocardium.

Cellular and Molecular Approach to Inflammation of the Reperfused Myocardium

In response to the more global approaches of the 1970s, many laboratories began utilizing more specific interventions to examine their effect on post-reperfusion myocardial injury. Initially, studies in animal models demonstrated the efficacy of approaches that reduced neutrophils or neutrophil function such as the use of anti-neutrophil antibodies [6], neutrophil depletion with anti-metabolites [7], the use of neutrophil filters [8] and monoclonal antibodies to adhesion molecules known to influence neutrophil trafficking such as CD11b [9, 10], CD18 [11], L-selectin [12], P-selectin [13], and intracellular adhesion molecule-1 (ICAM-1) [14]. The almost universal success of this approach suggests an adhesion-molecule-mediated inflammatory injury of the reperfused myocardium. Studies carried out by ourselves and others have sought to specifically characterize the steps involved in inflammatory induction.

Cellular Basis for Leukocyte Localization in the Ischemic and Reperfused Myocardium

The early work of Hill and colleagues demonstrated that the activation of complement occurred in a model for myocardial ischemia [15]. Thus, activation of the complement cascade may lead to neutrophil activation, shape change, homotypic aggregation, and neutrophil endothelial cell adhesion, all of which promote the observed neutrophil margination and microvascular plugging associated with reperfusion. Studies in our laboratory have suggested that complement activation precedes reperfusion [16] and results in the presence of C5a in the extracellular fluid during the first several hours of reperfusion [17]. This complement activation appears to emanate from complement fixation upon C1q binding proteins of mitochondrial origin that are extruded from infarcted myocardium [18]. Within the first hour, most of the leukocyte accumulation in the previously ischemic myocardium relates to intravascular margination which is rapidly followed by transendothelial migration of both neutrophils and monocytes [19]. As described above, this transendothelial migration is associated with specific adhesion molecules; initially the selectins [20, 21] promote leukocyte margination followed by leukocyte integrin activation and adhesion to endothelial ICAM-1 [22–24].

Our laboratory examined the hypothesis that neutrophils directly injure cardiac myocytes by adhesion-molecule-dependent interactions. We demonstrated that activated neutrophils adhere to isolated cardiac myocytes only if the latter has undergone induction of ICAM-1 by cytokines [25]. This adhesion is accompanied by a highly toxic reaction in which neutrophil-induced myo-cardial cell destruction occurs by a highly compartmentalized transfer of re-active oxygen from neutrophils to cardiac myocytes [26]. Thus, in the presence of activated neutrophils that have transmigrated from the vascular compart-ment, the presence of ICAM-1 on cardiac myocytes renders them vulnerable to neutrophil-induced myocardial injury. This has lead to a series of investiga-tions in our laboratory of factors that control myocardial ICAM-1 induction during myocardial ischemia and reperfusion. This cellular and molecular control of the cytokine cascade responsible for ICAM-1 induction of the myocardium is discussed below.

Myocardial ICAM-1 Induction in the Ischemic Myocardium – An Introduction

After the discovery of the critical role of ICAM-1 on the cardiac cell, we began to examine its relevance in ischemia and reperfusion. Our experiments dem-onstrated that in cardiac lymph collected from an animal in which the cardiac lymph duct had been chronically cannulated [27] cytokine activity was present upon reperfusion of the ischemic myocardium. This cytokine activity was capable of inducing ICAM-1 formation in isolated cardiac myocytes, and sig-nificant cytokine activity persisted for 72 hours [28]. Subsequent experiments demonstrated that a neutralizing antibody to IL-6 completely inhibited ICAM-1 induction by cardiac lymph in cardiac myocytes [28]. However, induction by cardiac lymph of ICAM-1 in endothelial cells was not altered by neutralizing antibodies to IL-6, suggesting the presence of other cytokines within the post-ischemic cardiac lymph. The relationship between IL-6 and cardiac ICAM-1 induction was further supported by the observation that IL-6 is almost a thousand times as potent as other cytokines in the induction of cardiac myocyte ICAM-1 [28].

Subsequent experiments demonstrated the rapid induction of ICAM-1 in previously ischemic myocardium only and also found a close correlation be-tween the degree of ischemia and the amount of ICAM-1 mRNA present after between 1 and 3 h of reperfusion [29]. Utilizing in situ hybridization, we demonstrated that ICAM-1 induction occurred in viable myocytes on the border of the infarcted myocardium [30]. These latter studies also demon-strated that ICAM-1 induction did not occur in the ischemic myocardium unless reperfusion was instituted [30, 31]. Because of the observed relationship between IL-6 and ICAM-1 induction, similar studies were performed with molecular probes for IL-6. IL-6 induction appeared to precede that of ICAM-1, but within the first 3 h, it was present in the same ischemic segments [31]. Moreover, as observed with ICAM-1 induction, the induction of IL-6 was also reperfusion-dependent within the first 3 h [31]. However, at 24 h, IL-6 in-duction was seen in the previously ischemic myocardium even in the absence of reperfusion [31]. This led to the suggestion that early induction of IL-6 and ICAM-1 in the previously ischemic area upon reperfusion depended upon the influx of leukocytes into the ischemic myocardium and that the leukocytes were involved in this induction. Thus, in the presence of reperfusion, induction occurred almost immediately; without reperfusion, influx of leukocytes and appearance of ICAM-1 mRNA is delayed until 18–24 h. Our recent investigations of the reperfusion-dependent cytokine cascade that results in the induction of ICAM-1 on the viable ischemic myocardial cell are described below.

Methods

Ischemic Protocol

Healthy mongrel dogs (15–25 kg) of either sex were used in this study. Each animal was anesthetized with sodium pentobarbital (30 mg/kg), intubated, and ventilated with room air by a respirator. A midline thoracotomy provided access to the heart and mediastinum. Using techniques previously described, cannulation of the cardiac lymph duct was then performed. Briefly, injection of the wall of the left ventricle allowed lymphatic vessel definition. The largest vessel was selected and cannulated at a site proximal to the cardiac lymph node and 2–5 cm from the base of the heart. Accessory noncardiac lymphatic vessels and tracheobronchial lymphatic connections in this region were ligated. Subsequently, a hydraulically activated occluding device and a Doppler flow probe designed and fabricated by our laboratory were secured around the circumflex coronary artery just proximal or just distal to the first distal branch. The choice of location depended on the proximity and anatomical arrangement of lymphatic vessels adjacent to the coronary vessels so that subsequent dissection would not damage the lymphatic system. To prevent damage of lymphatic vessels in close proximity to the coronary vasculature, dissection of adipose tissue adjacent to the coronary vessel at two sequential 3–4 mm sections was carefully performed. Subsequently the occluding device and flow probe were placed. In animals selected for experimental assessments of cardiac lymph, intact lymphatic vessels draining the regions of ischemic myocardium were identified by injecting Evans blue (0.05 ml) into the free wall of the left ventricle after the occluder and flow probe were in place. The appearance of Evans blue in the cardiac lymph cannula confirmed the patency of the lymph vessel architecture. Cannulas were also placed in the right and left atria to allow blood sampling when needed.

The animal was allowed to recover for at least 72 h before occlusion. The protocol used in these studies involved a 1 h occlusion of the left circumflex coronary artery followed by reperfusion for up to 72 h. During occlusion and reperfusion, ischemia was verified by the Doppler probe and characteristic electrocardiograph changes detected with standard limb lead electrodes. Blood flow in the circumflex was continuously monitored with flow probes to assure occlusion and reperfusion. Lymph samples (1 ml) were collected from the cannula tubing in tubes containing 10 U heparin. The samples were spun in a table-top centrifuge at 13 000 g for 5 min. The supernatant was taken, aliquoted, frozen in liquid nitrogen, and stored at –70 °C until use. Once thawed, lymph samples were used immediately and never refrozen or stored thawed. Cell pellets were fixed in 10% buffered formalin and used for histological studies or for RNA isolation. After the reperfusion periods, the hearts were stopped by rapid intravenous infusion of 30 mEq of KCl and removed from the chest for sectioning from apex to base into four transverse rings 1 cm in thickness. The posterior papillary muscle and the posterior free wall were identified. Tissue samples were isolated from infarcted or normally perfused myocardium based on visual inspection. Myocardial segments were fixed in 10% buffered formalin, Carnoy's fixative or B*5 fixative for histological analysis and in situ hybridization studies. Duplicate samples were also processed for blood flow determinations using radiolabeled microspheres as previously described [19, 32]. Samples described as ischemic were all from areas where ischemic blood flow was less that 20%. Samples of control tissues were taken from the anterior septum and had normal blood flow during coronary occlusion.

The methods used for in situ hybridization were identical to those previously described for ICAM-1 [30]. The IL-6 probe was a digoxigenin labelled oligonucleotide prepared from the canine IL-6 sequence.

Immunostaining

Sequential sections (2–6 μm) were cut using an ultramicrotome and stained with toluidine blue or for tryptase using an enzymatic stain as described by Caughey [33]. Immunostaining for TNF-α was performed using the Elite ABC kit from Vector laboratories using a polyclonal anti human TNF-α antibody from Genzyme. Briefly, sections were deparaffinized and rehydrated through a series of graded alcohols. The sections were blocked with 1% normal goat serum in PBS for 30 min followed by incubation in primary antibody at a 1:500 dilution in PBS containing 1% goat serum. The sections were washed twice in PBS for 15 min and incubated for 30 min with a secondary antibody conjugated with peroxidase. Following washing in PBS the sections were stained using either diaminobenzidine (DAB) or 3-amino-9-ethyl-carbazole (AEC) as substrates to identify the peroxidase-conjugated secondary antibody. Hematoxylin and eosin staining followed immunostaining where indicated. Additional sections were stained with FITC-labeled avidin as described by Bergstresser [34] and visualized with a fluorescent microscope. In double fluorescent immunohistochemistry, TNF-α was examined using a rhodamine-conjugated secondary antibody and counterstaining with FITC-labeled avidin.

TNF-α Bioassay

Cardiac lymph samples were assayed for TNF-α activity using the WEHI 164 subclone 13 fibroblast cytotoxicity assay as previously described [35]. The WEHI 164 cells are very sensitive to the lytic effects of TNF, detecting as little as 2 pg/ml.

Results

IL-6 Production in the Reperfused Myocardium

cDNA corresponding to IL-6 mRNA was cloned and sequenced [31]. To identify the site of origin of IL-6 induction in the ischemic myocardium, we utilized an oligonucleotide probe and performed the in situ hybridization studies shown in Fig. 1A and 1B. These studies show that IL-6 mRNA was rapidly induced in infiltrating mononuclear cells in the previously ischemic reperfused segment after 3 h of reperfusion. Figure 1C shows immunohisto-chemical staining for IL-6 using an AEC-peroxidase detection system. Figure 1B shows the same cell after destaining and restaining with an antibody to CD64 using the DAB detection system. IL-6 production appears to occur primarily in monocytes. Similar studies done at 1 hour of reperfusion yielded the same results.

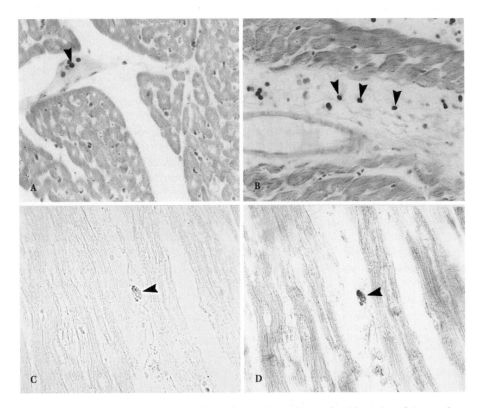

Fig. 1 A and **B** In situ hybridization with anti-sense IL-6 oligonucleotide probe of tissue taken following 1 h occlusion and 3 h reperfusion. **C** Immunostain for IL-6 on mononuclear cells with AEC-peroxidase detection system. **D** Same section as C destained and restained with Mab to CD64 using DAB detection system

As observed previously, the induction of IL-6 occurred only in the ischemic and reperfused myocardium, and our previous studies with cardiac lymph [28] suggested that IL-6 appeared in the first hour of reperfusion. This has led to our hypothesis that IL-6 induction in cardiac monocytes occurs as a result of a pre-existing "upstream" cytokine which the cell encounters in entering previously ischemic myocardium upon reperfusion. This hypothesis is strengthened by the observations described above regarding the presence of an additional cytokine in post-ischemic cardiac lymph which is capable of inducing endothelial ICAM-1 during the first hour of reperfusion [28]. Because we had ruled out the significance of IL-1 as an inducing cytokine in post-ischemic cardiac lymph [28], we decided to concentrate our efforts on the possible presence of a preformed pool of TNF-α.

The Cardiac Mast Cell as a Source of TNF-α

Mast cells occur in cardiac tissue and have been reported in the past to be a source of preformed cytokines [36, 37]. Examination of normal myocardial tissue revealed the presence of mast cells. Figure 2A shows a cardiac mast cell within the myocardium stained with toluidine blue. In Fig 2B the same mast cell is examined in a serial section 2 μm thick which has been stained with the enzymatic stain for tryptase activity typical of mast cells. In Fig 2C, the same mast cell has been stained with a polyclonal antibody to TNF-α with known cross-reactivity for canine TNF-α. Figure 2D shows an electron micrograph of a cardiac mast cell. No other cell in the normal myocardium is seen to contain such a significant amount of TNF-α. In additional studies, fluorescent immunohistochemistry was performed utilizing both FITC-avidin and antibodies against TNF-α. The former specifically stains heparin in mast cells and is used to identify them in tissue [34]. This experiment demonstrated that TNF-α immunoreactivity was confined exclusively to FITC-avidin-labeled cells (data not shown). Studies done by us and by others show that the distribution of cardiac mast cells appears to put them in a unique position for interacting with venular endothelial cells and infiltrating leukocytes; they are lined up along the outside of the small veins and venules which support leukocyte transendothelial migration.

Degranulation of Cardiac Mast Cells

In Fig. 3A, we show that TNF-α is released into the cardiac lymph within the first 30 minutes of reperfusion following a 1-h cardiac occlusion. The rapid appearance of TNF-α immediately upon reperfusion is similar to that observed for creatine kinase release from a reperfused myocardial infarct [38], suggesting that a source of preformed TNF-α was present; indeed, there would be insufficient time for de novo synthesis. As additional evidence of a mast cell origin, Fig. 3B shows that a similar time course of release into post-ischemic cardiac lymph is observed for TNF-α and histamine. This further suggests that

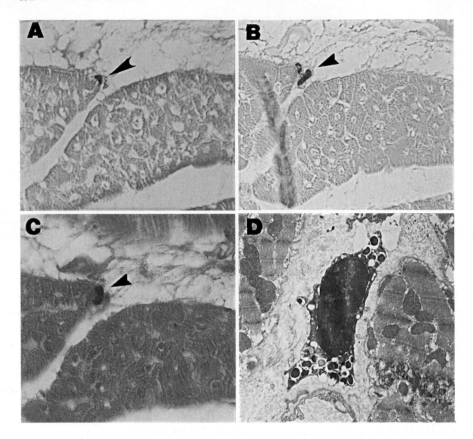

Fig. 2. Staining of normal canine cardiac tissue in 2 μm serial sections. **A** Stained with toluidine blue. **B** Stained for tryptase with an enzymatic stain. **C** TNF-α immunostaining. **D** Electron micrograph of a normal granulated cardiac mast cell

degranulation of cardiac mast cells has occurred. Figure 3C demonstrates a post-ischemic cardiac mast cell from the ischemic area; the presence of mast cell degranulation in the reperfused myocardium is clearly visible. No such degranulation was seen in control areas of myocardium from the stained heart (Fig. 3D).

Discussion

That an inflammatory response occurs within the myocardium following occlusion and reperfusion has been recognized for years. Strategies used in experimental animal models which limit the function of neutrophils have resulted in a decrease in infarct size and a salvage of viable myocardium [11]. We have previously demonstrated that leukocytes infiltrate the jeopardized zone very

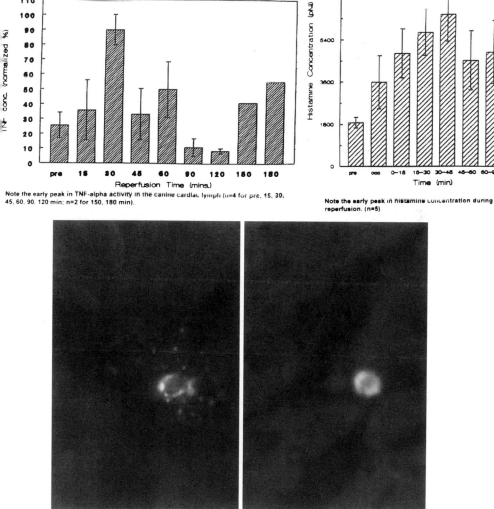

Fig. 3. A TNF-α activity in cardiac lymph collected before occlusion (*Pre*) or during reperfusion following 1 h of occlusion. **B** Histamine levels in cardiac lymph collected before occlusion (*Pre*) during occlusion (*Occ*) or during reperfusion. **C** Avidin-FITC staining of a degranulating mast cell from tissue taken from the occluded myocardium. **D** Avidin-FITC staining of a non-degranulating mast cell in a control septal segment in the same animal

early in reperfusion and that up-regulation of ICAM-1 occurs at the same time. Our in vitro studies have shown that the up-regulation of ICAM-1 on myocytes is necessary for adhesion of neutrophils and that the neutrophils can cause myocardial cell death following adhesion [39]. We have also obtained results which show that both the ICAM-1 and IL-6 up-regulation appear early in reperfusion and are dependent on reperfusion of the occluded myocardium [29, 30, 40]. Our demonstration here of IL-6 production by the infiltrating monocyte in early reperfusion is in accordance with these previous results. The exquisite sensitivity of the myocyte to IL-6 which results in ICAM-1 up-regulation is also in accordance with results previously published [28]. Although in vitro studies have shown that many cells, including endothelial cells, are capable of IL-6 production, our studies indicate that it is the mononuclear cells (primarily monocytes) which produce IL-6 in the first few hours of reperfusion, indicating that other regulatory mechanisms probably exist which cause a cell specific up-regulation of IL-6. Thus, it seems likely that margination and up-regulation of monocytes following occlusion and reperfusion is a necessary step for ICAM-1 up-regulation in the viable myocytes found in a border zone surrounding the necrotic region. The up-regulation of ICAM-1 may then support neutrophil adhesion and subsequent death of the myocardial cell thus extending the infarcted region to otherwise salvageable tissue.

Lymph from the ischemic myocardium also induces ICAM-1 formation in the endothelium by a mechanism which is not related to the presence of IL-6. We have previously demonstrated the presence of excess IL-1 inhibitor in cardiac lymph which precludes IL-1 as the inducer of endothelial cell ICAM-1 [28]. We postulated that TNF-α was a likely source of cytokine activity with has been shown in vitro to be capable of up-regulating endothelial cell ICAM-1 [28]. The very early induction of IL-6 from monocytes also suggested the presence of another cytokine that was preformed and, potentially, released even before reperfusion.

Previously we found that both C5a and thromboxane B2 are present in the cardiac lymph [17, 14]. Ito et al. demonstrated in the pig heart that when exposed to C5a, cardiac mast cells were rapidly degranulated and released histamine and thromboxane B2 [42]. This suggested to us that the degranulation of cardiac mast cells may be occurring and that they may play a critical role in reperfusion injury. There were also data in the literature suggesting that preformed cytokines including TNF-α are present in various mast cell populations [36, 37]. Therefore, we examined the role of the cardiac mast cell and specifically the presence and release of TNF-α in response to myocardial ischemia/reperfusion. This is the first study to demonstrate the presence of preformed TNF-α in the myocardium localized in resident cardiac mast cells and its rapid release during myocardial ischemia and reperfusion. We have presented evidence for mast cell degranulation and the release of TNF-α and histamine following reperfusion of the previously ischemic heart.

We propose the following model (Fig. 4) for the cytokine cascade leading to post reperfusion inflammatory injury of the myocardium. C5a, reactive oxygen, or adenosine, generated during occlusion, stimulate degranulation of the cardiac mast cell before or upon reperfusion. Histamine and TNF-α are released

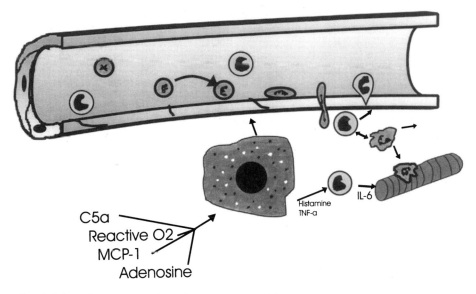

Fig. 4. Schematic representation of events suggested by current data. See text for details

from granular stores and are instrumental in the induction of infiltrating mononuclear cells to produce IL-6. IL-6 acts as a stimulus for ICAM-1 production by the myocyte, rendering them susceptible to neutrophil adhesion and neutrophil-mediated cytotoxicity. This cytotoxic effect extends the necrotic zone and increases infarct size.

Acknowledgement. This work was supported in part by NIH grants HL-42250, ES 06091, and AI 19031.

References

1. Mallory GK, White PD, Salcedo-Salgar J (1939) The speed of healing of myocardial infarction. A study of the pathologic anatomy in seventy-two cases. Am Heart J 18: 647–671
2. Hirayama A, Adachi T, Asada S, Mishima M, Nanto S, Kusuoka H, Yamamoto K, Matsumura Y, Hori M, Inoue M, Kodama K (1993) Late reperfusion for acute myocardial infarction limits the dilatation of left ventricle without the reduction of infarct size. Circulation 88: 2565–2574
3. Morita M, Kawashima S, Ueno M, Kubota A, Iwasaki T (1993) Effects of late reperfusion on infarct expansion and infarct healing in conscious rats. Am J Pathol 143: 419–430
4. Roberts R, DeMello V, Sobel BE (1976) Deleterious effects of methylprednisolone in patients with myocardial infarction. Circulation 53 (Suppl I): 204–206
5. Hammerman H, Kloner RA, Hale S, Schoen FJ, Braunwald E (1983) Dose-dependent effects of short-term methylprednisolone on myocardial infarct extent, scar formation, and ventricular function. Circulation 68: 446–452

6. Romson JL, Hook BG, Kunkel SL, Abrams GD, Schork MA, Lucchesi BR (1983) Reduction of the extent of ischemic myocardial injury by neutrophil depletion in the dog. Circulation 67: 1016–1023

7. Mullane KM, Read N, Salmon JA, Moncada S (1984) Role of leukocytes in acute myocardial infarction in anesthesthized dogs. Relationship to myocardial salvage by anti-inflammatory drugs. J Pharmacol Exp Ther 228: 510–522

8. Engler RL, Dahlgren MD, Morris DD, Peterson MA, Schmid-Schonbein GW (1986) Role of leukocytes in response to acute myocardial ischemia and reflow in dogs. Am J Physiol 251: H314–323

9. Simpson PJ, Todd III, Fantone JC, Mickelson JK, Griffin JD, Lucchesi BR (1988) Reduction of experimental canine myocardial reperfusion injury by a monoclonal antibody (anti-Mol, anti-CD11b) that inhibits leukocyte adhesion. J Clin Invest 81: 624–629

10. Williams FM, Collins PD, Nourshargh S, Williams TJ (1988) Suppression of 111In-neutrophil accumulation in rabbit myocardium by MoA ischemic injury. J Mol Cell Cardiol 20: S33

11. Lefer DJ, Suresh ML, Shandelya ML, Serrano CV, Becker LC, Kuppusamy P, Zweier JL (1993) Cardioprotective actions of a monoclonal antibody against CD-18 in myocardial ischemia-reperfusion injury. Circulation 88: 1779–1787

12. Ma X-L, Weyrich AS, Lefer DJ, Buerke M, Albertine KH, Kishimoto TK, Lefer AM (1993) Monoclonal antibody to L-selectin attenuates neutrophil accumulation and protects ischemic reperfused cat myocardium. Circulation 88: 649–658

13. Weyrich AS, Ma X-L, Lefer DJ, Albertine KH, Lefer AM (1993) In vivo neutralization of P-selectin protects feline heart and endothelium in myocardial ischemia and reperfusion injury. J Clin Invest 91: 2620–2629

14. Ma XL, Lefer DJ, Lefer AM, Rothlein R (1992) Coronary endothelial and cardiac protective effects of a monoclonal antibody to intercellular adhesion molecule-1 in myocardial ischemia and reperfusion. Circulation 86: 937–946

15. Hill JH, Ward PA (1971) The phlogistic role of C3 leukotactic fragment in myocardial infarcts of rats. J Exp Med 133: 885–900

16. Dreyer WJ, Michael LH, Nguyen T, Smith CW, Anderson DC, Entman ML, Rossen RD (1992) Kinetics of C5a release in cardiac lymph of dogs experiencing coronary artery ischemia-reperfusion injury. Circ Res 71: 1518–1524

17. Dreyer WJ, Michael LH, Rossen RD, Nguyen T, Anderson DC, Smith CW, Entman ML (1991) Evidence for C5a in post-ischemic canine cardiac lymph. Clin Res 39: 271A (Abstract)

18. Rossen RD, Michael LH, Hawkins HK, Youker K, Dreyer WJ, Baughn RE, Entman ML (1994) Cardiolipin–protein complexes and initiation of complement activation after coronary artery occlusion. Circ Res 75: 546-555

19. Dreyer WJ, Michael LH, West MS, Smith CW, Rothlein R, Rossen RD, Anderson DC, Entman ML (1991) Neutrophil accumulation in ischemic canine myocardium: Insights into the time course, distribution, and mechanism of localization during early reperfusion. Circulation 84: 400–411

20. Abbassi O, Kishimoto TK, McIntire LV, Anderson DC, Smith CW (1993) E-Selectin supports neutrophil rolling in vitro under conditions of flow. J Clin Invest 92: 2719-2730

21. Dore M, Korthuis RJ, Granger DN, Entman ML, Smith CW (1993) P-selectin mediates spontaneous leukocyte rolling in vivo. Blood 82: 1308–1316

22. Smith CW, Marlin SD, Rothlein R, Toman C, Anderson DC (1989) Cooperative interactions of LFA-1 and Mac-1 with intercellular adhesion molecule-1 in facilitating adherence and transendothelial migration of human neutrophils in vitro. J Clin Invest 83: 2008–2017

23. Smith CW, Anderson DC, Taylor AA, Rossen RD, Entman ML (1991) Leukocyte adhesion molecules and myocardial ischemia. Trends Cardiovasc Med 1: 167–170

24. Dore M, Simon SI, Hughes BJ, Entman ML, Smith CW (1995) P-selectin- and CD18-mediated recruitment of canine neutrophils under conditions of shear stress. Vet Pathol 32: 258–268

25. Smith CW, Entman ML, Lane CL, Beaudet AL, Ty TI, Youker KA, Hawkins HK, Anderson DC (1991) Adherence of neutrophils to canine cardiac myocytes in vitro is dependent on intercellular adhesion molecule-1. J Clin Invest 88: 1216–1223

26. Entman ML, Youker KA, Shappell SB, Siegel C, Rothlein R, Dreyer WJ, Schmalstieg FC, Smith CW (1990) Neutrophil adherence to isolated adult canine myocytes: Evidence for a CD18-dependent mechanism. J Clin Invest 85: 1497–1506
27. Dreyer WJ, Smith CW, Michael LH, Rossen RD, Hughes BJ, Entman ML, Anderson DC (1989) Canine neutrophil activation by cardiac lymph obtained during reperfusion of ischemic myocardium. Circ Res 65: 1751–1762
28. Youker KA, Smith CW, Anderson DC, Miller D, Michael LH, Rossen RD, Entman ML (1992) Neutrophil adherence to isolated adult cardiac myocytes. Induction by cardiac lymph collected during ischemia and reperfusion. J Clin Invest 89: 602–609
29. Kukielka GL, Hawkins HK, Michael LH, Manning AM, Lane CL, Entman ML, Smith CW, Anderson DC (1993) Regulation of intercellular adhesion molecule-1 (ICAM-1) in ischemic and reperfused canine myocardium. J Clin Invest 92: 1504–1516
30. Youker KA, Hawkins HK, Kukielka GL, Perrard JL, Michael LH, Ballantyne CM, Smith CW, Entman ML (1994) Molecular evidence for induction of intercellular adhesion molecule-1 in the viable border zone associated with ischemia-reperfusion injury of the dog heart. Circulation 89: 2736–2746
31. Kukielka GL, Youker KA, Hawkins HK, Perrard JL, Michael LH, Ballantyne CM, Smith CW, Entman ML (1994) Regulation of ICAM-1 and IL-6 in myocardial ischemia: Effect of reperfusion. Ann N Y Acad Sci 723: 258–270
32. Heymann MA, Payne BD, Hoffman JIE, Rudolph AM (1977) Blood flow measurements with radionucleotide-labeled particles. Prog Cardiovasc Dis XX: 55–78
33. Caughey GH, Viro NF, Calonico LD, McDonald DM, Lazarus SC, Gold WM (1988) Chymase and tryptase in dog mastocytoma cells: asynchronous expression as revealed by enzyme cytochemical staining. J Histochem Cytochem 36: 1053–1060
34. Bergstresser PR, Tigelaar RE, Tharp MD (1984) Conjugated avidin identifies cutaneous rodent and human mast cells. J Invest Dermatol 83: 214–218
35. Ignatowshi TA, Spengler RN (1994) Tumor necrosis factor-alpha: presynaptic sensitivity is modified after antidepressant drug administration. Brain Res 665: 293–299
36. Gordon JR, Galli SJ (1990) Mast cells as a source of both preformed and immunologically inducible TNF-alpha/cachectin. Nature 346: 274–276
37. Walsh LJ, Trinchieri G, Waldorf HA, Whitaker D, Murphy GF (1991) Human dermal mast cells contain and release tumor necrosis factor alpha, which induces endothelial leukocyte adhesion molecule 1. Proc Natl Acad Sci USA 88: 4220–4224
38. Michael LH, Hunt JR, Weilbaecher D, Perryman MB, Roberts R, Lewis RM, Entman ML (1985) Creatine kinase and phosphorylase in cardiac lymph: Coronary occlusion and reperfusion. Am J Physiol 248: H350–H359
39. Entman ML, Youker KA, Shoji T, Kukielka GL, Shappell SB, Taylor AA, Smith CW (1992) Neutrophil induced oxidative injury of cardiac myocytes: A compartmented system requiring CD11b /CD18-ICAM-1 adherence. J Clin Invest 90: 1335–1345
40. Kukielka GL, Youker KA, Michael LH, Kumar AG, Ballantyne CM, Smith CW, Entman ML (1995) Role of early reperfusion in the induction of adhesion molecules and cytokines in previously ischemic myocardium. Mol Cell Biochem 147: 5–12
41. Michael LH, Zhang Z, Hartley CJ, Bolli R, Taylor AA, Entman ML (1990) Thromboxane B2 in cardiac lymph: effect of superoxide dismutase and catalase during myocardial ischemia and reperfusion. Circ Res 66: 1040–1044
42. Ito BR, Engler RL, Del Balzo U (1993) Role of cardiac mast cells in complement C5a-induced myocardial ischemia. Am J Physiol 264: H1346–H1354

Molecular Mechanisms of Adhesion of *Staphylococcus aureus* to Cardiac Surfaces and Vegetations

C.M. Johnson

Introduction

The initial event in many infectious processes is the attachment of the invading micro-organism to the host tissues. The ability of a particular micro-organism to adhere to host tissues is an important attribute determining its pathogenicity relative to other strains of bacteria. The organ specificity of many infectious processes suggests that there often exists a special propensity for particular organisms to interact with and adhere to selected host cells. There are many examples that serve to illustrate this viewpoint: for example, group A streptococci possess special cell-surface determinants, or adhesions, which mediate attachment of the bacteria to oral epithelial cells [1]; enterotoxigenic strains of *Escherichia coli* possess adhesions that bind to specific receptors found on the surfaces of intestinal epithelial cells [2]; whereas *E. coli* strains that are associated with urinary tract infections possess adhesions that bind to uroepithelial cells [3]. These and many similar observations suggest that the pathophysiological basis for the relative organ specificity exhibited by many clinical infections may result from specific binding interactions between adhesions on the surface of the micro-organism and receptors on the host cell-surface.

Infective endocarditis, an endovascular infection involving the cardiac valves, endocardial surface, or intra-cardiac prosthetic material, is a particularly intriguing example of the potential usefulness of such a paradigm in understanding the early events in microbial invasion. Infective endocarditis is caused by a fairly restricted group of bacteria, primarily oral streptococci, enterococci, and staphylococci [4]. The pathogenesis of endocarditis is generally presumed to begin with colonization of cardiac tissues by bacteria that gain access to the circulation during brief bacteremias. In most instances, such colonization appears to occur initially in regions of the heart that have previously been rendered abnormal by mechanical or immunological damage, as occurs following such events as cardiac surgery or rheumatic carditis. Previous damage may leave deposits of activated platelets and fibrin on the cardiac surface, a lesion termed non-bacterial thrombotic endocarditis. Abundant experimental work, both in animal model systems [5–8] and in vitro [9–11] has

Section of Critical Care, Department of Pediatric and Adolescent Medicine,
Mayo Clinic and Mayo Foundation, Rochester, MN 55905, USA

shown that bacterial strains that are often associated with endocarditis exhibit a particular propensity to bind to platelets and fibrin. There are limited observations in humans that support this viewpoint [12]. It remains unknown, however, which of the multiple possible adherence events – bacteria to platelets, bacteria to cardiac cells, bacteria to fibrin – are key to the initial pathogenesis of infection. The inherently complicated nature of most experimental endocarditis model systems makes it difficult to study potentially important binding events in isolation.

Staphylococcal infective endocarditis, particularly when caused by *Staphylococcus aureus*, may differ in its pathogenesis from infection caused by other organisms, at least in regard to the initial adherence events discussed above. It has long been appreciated clinically that endocarditis typically occurs in patients whose cardiac anatomy is abnormal as a result of congenital or acquired heart disease. This may reflect a tendency for previous cardiac injury to induce the platelet and fibrin deposits that may favor subsequent bacterial attachment. Endocarditis caused by *S. aureus*, however, often occurs in patients who have no previous history of cardiac disease [13]. In such instances the key adherence events may be between the bacteria and the endothelial cells covering the cardiac valve. We have chosen to study the pathogenesis of *S. aureus* cardiac infection, in part because of this potential for reducing the number of potential adherence events in a complicated biological system, but also because endocarditis caused by this organism is emerging as a common clinical entity. Among children, for example, *S. aureus* endocarditis has become the most common form of the infection [14]. We have selected a porcine experimental model system for our investigations because pigs naturally contract a form of endocarditis that clinically mimics the human disease [15]. We have established a porcine clinical model for infective endocarditis that offers the opportunity for testing in vivo the relevance of any observations made on in vitro cell culture systems [16].

Cell Culture and Bacterial Binding Assay

We have previously described in detail our technique for isolation of endothelial cells derived from porcine vascular sites, including the aortic valve [17]. Following collagenase digestion of the tissue, the primary cell suspensions are inoculated into 96-well plates at limiting dilution. This results in wells containing cell populations derived from a single initial endothelial cell growth focus. Such wells are then expanded to produce pure cell lines of cardiac valve endothelial cells, which are then frozen at third passage in liquid nitrogen for use in later experiments. The strains of *S. aureus* used in these experiments were first isolated from clinical cases of infective endocarditis and had been kept frozen in aliquots. Before use an aliquot of bacteria is grown overnight to late stationary phase in L-broth.

We have also previously described in detail our method for establishing binding assays between cardiac endothelial cells and bacteria [18]. The endothelial cells are grown to confluence in 12-well plates, following which they are briefly fixed with dilute formalin. The bacteria are endogenously labeled with [35][S] methionine. They are washed, suspended in assay buffer, and added to the wells containing the endothelial cells. The bacteria are allowed to bind to the endothelial cells both in the presence and absence of an excess of unlabeled bacteria. Binding that occurs in the presence of excess unlabeled organisms is deemed non-specific and is subtracted from total binding values. Specific binding is defined as the total binding value with non-specific binding subtracted; specific binding is normalized to allow comparisons between different assays by expressing the number of colony forming units of *S. aureus* bound per endothelial cell. This assay demonstrates attributes highly suggestive of receptor-mediated interactions [19], in that it is saturable with respect to bacterial concentration (Fig. 1) and incubation time (Fig. 2). Having established this observation, we next endeavored to identify and isolate the putative endothelial cell-surface receptor. If successful, this approach offers the possibility of inhibiting the binding interaction in clinically useful ways.

Identification of Endothelial Receptor for *S. aureus*

We first evaluated ways of extracting the receptor from endothelial membranes. We determined that a detergent digest (1% CHAPS) of cultured en-

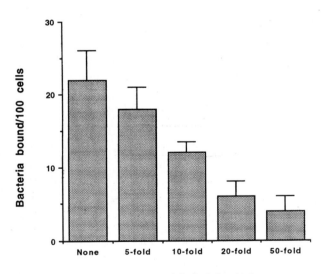

Fig. 1. Competitive binding assay. Radiolabeled *S. aureus* were allowed to compete in a binding assay with unlabeled bacteria as described in the text and in [18]. The number of bacteria bound specifically per 100 porcine aortic valve endothelial cells is indicated *on the y-axis*; the relative quantity of excess unlabeled bacteria is indicated *on the x-axis*. Values are expressed as mean ± standard error for triplicate assay wells. It can be seen that this assay system exhibits competition for binding between labeled and unlabeled bacteria

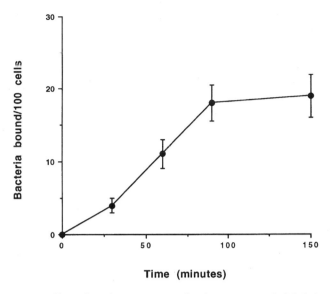

Fig. 2. Effect of incubation time on binding assay. Radiolabeled *S. aureus* were added to the binding wells as described in the text and in [18]. Triplicate wells were digested at serial times, as indicated *on the x-axis*. Specific bacterial binding per 100 endothelial cells is indicated *on the y-axis* as the mean ± standard error of triplicate assay wells. It can be seen that the assay system reached a steady state at approximately 90 minutes of incubation, indicating saturability with respect to time

dothelial cells significantly inhibited specific binding of *S. aureus* to the endothelial cell monolayers. This indicated that a putative cellular receptor for the bacteria could be extracted from the endothelial cells in active form. The extracellular matrix remaining following detergent extraction of the cells also exhibited specific binding to *S. aureus*, although this accounted for only 20% of the specific binding to intact endothelial monolayers. We next reasoned that, since many cell-surface receptors are glycoproteins, one or more lectins could modify specific bacterial binding by competing with *S. aureus* for the receptor. Our results showed that concanavalin A exhibited such inhibition by blocking approximately 50% of specific bacterial binding. This observation suggested that there were at least two forms of receptors mediating specific binding, one of which was a mannose containing glycoprotein. It also suggested that lectin affinity chromatography might allow partial purification of one of these endothelial receptors for *S. aureus*. Accordingly, we passed detergent extracts of endothelial cells through an affinity resin consisting of concanavalin A linked to 4% agarose. The resin was eluted with methyl α-D-mannopyranoside, the carbohydrate ligand for concanavalin A. The resulting fractions, consisting of the starting stock detergent extract, material flowing through the column without binding to the affinity resin, and eluate from the resin, were then tested for their ability to inhibit specific bacterial binding. As can be seen in Fig. 3, this technique appeared to accomplish partial purification of one of the species of endothelial receptor for *S. aureus*.

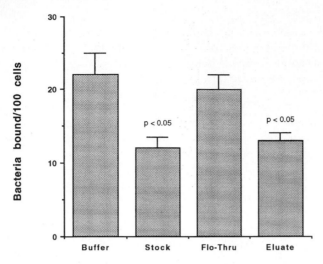

Fig. 3. Effect of partially purified receptor on *S. aureus* binding to aortic valve endothelial cells. Affinity chromatography of endothelial cell extract over concanavalin A-agarose was carried out as described in the text and in [18]. Binding of *S. aureus* to endothelial cells was then measured in the presence of various fractions from the affinity resin. The number of bacteria bound per 100 cells is indicated *on the y-axis*. The effects of the various column fractions on specific binding are noted *on the x-axis*: *buffer*, control conditions; *stock*, endothelial extract before chromatography; *flo-thru*, material flowing through the column without binding; *eluate*, material eluted by the mannose analog. It can be seen that the eluate from the lectin column contained virtually all of the receptor activity identified in the starting endothelial cell extract. Results are expressed as mean ± standard error of triplicate assay wells, with statistically significant reductions in binding noted

We next attempted to identify the receptor by using a technique of selective radiolabeling of cell-surface proteins. We have previously described in detail the application of this technique to the surface-labeling of endothelial cell proteins [20]. In brief, the intact endothelial cells were radiolabeled with ^{125}[I] using the glucose oxidase/lactoperoxidase method under mild conditions. This technique confines the labeling reaction to those proteins on the apical surface of the cells that present an available tyrosine residue. The radiolabeled cells were then extracted in detergent and the labeled cell extract subjected to concanavalin A affinity chromatography as described above. The resulting fractions were then analyzed by fluoroautoradiography after separation by sodium dodecyl sulfate polyacrylamide electrophoresis on 10% gels. This technique successfully identified a single protein migrating at an approximate apparent mass of 130 kD [18].

Conclusions and Future Directions

The pathogenesis of endovascular infections, particularly infective endocarditis, provides an example of the importance of adherence events between micro-organisms and host tissues. It appears that the unusual propensity of certain bacteria, particularly gram positive cocci, to cause endocarditis is linked to their ability to bind with high affinity to fibrin and to cellular determinants on cardiac cells and platelets. We have shown that aortic valve endothelial cells express on their apical surface a 130 kD glycoprotein that exhibits properties expected for a specific receptor.

The morbidity and mortality of infective endocarditis caused by *S. aureus* is high in spite of appropriate antibiotic therapy; thus additional therapeutic modalities could prove useful in treating this infection. We have directed our efforts at identifying determinants on cardiac tissues that could serve as bacterial receptors because we believe that this approach offers the possibility of therapies aimed at blocking bacterial binding. We are presently endeavoring to use molecular cloning techniques to identify the 130 kD putative receptor as a first step in this line of investigations.

References

1. Gibbons RJ, van Houte J (1971) Selective bacterial adherence to oral epithelial surfaces and its role as an ecological determinant. Infect Immun 3: 367–373
2. Evans DG, Evans DJ (1978) New surface-associated heat-labile colonization factor antigen (CFA/II) produced by enterotoxigenic *Escherichia coli* of serogroups 06 and 08. Infect Immun 21: 638–647
3. Kallenius G, Mollby R, Winberg J (1980) In vitro adhesion of uropathogenic *Escherichia coli* to human periurethral cells. Infect Immun 28: 972 980
4. Durack DT (1986) Infective and noninfective endocarditis. In: Hurst JW (ed) The heart. McGraw Hill, New York, p 1130
5. Garrison PK, Freedman LR (1970) Experimental endocarditis. I. Staphylococcal endocarditis in rabbits resulting from placement of a polyethylene catheter in the right side of the heart. Yale J Biol Med 42: 394–410
6. Perlman BB, Freedman LR (1971) Experimental endocarditis. II. Staphylococcal infection of the aortic valve following placement of a polyethylene catheter in the left side of the heart. Yale J Biol Med 44: 206–213
7. Durack DT, Beeson PB (1972) Experimental endocarditis. I. Colonization of a sterile vegetation. Br J Exp Pathol 53: 44–49
8. Durack DT, Beeson PB, Petersdorf RG (1973) Experimental endocarditis. III. Production and progress of the disease in rabbits. Br J Exp Pathol 54: 142–151
9. Clawson CC, White JG (1971) Platelet interactions with bacteria. I. Reaction phases and effects of inhibitors. Am J Pathol 65: 367–380
10. Hook EW, Sande MA (1974) Role of the vegetation in experimental *Streptococcus viridians* endocarditis. Infect Immun 10: 1433–1438
11. Scheld WM, Valone JA, Sande MA (1978) Bacterial adherence in the pathogenesis of endocarditis. Interaction of bacterial dextran, platelets, and fibrin. J Clin Invest 61: 1394–1404
12. Angrist A, Oka M, Nakao K (1967) Vegetative endocarditis. Pathol Annu 2: 155–212
13. Thompson RL (1982) Staphylococcal infective endocarditis. Mayo Clin Proc 57: 106–114
14. Johnson CM, Rhodes KH (1982) Pediatric endocarditis. Mayo Clin Proc 57: 86–94
15. Jones JET (1980) Bacterial endocarditis in the pig with special reference to streptococcal endocarditis. J Comp Pathol 90: 11–28
16. Johnson CM, Bahn RC, Fass DN (1986) Experimental porcine infective endocarditis: description of a clinical model. Vet Pathol 23: 780–782
17. Johnson CM, Fass DN (1983) Porcine cardiac valve endothelial cells in culture: a relative deficiency of fibronectin synthesis in vitro. Lab Invest 49: 589–598

18. Johnson CM (1993) *Staphylococcus aureus* binding to cardiac endothelial cells is partly mediated by a 130 kilodalton glycoprotein. J Lab Clin Med 121: 675– 682
19. Johnson CM, Hancock GA, Goulin GD (1988) Specific binding of *Staphylococcus aureus* to cultured porcine cardiac valvular endothelial cells. J Lab Clin Med 112: 16–22
20. Campbell KM, Johnson CM (1990) Identification of *Staphylococcus aureus* binding proteins on isolated porcine cardiac valve cells. J Lab Clin Med 115: 217–223

Endotoxins as Potential Mediators of Myocardial Depression

U. Müller-Werdan[1], R. Witthaut[2], and K. Werdan[2]

Endotoxins: The Molecules

Among the numerous toxins from germs pathogenic in humans, the endotoxin of gram-negative bacteria is of foremost importance in sepsis and septic shock. It is a central trigger which substantially contributes to the impairment of cardiovascular function in sepsis and septic shock, frequently resulting in vasodilatation and myocardial depression refractory to therapy.

Endotoxin is a lipopolysaccharide (LPS) localized in the outer cell membrane of gram-negative bacteria. The molecule consists of a uniform lipid component, lipid A, anchored in the cell membrane, a carbohydrate chain with an outer and inner core oligosaccharide integrated in the cell membrane, and a variable O-specific chain of sugars, protruding from the cell membrane like a hair (Loppnow et al. 1993; Schumann and Rietschel 1995). Endotoxin either reaches the blood by decay of intravasal bacteria – which to some extent may also be caused by the administration of antibiotics – or by translocation of bacteria and endotoxin from the primary site of infection or from the gut into the blood stream. It may be detectable in the peripheral blood as soon as the clearance capacity of the reticulo-endothelial system for endotoxin is exhausted ("spillover"). Thus, in patients with gram-negative septic shock, endotoxin plasma levels may reach 10–200 pg/ml.

Once systemic endotoxemia prevails, the following diverse reactions are prompted by endotoxins: (a) the pyrogenic reaction; (b) the stimulation of a humoral response; (c) the activation of the coagulation, complement and kallikrein-kinin systems, and (d) the release of various products into the interstitial tissue (biogenic amines, proteases, peptides, and eicosanoids), partly mediated by the cytokines tumor necrosis factor-α (TNF-α) and interleukins 1, 6 and 8 (IL-1, -6, -8; Loppnow et al. 1993; Schumann and Rietschel 1995).

Endotoxin unequivocally is one of the factors determining the poor prognosis of gram-negative shock. However, it must not be forgotten that endotoxin in low concentrations via a moderate mediator release may actually be beneficial for defence against infections.

[1]Martin-Luther-Universität Halle-Wittenberg, Klinikum Kröllwitz, Klinik für Innere Medizin III, Ernst-Grube-Str. 40, 06097 Halle/Saale, Germany
[2]Martin-Luther-Universität Halle-Wittenberg, Klinikum Kröllwitz, Lehrstuhl für Kardiologische Intensiv medizin an der Klinik für Innere Medizin III, Ernst-Grube-Str. 40, 06097 Halle/Saale, Germany

Endotoxin Receptors

Endotoxin effects are brought about by specific, receptor-mediated binding of the molecule to target cells (Schumann and Rietschel 1995) prompting cell-specific protein expression. The circulating endotoxin molecules first combines with LPS binding proteins (LBPs) circulating in the blood. This LPS–LBP complex binds to endotoxin receptors on monocytes/macrophages, which consist of the CD14 molecule and an additional receptor component not yet fully characterized. If the target cell lacks a membrane-based CD14 molecule, the circulating LPS–LBP complex can only attach to the target cell, e.g. an endothelial cell, after combining with a soluble CD14 molecule present in the circulation. Endotoxin-receptor binding in monocytes/macrophages is followed by an induction of cytokine expression and the release of TNF-α and interleukin-1β. In endothelial cells the expression of adhesion molecules is triggered; these adhesion molecules are required for the attachment of blood cells to the endothelium.

In muscle cells endotoxin may trigger specific receptor-mediated effects. Only in the case of smooth muscle cells, the endotoxin–receptor interaction has been revealed (Loppnow et al. 1995). These cells are devoid of a cell-membrane-bound LPS receptor; LPS binds to smooth muscle cells after combining with a soluble CD14 molecule, which results in the cellular production of cytokines (Loppnow et al. 1995). Endotoxin produces specific effects also in heart muscle cells; however, the receptor mechanism involved has not yet been identified.

Septic Cardiomyopathy

In gram-negative and in gram-positive sepsis and septic shock, characteristic cardiovascular changes are induced. A fall in blood pressure occurs due to an extensive vasodilatation with lowering of the systemic vascular resistance down to 30% of the normal level. To a certain degree, blood pressure can be kept within physiological ranges by an increase in cardiac output. However, a full compensation – a two- to threefold rise in cardiac output – is only rarely observed in patients with septic shock. The rather inadequate rise in pressure is explained by the reversible, multifactorial septic cardiomyopathy, characterized by a dilatation of both ventricles, reduced ejection fractions, and global as well as regional, systolic pump and diastolic relaxation failure. Surprisingly there is an increase in ventricular compliance which is responsible for the pathological expansion in heart size after volume substitution. Finally, coronary arteries are dilated and coronary blood flow is high (for a review see Müller-Werdan et al. 1996).

The mechanisms underlying septic cardiomyopathy are manifold, including the cardiodepressive effects of excess catecholamines, bacterial toxins, sepsis mediators, and cardiodepressant factors (for a review see Müller-Werdan et al. 1996).

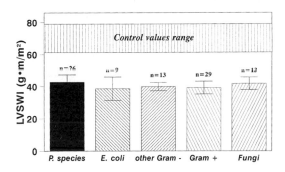

Fig. 1. Decreased left ventricular stroke work indices (LVSWI) in various forms of gram-negative, gram-positive, and fungal sepsis. *P.*, *Pseudomonas*. Adapted from Pilz et al., 1994

Many experimental and clinical findings (see below) support the view that endotoxin plays a very prominent role in this myocardial depression in sepsis, but it is certainly not the only trigger substance. Patients with various forms of gram-negative (*Pseudomonas, Escherichia coli,* and other gram-negative bacteria), gram-positive, and fungal sepsis suffer from similar degrees of septic cardiomyopathy, as measured by a reduction in left ventricular stroke work index (Fig. 1; Pilz et al. 1994). Furthermore, infectious agent-specific differences cannot be discerned for some sepsis subgroups, e.g., septic patients with or without culture-proven bacteremia, with or without septic shock and also with or without pre-existing cardiovascular disease (Pilz et al. 1994).

Considering these results, one may hypothesize that not the specific virulence factors, but rather the mediators of the common final pathway determine the occurrence and severity of septic cardiomyopathy. In the case of endotoxin, not only should the direct effects of this toxin be taken into account; at least as important is the fact that endotoxin may also trigger a cascade of mediators leading finally to cardiodepression (see below).

Cardiovascular Effects of Endotoxin in Man

Bacterial endotoxin is believed to be one of the principal mediators of cardiovascular dysfunction in human septic shock. In healthy human beings, an intravenous bolus dose of *E. coli* endotoxin (4 ng/kg of body weight) mimics within hours the cardiac impairment seen in septic shock: an increase in volume indices, a decrease in ejection fraction, and a depression of performance (ratio of peak systolic pressure to the end-systolic volume index) of the left ventricle (Suffredini et al. 1989). Since endotoxin injection in man induces a well-documented rise in serum levels of TNF-α (Michie et al. 1988; Martich et al. 1993), the myocardial depression induced by endotoxin might be mediated by this cytokine, the cardiodepressive effect of which is well known (Fig. 2; see also below; for a review see Müller-Werdan et al. 1996).

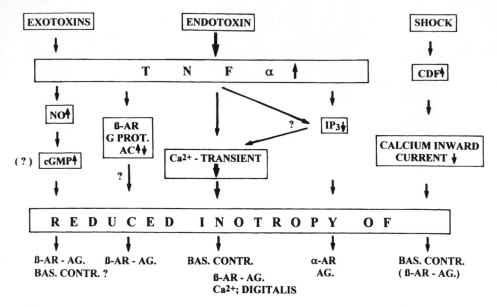

Fig. 2. Cardiodepression in sepsis: the "most proven concepts" in perspective. *NO*, nitric oxide; *cGMP*, cyclic guanosine monophosphate; *G Prot.*, G protein; *AC*, adenylyl cyclase; *AR-AG.*, adrenoceptor agonist; *IP₃*, inositol triphosphate; *CDF*, cardiodepressant factor; *BAS. CONTR.*, basal contractility; *TNFα*, tumor necrosis factor alpha. From Müller-Werdan et al., 1996

Cardiovascular Effects of Endotoxin: Animal Studies and Cardiomyocytes from Endotoxin-Treated Animals

The cardiodepressive effect of endotoxin has been documented in a number of experimental settings (for review see Hinshaw 1985; Abel 1989; Müller-Werdan et al. 1996). Endotoxin injection in dogs clearly impairs cardiac function, with the maximum reduction in ejection fraction occurring 48 h after endotoxin clot implantation (Natanson et al. 1989).

In endotoxin-treated rabbits, both hearts in vivo and cardiomyocytes (CMs) ex vivo-in vitro exhibit depressed contractility (Hung and Lew 1993; Brady et al. 1992). Moreover, endotoxin results in a shortening of the action potential of the CMs, an impaired sarcoplasmic reticulum Ca^{2+}-ATPase activity, a reduced Ca^{2+}-induced Ca^{2+} release of the sarcoplasmic reticulum, an altered Na^{2+}–Ca^{2+} exchange, and an inhibition of $(Na^{+}+K^{+})$-ATPase. The latter two effects are probably due to changes in the cell membrane microenvironment in response to phospholipase A activation (Hung and Lew 1993; Liu 1990).

In neonatal rat CMs, serum from rats treated with a sublethal dose of *E. coli* endotoxin depresses contractile activity (decrease in deflection amplitude of about 35%) and induces arrhythmias when perfusion is prolonged. It also attenuates the chronotropic effect of isoprenaline (10^{-7}M) by 40% (25 °C). These effects are only seen when the sera are collected within 2–16 h after endotoxin administration to the rats (Carli et al. 1981). This depression of contractility is, however, not a direct effect of endotoxin itself nor of non-esterified fatty acids, but rather is attributed to an endotoxin-induced early and prolonged (up to 14–16 h) induction of one or more humoral lipid-soluble cardiodepressant factors (Carli et al. 1981).

A direct depressive effect of endotoxin on cardiac muscle without the release of a substance elsewhere in the body was proven by a comparison of the direct effects of endotoxin on the contractile response of feline papillary muscles to calcium with that seen after administration to the intact animal (Starr et al. 1995). The contractile state of the muscle was assessed by monitoring the tension which developed as extracellular calcium concentrations were raised from 0.5 to 8.0 mM. After endotoxin was administered to the intact animal and given to the muscle directly in the bathing solution, endotoxin-exposed muscles showed smaller increases in contractile tension with increasing calcium concentrations than control muscles after 70–85 min. NaOH-inactivated endotoxin produced results similar to the control experiments (Starr et al. 1995).

Acute and Chronic Effects of Endotoxin on Beating of Cardiomyocytes

Acute exposure of neonatal rat CMs to endotoxin (*E. coli*, *Pseudomonas aeruginosa*) does not depress CM contraction or the amplitude of pulsation, even in concentrations substantially higher (1–200 μg/ml) than those measured during human septic shock (Carli et al. 1981; Brenner et al. 1987; Hollenberg et al. 1989; Snell and Parrillo 1991). Also, the beating frequency of these cells is neither impaired during acute exposure with 0.001–10 μg/ml endotoxin (*P. aeruginosa* LPS, Fisher types I, II and VII) in serum-free medium (Müller-Werdan et al. 1996) nor is it impaired with *E. coli* endotoxin in rat serum (Carli et al. 1981).

In cell cultures of neonatal rat CMs, even high concentrations (0.001–10 μg/ml) of endotoxin (*P. aeruginosa* LPS, Fisher types I, II and VII) in serum-free medium neither impair spontaneous beating and beating frequency of the cells during a 72-h incubation period nor influence – in concentrations up to 100 μg/ml – gross morphology and cell viability (cell potassium, cell protein/well, lactate dehydrogenase release) of these CMs (Müller-Werdan et al. 1996). This suggests that the toxin exerts its detrimental effects on the heart mainly by indirect action; TNF-α and IL-1 liberated from endotoxin-activated mediator cells are most likely involved.

However, at least under two experimental conditions, endotoxin directly induces contractile dysfunction of CMs. Firstly, in the absence of glucocorticoids, endotoxin suppresses the "positive inotropic" effect of the β-adrenoceptor agonist isoproterenol (Werdan et al., 1995; Müller-Werdan et al. 1996). When neonatal rat CMs are cultured in a well-defined, serum-free medium in the absence of dexamethasone, with which it is regularly supplemented, the addition of endotoxin (10 μg/ml) for 24 h suppresses the "positive inotropic" effect of isoproterenol (Fig. 3, upper graph). The enhanced production of nitrite – an end product of nitric oxide (NO) formation – by the cells under the

WITHOUT DEXAMETHASONE

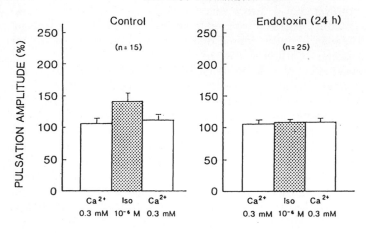

WITH DEXAMETHASONE (10^{-7} M)

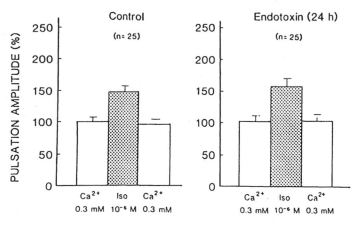

Fig. 3. Endotoxin-induced depression of the "positive inotropic" effect of isoproterenol in neonatal rat cardiomyocytes: effect of dexamethasone. Neonatal rat cardiomyocytes were cultured for 24 h in serum-free medium, in the presence or in the absence of endotoxin (10 μg/ml) and dexamethasone (0.1 μmol/l). After the incubation period, the "positive inotropic" effect of isoproterenol (10^{-6} M, Iso) was measured. For further details see Müller-Werdan et al. 1996

very same conditions (Table 1) strongly argues for a NO-mediated depression of this catecholamine "inotropy" by endotoxin in the absence of glucocorticoids (Werdan et al. 1995; Müller-Werdan et al. 1996). When, however, dexamethasone (10^{-7} mol/l), which suppresses the formation of the inducible NO synthase (iNOS), is added to the culture medium, the endotoxin effect is clearly abolished (Fig. 3, lower graph). It remains to be clarified whether only the β-adrenoceptor-agonist-triggered positive inotropy is impaired by endotoxin in a specific manner or – as in the case of TNF-α (see below) – whether other inotropic pathways are also altered (such as Na^+/K^+-ATPase inhibition by ouabain, α-adrenoceptor stimulation, or high calcium).

Secondly, incubation of adult rat CMs for 6 h with 10–100 ng/ml endotoxin resulted in a progressive time- and protein-synthesis-dependent decrease in electrically stimulated twitch magnitudes and increased contraction and relaxation times (Tao and McKenna 1994). Serum was not required for the endotoxin-induced hypocontractility. The endotoxin-induced defect in contractility was reversed over time; myocytes continuously incubated with endotoxin for 24 h exhibited normal contractility. In contrast, control cells incubated for 18 h were suppressed by a subsequent 6-h exposure to endotoxin. Superfusion of endotoxin-incubated cells with N-nitro-L-arginine methyl ester restored contractile function, whereas superfusion with L-arginine reimposed abnormal contractility. Control myocytes superfused with 8-bromoguanosine 3′, 5′-cyclic monophosphate expressed contractile defects similar to those induced by endotoxin. These findings demonstrate that endotoxin has direct negative effects on cardiac cell contractile function and that the induction of NO synthase (NOS) activity is a primary intracellular mediator of the diminished contractility (Tao and McKenna 1994).

Nitric Oxide Production in Neonatal Rat Cardiomyocytes by Endotoxin

CMs express a constitutive as well as an inducible NOS (Schulz et al. 1992; Balligand et al. 1993a; Balligand et al. 1993b). Formation of nitric oxide can be determined by measuring nitrite production with the Grieß reaction. In the

Table 1. Nitrite production by cultured muscle and non-muscle cells from neonatal rat hearts[a]

Incubation (24 h)	Nitrite Production [nmol/mg protein/24 h]	
	Cardiomyocytes	Non Muscle Cells
Basal	30.5 ± 5.8	30.2 ± 20.8
TNF 10 U/ml	25.7 ± 3.3	18.5 ± 0.7
TNF 100 U/ml	20.2 ± 2.4	22.1 ± 4.8
IL-1 20 U/ml	36.8 ± 4.5	32.3 ± 5.0
LPS 10 µg/ml	139.0 ± 15.0	180.9 ± 39.4
LPS 10 µg/ml + TNF 100 U/ml	153.8 ± 44.7	208.9 ± 46.5
LPS 10 µg/ml + IL-1 20 U/ml	253.8 ± 80.9	

[a]Neonatal rat heart muscle cells (cardiomyocytes) were cultured in serum-free medium without dexamethasone; in the case of non-muscle cells, the medium was supplemented with 10% calf serum. Recombinant human tumor necrosis factor α (*TNF*), interleukin-1α (*IL-1*; recombinant human, Sigma I 6011), endotoxin (lipopolysaccharide, *LPS*), or the combinations of these substances indicated were added to the medium. After the incubation period, the accumulated nitrite was determined photometrically (Grieß reaction), with the nitrite accumulated being a measure of nitric oxide produced during the incubation period. Data are given as mean ± SD; $n = 3$. For further details see Müller-Werdan et al. 1996.

absence of dexamethasone, endotoxin is a strong stimulator of nitrite production in neonatal rat cardiomyocytes during a 24-h incubation period (Table 1).

In contrast to endotoxin, TNF-α – at concentrations up to 100 U/ml – does not induce any measurable nitrite production above the basal level (Table 1). Interferon γ (recombinant human, 100 U/ml) also did not induce nitrite production (data not shown). Both dexamethasone (0.1 μM) and N^G-monomethyl-L-arginine (L-NMMA), an inhibitor of NO synthase, suppress the endotoxin-triggered nitrite production down to basal levels or even lower (Werdan et al. 1995; Müller-Werdan et al. 1996).

Primary cultures of neonatal rat cardiomyocytes are contaminated by about 10%–20% with non-muscle cells, which also are likely candidates for NO production in the heart. These non-muscle cells can be cultured and investigated separately from the muscle cells. Measurement of nitrite production in both primary cardiomyocyte cultures and pure cultures of cardiac non-muscle cells reveals similar production rates (Table 1). Therefore one may assume that in primary cultures of neonatal rat CMs NO is produced mainly by the muscle cells, with some additional amount released from the contaminating non-muscle cells. In both cell types, endotoxin is a strong stimulus, while TNF-α and IL-1 at the concentrations chosen are not. However, a combination of endotoxin and either TNF-α or IL-1 boosts nitrite production (Table 1).

In the case of adult rate CMs, NOS activity is increased after a 6-h treatment with endotoxin (10–100 ng/ml) as evidenced by a dose-dependent enhanced conversion of [^{3}H]arginine to [^{3}H]citrulline and by elevated guanosine-3', 5'-cyclic monophosphate levels (Tao and McKenna 1994).

Mechanism of Endotoxin-Induced Myocardial Depression

The currently most attractive "mechanism of myocardial depression in sepsis hypothesis" is the following (Fig. 2): circulating endotoxin triggers mediator cells to release TNF-α and IL-1, either into the circulation or into the myocardium. TNF-α and IL-1 then trigger the expression of iNOS in the heart, with the consequence of an accelerated release of NO from arginine. NO might then stimulate the activity of the soluble and probably also the particulate form of the guanylyl cyclase of the cardiomyocyte, and the subsequent rise in cyclic guanosine monophosphate (cGMP) could finally lead to an attenuation of the systolic and diastolic function of the heart (for a detailed discussion see Kumar and Parrillo 1995; Müller-Werdan et al. 1996). The question of whether the cardiodepressive effect is mediated exclusively via cGMP elevation still remains to be answered. There is increasing evidence that the cardiodepressive effects of cytokines are not mediated exclusively by NO (Fig. 2; for further discussion see Müller-Werdan et al. 1996). In the case of a direct endotoxin action on the heart the NO–cGMP pathway seems to be the most important one. This statement is supported by many findings:

1. In neonatal rat CMs dexamethasone, which suppresses the formation of iNOS, both inhibits endotoxin-induced synthesis of nitrite (see above) and

overcomes endotoxin-mediated attenuation of isoproterenol-inotropy (Fig. 3).

2. In adult rat CMs, inhibitors of NOS restore the endotoxin-induced direct depression of contractility (see above; Tao and McKenna 1994).

3. Baseline contraction of guinea pig cardiac ventricular CMs is reduced by 46% after endotoxin pretreatment of the animals (Brady et al. 1992). This effect of endotoxin is abolished by pretreatment with the NOS inhibitor N-nitro-L-arginine methyl ester (L-NAME), dexamethasone, or methylene blue, an inhibitor of guanylyl cyclase (Brady et al. 1992).

4. In endothelium-myocyte coculture experiments, 10^{-7} M bradykinin reduces guinea pig CM shortening by 11%. This effect is inhibited by the presence of the L-arginine analogue N^G-monomethyl-L-arginine (L-NMMA). Sodium nitroprusside (3×10^{-5} M) reduces CM shortening by 23% (reversal by methylene blue). Superfusion with NO solution and 8-bromo-guanosine 3' 5'-cyclic monophosphate has an effect similar to sodium nitroprusside.

These experiments show that CM contractility can be attenuated by NO, which appears to act via the production of cGMP within the cells (Brady et al. 1993).

Impairment of Adrenergic Responsiveness of Cardiomyocytes by Endotoxin

Isoproterenol- and forskolin-stimulated cAMP accumulation is decreased in CMs prepared from the hearts of rats pretreated with endotoxin 4 h in advance (Shepherd et al. 1987). The extent of this suppression depends on the endotoxin-dose applied (10–100 μg); isoproterenol-stimulated cAMP production is more sensitive to the endotoxin effect than forskolin-stimulated cAMP production. Catecholamine desensitization is accompanied by a 25% reduction in β-adrenoceptor density of the cells. The authors conclude that the blunted CM hormonal responsiveness following endotoxin challenge appears to be related to the decreased activity of the adenylyl cyclase system which may be attributed to alterations in both receptor density and in the adenylyl cyclase itself.

Following infusion of endotoxin, the basal rate pressure product, the rate of contraction, the rate of relaxation, and cAMP concentrations in isolated rat heart preparations remain unaffected (Bensard et al. 1994). Endotoxin impairs increases in the rate pressure product, the rate of contraction and relaxation, and cAMP in response to isoproterenol, but the effect of the direct adenylyl cyclase activator forskolin is unaffected by endotoxin (Bensard et al. 1994).

A possible mechanism of the disruption of β-adrenergic signal transduction by endotoxin in the heart is suggested by the work of Balligand et al. (1993b). These investigators showed that the depression of the contractile response of adult rat ventricular CMs to β-adrenergic agonists by exposure to soluble inflammatory mediators is mediated at least in part by induction of an autocrine NO signalling pathway. Following preincubation of ventricular CMs from adult rat hearts for 24 h in medium conditioned by endotoxin-activated rat alveolar macrophages, the subsequent inotropic response to isoproterenol is reduced from 225% to 155% of baseline amplitude of shortening. Addition of L-NMMA completely restores the positive inotropic response to isoproterenol in CMs preincubated in activated macrophage medium, while the response of control CMs to isoproterenol is unaffected. The release of NO by ventricular CMs following exposure to activated macrophage medium can be detected as an increase in cGMP content in a reporter cell bioassay and also as an increase in nitrite content in macrophage-conditioned medium (Balligand et al. 1993b). In neonatal rat CMs, the negative chronotropic effect of the muscarinic cholinoceptor agonist carbachol is inhibited by L-NMMA and by methylene blue, an inhibitor of guanylyl cyclase. This suggests that the physiologic response to muscarinic cholinergic stimuli is also mediated, at least in part, by products of an endogenous NOS (Balligand et al. 1993a).

Beneficial Effects of Endotoxin in Ischemia/Reperfusion

From the viewpoint of a cardiologist, endotoxin still offers some moments of surprise: besides the deleterious direct and indirect cardiodepressive action (see above), protective effects on the heart have been documented.

In rats, deleterious ventricular arrhythmias after coronary ligation are markedly reduced by pretreatment of the animals with endotoxin (Song et al. 1994). This protective effect is ascribed to the induction of iNOS (see above). A non-toxic lipid A-analogue reduces the infarct size after coronary ligation in rabbits (Yao et al. 1993). Although endotoxin pretreatment of rabbits has a moderate cardiodepressive effect, after coronary ligation, the heart function almost completely recovers during the succedent reperfusion phase, while in the control group heart function remains substantially impaired (McDonough et al. 1995). The increase in coronary perfusion by endotoxin is thought to contribute to this protective effect.

Summary and Conclusion

There is no doubt that endotoxin can depress contractility and attenuate the inotropic catecholamine response of the heart, both in a direct and indirect, cytokine-mediated manner. The receptor mechanism by which endotoxin binds to the CM remains to be determined, while the signal cascade which is consequently induced (iNOS-induction resulting in a rise in NO levels and subsequently in cGMP levels in the CM) is well understood. The direct endotoxin effect impairs basal contractility and β-adrenoceptor-mediated positive inotropy. The indirect, cytokine-mediated endotoxin effects can additionally attenuate other inotropic mechanisms such as that mediated by α-adrenoceptor stimulation (Fig. 2).

The relative contributions of the direct and indirect effects of endotoxin to myocardial depression in sepsis remains to be determined. The induction of myocardial iNOS and an increased cGMP level in the hearts of patients in septic shock (Thoenes et al. 1995) provide evidence for a direct endotoxin action in septic cardiomyopathy. However, activation of the same signal transduction pathway – endotoxin, NO, and cGMP – may be beneficial in myocardial ischemia and reperfusion injury (Song et al. 1994; Pabla et al. 1995).

If endotoxin plays a role in the pathophysiology of septic cardiomyopathy, then neutralization of this toxin by antibodies should improve cardiac function. This, however, was not achieved with the anti-endotoxin antibody HA-1A. In observational studies of patients with septic shock, no change in the depressed left ventricular stroke work index was observed (Werdan 1995; Müller-Werdan et al. 1996). In fact, in a canine model of gram-negative septic shock, the administration of HA-1A antibodies even further suppressed the left ventricular stroke work index (Quezado et al. 1993). Although a lot is known about the deleterious mechanisms of endotoxin in septic shock, the development of therapeutic approaches to effectively neutralize its action in the clinical arena is still in the initial stages.

References

Abel FL (1989) Myocardial function in sepsis and endotoxin shock. Am J Physiol 257: R1265–R1281

Balligand J-L, Kelly RA, Marsden PA, Smith TW, Michel T (1993a) Control of cardiac muscle cell function by an endogenous nitric oxide signaling system. Proc Natl Acad Sci USA 90: 347–351

Balligand J-L, Ungureanu D, Kelly RA, Kobzik L, Pimental D, Michel T, Smith TW (1993b) Abnormal Contractile Function due to Induction of Nitric Oxide Synthesis in Rat Cardiac Myocytes Follows Exposure to Activated Macrophage-conditioned Medium. J Clin Invest 91: 2314–2319

Bensard DD, Banerjee A, McIntyre Jr RC, Berens RL, Harken AH (1994) Endotoxin Disrupts β-Adrenergic Signal Transduction in the Heart. Arch Surg 129: 198–205

Brady AJB, Poole-Wilson PA, Harding SE, Warren JB (1992) Nitric oxide production within cardiac myocytes reduces their contractility in endotoxemia. Am J Physiol 263: 1963–1966

Brady AJB, Warren JB, Poole-Wilson PA, Williams TJ, Harding SE (1993) Nitric oxide attenuates cardiac myocyte contraction. Am J Physiol 265: H176–H182

Brenner M, Doerfler M, Danner RL, Reilly JM, Weideman MM, Parrillo JE (1987) Determination of direct myocardial contractile effects of eicosanoids, endotoxin, tumor necrosis factor and other mediators using a newly designed quantitative cellular contractile assay. Clin Res 35: 785A

Carli A, Auclair M-C, Benassayag C, Nunez E (1981) Evidence for an Early Lipid Soluble Cardiodepressant Factor in Rat Serum After a Sublethal Dose of Endotoxin. Circ Shock 8: 301–312

Hinshaw LB (1985) Cardiodepressant effects of endotoxin. In: Hinshaw LB (ed) Pathophysiology of endotoxin. Elsevier, Amsterdam, pp 16–35 (Handbook of Endotoxin, vol 2)

Hollenberg SM, Cunnion RE, Lawrence M, Kelly JL, Parrillo JE (1989) Tumor necrosis factor depresses myocardial cell function: Results using an in vitro assay of myocyte performance. Clin Res 37: 528A

Hung J, Lew WYW (1993) Cellular mechanisms of endotoxin-induced myocardial depression in rabbits. Circ Res 73: 125–134

Kumar A, Parrillo JE (1995) Nitric Oxide and the Heart in Sepsis. In: Fink MP, Payen D (eds) Role of Nitric Oxide in Sepsis and ARDS (Update in Intensive Care and Emergency Medicine 24). Springer, Berlin Heidelberg New York, pp 73–99

Liu M-S (1990) Mechanism of myocardial membrane alterations in endotoxin shock: roles of phospholipase and phosphorylation. Circ Shock 30: 43–49

Loppnow H, Flad H-D, Rietschel ET, Brade H (1993) The Active Principle of Bacterial Lipopolysaccharides (Endotoxins) for Cytokine Induction. In: Schlag G, Redl H (eds) Pathophysiology of Shock, Sepsis, and Organ Failure. Springer, Berlin Heidelberg New York, 405–416

Loppnow H, Stelter F, Schönbeck U, Schlüter C, Ernst M, Schütt C, Flad H-D (1995) Endotoxin activates human vascular smooth muscle cells despite lack of expression of CD14 mRNA or endogenous membrane CD14. Infect Immun 63: 1020–1026

Martich GD, Boujoukos AJ, Suffredini AF (1993) Response of Man to Endotoxin. Immunobiology 187: 403–416

McDonough KH, Giaimo ME, Miller HI (1995) Effects of endotoxin on the guinea pig heart response to ischemia reperfusion injury. Shock 4: 139–142

Michie HR, Manogue KR, Spriggs DR, Revhaug A, O'Dwyer S, Dinarello CA, Cerami A, Wolff SM, Wilmore DW (1988) Detection of Circulating Tumor Necrosis Factor after Endotoxin Administration. N Engl J Med 318: 1481–1486

Müller-Werdan U, Reithmann C, Werdan K (1996) Cytokines and the Heart - Molecular Mechanisms of Septic Cardiomyopathy. Landes, Georgetown/Chapman and Hall, New York/Springer-Verlag, Berlin Heidelberg New York

Natanson C, Eichenholz PW, Danner RL, Eichacker PQ, Hoffman WD, Kuo GC, Banks SM, MacVittie TJ, Parrillo JE (1989) Endotoxin and tumor necrosis factor challenges in dogs simulate the cardiovascular profile of human septic shock. J Exp Med 169: 823–832

Pabla R, Bland-Ward P, Moore PK, Curtis MJ (1995) An endogenous protectant effect of cardiac cyclic GMP against reperfusion-induced ventricular fibrillation in the rat heart. Br J Pharmacol 116: 2923–2930

Pilz G, McGinn P, Boekstegers P, Kääb S, Weidenhöfer S, Werdan K (1994) Pseudomonas sepsis does not cause more severe cardiovascular dysfunction in patients than non-Pseudomonas sepsis. Circ Shock 42: 174–182

Quezado ZMN, Natanson C, Alling DW, Banks SM, Koev CA, Elin RJ, Hosseini JM, Bacher JD, Danner RL, Hoffman WD (1993) A controlled trial of HA-1A in a canine model of Gram-negative septic shock. JAMA 269: 2221–2227

Rietschel ET, Brade H (1992) Bacterial endotoxins. Sci Am Au 26–33

Schulz R, Nava E, Moncada S (1992) Induction and potential biological relevance of a Ca^{2+}-independent nitric oxide synthase in the myocardium. Br J Pharmacol 105: 575–580

Schumann RR, Rietschel ET (1995) Endotoxin - Structure, Recognition, Cellular Response and Septic Shock. Antiinfect Drugs Chemother 13: 115–124

Shepherd RE, Lang CH, McDonough KH (1987) Myocardial adrenergic responsiveness after lethal and nonlethal doses of endotoxin. Am J Physiol 252: H410–H416

Snell RJ, Parrillo JE (1991) Cardiovascular dysfunction in septic shock. Chest 99: 1000–1009

Song W, Furman BL, Parratt JR (1994) Attenuation by dexamethasone of endotoxin protection against ischaemia-induced ventricular arrhythmias. Br J Pharmacol 113: 1083–1084

Starr RG, Lader AS, Philips GC, Stroman CE, Abel FL (1995) Direct action of endotoxin on cardiac muscle. Shock 3: 380–384

Suffredini AF, Fromm RE, Parker MM, Brenner M, Kovacs JA, Wesley RA, Parrillo JE (1989) The cardiovascular response of normal humans to the administration of endotoxin. N Engl J Med 321: 280–287

Tao S, McKenna TM (1994) In vitro endotoxin exposure induces contractile dysfunction in adult rat cardiac myocytes. Am J Physiol 267: H1745–H1752

Thoenes M, Förstermann U, Rüdiger J, Scholz H, Starbatty J, Stein B (1995) Expression of inducible nitric oxide synthase in failing and non-failing human heart. Naunyn Schmiedebergs Arch Pharmacol 351: R112

Werdan K (1995) Towards a More Casual Treatment of Septic Cardiomyopathy. In: Vincent J-L (ed) Yearbook of Intensive Care and Emergency Medicine 1995. Springer, Berlin Heidelberg New York, pp 518–538

Werdan K, Müller-Werdan U, Reithmann C, Boekstegers P, Fuchs R, Kainz I, Stadler J (1995) Nitric-oxide-dependent and nitric-oxide-independent effects of tumor necrosis factor α on cardiomyocyte's beating activity and signal transduction pathways. In: Schlag G, Redl H (eds) 4th Wiggers Bernard Conference: Shock, sepsis, and organ failure – nitric oxide. Springer, Berlin Heidelberg New York, 286–309

Yao Z, Auchampach JA, Pieper GM, Gross GJ (1993) Cardioprotective effects of monophosphoryl lipid A, a novel endotoxin analogue, in the dog. Cardiovasc Res 27: 832–838

Immunological Mediators in Arteriosclerosis

Transplant Associated Coronary Artery Disease

C.H. Wheeler, A.D. Collins, M.J. Dunn, S.J. Crisp, M.H. Yacoub, and M.L. Rose

Introduction

Heart transplantation is the clinically acceptable treatment for end-stage heart failure. Since the development of better immunosuppressive regimes and particularly the introduction of Cyclosporin A in 1983, which combats cellular rejection, short-term survival for heart transplant recipients has increased steadily with survival at 1 year being in the order of 85% (Kriett and Kaye 1990). The major medium to long-term complication is development of a proliferative occlusive disease of the vasculature of the allograft. This disease, variously described as transplant associated coronary artery disease (TxCAD; Rose and Dunn 1993), cardiac allograft vasculopathy (CAV; Hosenpud et al. 1992), accelerated coronary artery sclerosis (ACS; Yacoub and Rose, 1994) and graft coronary artery sclerosis (GCA; Schoen and Libby 1991), is a rapidly progressing disease which causes blockage of the coronary arteries. The incidence of TxCAD varies between heart transplant centres. Harefield Hospital, U.K. has an incidence of 6% at 1 year increasing to 17% at 3 years (see Dunn and Rose, 1993), however, other centres have reported incidences as high as 10%–20% at 1 year, 25%–40% at 3 years and at least 40%–50% at 5 years (Gao et al. 1989; Uretsky et al. 1987).

The development of TxCAD can be extremely rapid and in some patients is detectable within months of transplantation. Studies on transplant recipients at Stanford University suggest that the earlier the onset and more rapid the progression of the disease the worse the prognosis (Schroeder and Gao 1995; Gao et al. 1994). The variability in the onset and severity of the disease may suggest a subtle difference in pathogenesis between different patient groups.

Diagnosis of TxCAD

The diagnosis of TxCAD is problematic because the disease is frequently asymptomatic in its early stages and angina pectoris is usually absent due to denervation of the allograft. In the longer-term TxCAD is characterised by

National Heart and Lung Institute, Heart Science Centre, Harefield Hospital, Harefield, Middlesex UB9 6JH, UK symptoms related to reduced cardiac output, congestive heart failure, myocardial infarction, sudden death or a combination of these events. TxCAD is generally diagnosed by routine coronary angiography (usually assessed on a yearly basis post-transplant), but difficulty in monitoring the diffuse and concentric nature of lesions within the coronary vasculature may lead to underdiagnosis of the frequency and severity of the disease (Johnson et al. 1991; Dressler and Miller 1992). Underdiagnosis is compounded in the early stages by the tendency for affected vessels to increase in size leading to little change in the luminal dimensions (Glagov et al. 1987; Pinto et al. 1993). Diagnosis can however be enhanced by measuring arterial dimensions very early after transplantation (Hosenpud et al. 1992) to give a baseline which allows more accurate quantification from subsequent angiograms.

Intracoronary ultrasound appears to be more sensitive in detecting TxCAD than coronary angiography, but has drawbacks due to its invasive nature. Using ultrasound, 13 out of 20 patients studied one month after transplantation were shown to have a "visible" coronary artery intima although angiographically they were "normal" (St. Goar et al. 1992). After one year, of 60 patients, 35% had minimal or mild, 28% moderate, and 35% severe intimal thickening by ultrasound imaging although 42 out of the 60 patients were angiographically normal. In fact 21 out of these 42 "normal" individuals exhibited moderate or severe intimal thickening as evidenced by ultrasound (St. Goar et al. 1992).

Another diagnostic strategy determines endothelial dysfunction by using coronary angiography to measure the effect of acetylcholine (or other vasorelaxants) on blood vessel dilatation. In normal vessels acetylcholine induces relaxation due to the release of endothelium derived relaxing factor (EDRF; nitric oxide). Paradoxically in vessels with compromised endothelia, vasoconstriction occurs either due to increased diffusion distances for EDRF between its sites of release and action (as a result of intimal thickening), or due to inactivation or uptake of EDRF (Fish et al. 1988). Impairment of the response to vasorelaxants may be a sensitive early marker for TxCAD. In a small study, 5 out of 10 transplant patients with angiographically normal coronary arteries exhibited a constrictive response when administered with ergonovine maleate (normally a vasorelaxant). After two years, four of these five patients developed detectable TxCAD whereas none of the patients who showed normal vasorelaxation developed the disease (Kushwaha et al. 1991).

The difficulties related to the diagnosis and monitoring of the disease suggest an on-going requirement for a convenient, sensitive, non-invasive method for the detection of TxCAD.

Morphology of TxCAD

TxCAD can affect both the coronary arteries and, to a lesser extent, veins (Oni et al. 1991), and has therefore been described as cardiac allograft vasculopathy (Hosenpud et al. 1992). At a gross level, lesions formed during TxCAD appear very different from those arising from conventional atherosclerosis (see Table 1).

Table 1. Comparison of atherosclerosis with transplant associated coronary artery disease

Disease characteristics	TxCAD	Typical atherosclerosis
Disease progression	Rapid (months to year)	Slow (many years)
Vessels affected	Epicardial and intramyocardial	Epicardial
Lesion	Usually concentric	Eccentric
	Distal	Proximal
	Diffuse	Focal
	Rarely complicated	Often complicated
Elastic laminar	Usually intact	Usually disrupted
Calcification	Rare	Common
Lipid deposition	Minimal	Ubiquitous
Cell types	Smooth muscle cells, macrophages, lymphocytes	Smooth muscle cells, macrophages, foam cells
Causation	Immunological insult	"Injury"
Treatment	Retransplantation	Revascularization by angioplasty or coronary bypass

The lesions tend to be distal rather than proximal and the disease affects both epicardial and intramyocardial vessels. The lesions are diffuse and concentric rather than focal and eccentric, they occlude the vessel lumen, and can affect the entire length of the arterial wall. TxCAD lesions can overlay pre-existing conventional atheroma in the donor heart (see Schoen and Libby 1991). Importantly, TxCAD only affects the allograft and never the recipient's own vessels. The time-course for development of TxCAD can be extremely rapid, in some cases only a few months, whereas normal atherosclerosis takes many years. However, due to the difficulty in diagnosis of TxCAD it is likely that the disease in many patients will have developed insidiously over a longer period than is apparent from angiographic measurement. The apparent differences in the development of lesions in TxCAD compared to those in normal atherosclerosis may be related more to their pathogenesis and time course of their development rather than to fundamental differences in the mechanism of plaque formation.

Lesions in TxCAD are due mainly to thickening of the vessel intima by proliferation of smooth muscle cells (SMCs) and secretion of matrix proteins, but T cells and macrophages are also present towards the lumen (Hruban et al. 1990; Salomon et al. 1991; Schoen and Libby 1991; Taylor et al. 1993). Foam cells are generally absent except in the latter stages of the disease and calcification is rare. Unlike conventional atheroma, the elastic lamina of affected vessels is generally intact, which may reflect reduced wall stress on the vessel due to the concentric nature of the lesion.

Normal atheroma are also composed of T lymphocytes and monocytes with proliferation of intimal cells, deposition of matrix proteins and eventually, accumulation of lipids and calcium. It can be argued therefore that both TxCAD and atherosclerosis are diseases resulting from the proliferation of components of the vessel intima and it is the chemotactic agents, growth factors (or lack of inhibitors) and inflammatory agents, which allow migration and proliferation of such cell types, which are responsible for the disease. Clearly, conditions for such growth do not exist in normal vessels and control of the signals which lead to this cell activation are a focus for research into the development of atherosclerosis in all its forms.

Pathogenesis of TxCAD

In common with the formation of normal atheroma (Rose and Glomset 1976; Ross 1986), TxCAD is believed to arise as a "response to injury". It is now generally accepted that this "injury" is mediated by an immunological insult to the transplanted organ and TxCAD has therefore been termed chronic rejection. Such an injury need not be cytotoxic. Sub-lethal damage by antibodies or cells could activate cells of the vessel wall which could stimulate cell migration and proliferation. Lesions similar to those in grafted hearts are formed in most solid organ allografts including lung, kidney, liver and pancreas which suggests a common mechanism for their initiation.

Circumstantial evidence for an immunological role in the pathogenesis of TxCAD is suggested by the localisation and ubiquitous nature of the disease in the transplanted organ. In studies to assess risk factors for TxCAD, incidence of the disease was not correlated with age, sex or ischaemic time. TxCAD is correlated with the degree of ischaemic damage (assessed histologically) in the post-transplant period (Gaudin et al. 1994) and with previous histories of cellular rejection (Uretsky et al. 1987; Zerbe et al. 1992). TxCAD is more frequent in patients who undergo repeat transplantation and such patients have lower survival rates than primary transplant recipients (Gao et al. 1988; Kriett and Kaye 1990). This could be due to a raised immunological status in the host leading to damage of the vessels of a subsequent allograft. Direct evidence for an immunological role in the genesis of TxCAD has been provided by animal models of the disease. Increased immunosuppression in rat and rabbit allograft models reduced the development of allograft vasculopathy (Laden 1972). In a non-transplant model, rabbits when "immunised" with injected foreign proteins and fed a high lipid diet developed lesions indistinguishable from those in transplant vasculopathy whereas rabbits fed only a high lipid diet did not develop the lesions (Minick and Murphy 1973). Considerable support for a humoral role in the development of TxCAD has been obtained using SCID mice. Allogeneic coronary arteries when grafted into SCID mice did not develop obstructive lesions, but when such mice were also injected regularly with antiserum against donor antigens, coronary artery disease did develop (Russell et al. 1994). Thus antibodies alone are capable of inducing lesions characteristic of coronary artery disease.

The endothelium, which presents an allogeneic barrier between the hosts immune system and the transplanted organ is likely to be a primary site for immunologically mediated injury. Integrity of the endothelium is essential to maintain normal vessel function. Physical injury to vessel endothelia by balloon catheterization alone can induce intimal thickening (see Shirotani et al. 1993). In animal models, it has been shown that proliferating endothelial cells secrete mitogens for smooth muscle cells (Castellot et al. 1987; Koo and Gottlieb 1989) whereas confluent endothelial cells in vitro secrete SMC growth inhibitors (Willems et al. 1982). SMC proliferation and migration cease only when endothelial regeneration is complete (Clowes et al. 1983, 1989a,b). Interestingly, there is evidence that normal atherosclerosis may in part be mediated immunologically also (see Wick et al. 1995). T cells are amongst the first cells to infiltrate arterial intima during the initial stages of atherosclerosis (Xu et al. 1990; Wick et al. 1995) and it has been shown in animal models that immunization with heat shock protein (HSP) 65 or adjuvants containing Mycobacterium tuberculosis, of which HSP65 is a major constituent, leads to the development of atherosclerosis (Xu et al. 1992). Expression of HSP60 (which exhibits a high degree of identity with HSP65), is increased in stressed aortic endothelial cells and 80% of cells are surface stained by antibodies towards HSP60 (Xu et al. 1994). Since serum antibodies towards heat shock 60 proteins are significantly increased in patients with carotid atherosclerosis (Xu et al. 1993) surface expression of the protein could mediate cytotoxic effects on the arterial endothelium.

Immunological Involvement in Chronic Rejection of Cardiac Allografts

Although it has been postulated that immunological factors may be responsible for endothelial damage in the genesis of TxCAD, until recently there has been little direct evidence for such damage. MHC (major histocompatibility complex) class I and class II molecules are constitutively expressed by capillaries and the main vessels in normal and diseased (cardiomyopathy) human hearts (Page et al. 1992; Salomon et al. 1991). Expression of both MHC class I and II molecules is upregulated on capillary endothelial cells during rejection of cardiac allografts (Rose et al. 1986). In addition, endothelial cells express unique endothelial/monocyte alloantigens (Cerilli et al. 1985; Schook et al. 1987) which are believed to be important in transplant rejection. The endothelium is therefore a potential primary target for both humoral and cell mediated immunity. There is some direct evidence for cell-mediated immune mechanisms in the development of TxCAD. In TxCAD lesions in vessels, CD4[+] and CD8[+] T-lymphocytes were found in equal numbers together with HLA-DR[+] macrophages immediately below the endothelium and were suggested to be responsible for a regional cell mediated immune response (Salomon et al. 1991). The possibility of such a response is supported by evidence which shows that cardiac and coronary artery endothelial cells also express accessory adhesion molecules including platelet endothelial cell adhesion molecule, intercellular adhesion molecule-1 and vascular cell adhesion molecule-1 (Taylor et al. 1992; 1993) which enable the tissue to act as a target for cytotoxic endothelial cells. However, activated (CD4[+], CD8[+], HLA-DR[+], interleukin-2R[+]) T lymphocytes are amongst the first cells to accumulate in the arterial intima at the development of normal atherosclerotic plaques (Emeson and Robertson 1988; Wick et al. 1995). The similarity in the molecular profile of lymphocytes in normal atheroma compared with those in TxCAD lesions suggests that it is unlikely that T-cells alone are responsible for the rapid progression of plaque formation seen in TxCAD.

There is perhaps more convincing evidence for a humoral role in the development of chronic transplant rejection. Immunofluorescence microscopy has shown that deposits of immunoglobulin (IgG and IgM), complement components (C3 or Clq), and fibrinogen are found in myocardial capillaries of biopsy specimens within 3 weeks of cardiac transplantation (Hammond et al. 1989). It was not determined whether the response was directed against donor HLA, endothelial or other tissue specific antigens (Hammond et al. 1989). Nevertheless, this vascular or humoral form of rejection was associated with lower survival rates compared with typical cellular rejection and suggested that induction of a humoral response could be linked to chronic graft failure.

Although anti HLA antibodies are formed after transplantation and these are associated with cell mediated rejection and poor long-term survival, there is no clear indication that these antibodies are associated with the appearance of TxCAD. The cause of death in patients with these antibodies include infection and cellular rejection as well as coronary artery disease (Rose et al. 1992). If anti-HLA antibodies were related to the occurrence of TxCAD it would be expected that HLA mismatching would be correlated with the disease. Although there is a clear correlation between the severity of rejection episodes after transplantation and the number of mismatches at the DR locus, a direct correlation between DR mismatching and TxCAD has not been demonstrated (Dunn and Rose, 1993; Pfeffer et al. 1988; Khaghani et al. 1989; Zerbe et al. 1991). The reasons for this anomaly suggest that acute cellular rejection (defined by a cellular infiltrate within the biopsy), which is influenced by the degree of HLA-DR incompatibility, is immunologically a different process to that which induces TxCAD in allografted coronary arteries (see Rose, 1996 for an explanation of this hypothesis). The endothelia within the heart are heterogeneous with respect to expression of cell surface antigens (Page et al. 1992) and it is possible that TxCAD is caused by an immune response to specific antigens expressed on larger vessel endothelia (Dunn et al. 1992; Dunn and Rose 1993). Alternatively, it may be that all donor endothelial cells are damaged chronically after transplantation, but the response to coronary vessels to damage differs from the response of microvessels, leading to a different histopathology.

Detection of Anti-endothelial Antibodies in Sera from Transplant Recipients

The presence of anti-endothelial antibodies in sera from heart transplant recipients has been investigated using sodium dodecyl sulphate-polyacrylamide gel electrophoresis (SDS-PAGE) and Western immunoblotting (Dunn et al. 1992). In an initial study, proteins derived from human umbilical vein endothelial cells (HUVEC) were separated according to size by SDS-PAGE and used to screen sera from cardiac transplant recipients to detect IgG and IgM anti-endothelial antibodies. Many patients possessed circulating antibodies, but when correlated with the development of TxCAD in these patients, 20 out of 21 patients with angiographically demonstrated TxCAD had circulating IgM antibodies, while only 9 out of 20 cases without TxCAD had such antibodies (see Fig. 1). In particular, 15 out of 21 sera from TxCAD$^+$ group reacted specifically with a doublet of proteins with molecular weights of 60–62 kDa, but they were present in only 1 patient without TxCAD (Dunn et al. 1992). These antibodies were present in only three patients prior to transplantation suggesting that they are raised concurrently with the development of TxCAD. Sera from TxCAD$^+$ patient's were also shown by indirect immunofluorescence to stain the endothelium and media of diseased and normal coronary arteries, but not the endothelium of microvasculature in sections of human atrium (Dunn et al. 1992). The distribution of this staining suggests that these antigens are re-

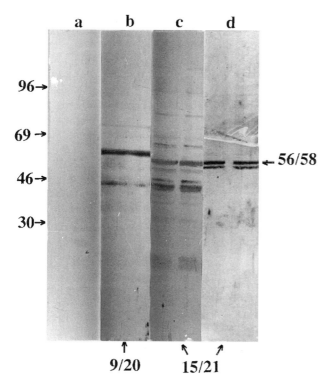

Fig. 1. Western blotted human umbilical vein endothelial cell proteins probed with patient's or control serum to show IgM reactive proteins as described in Dunn et al. (1992). The *left-hand track* of each pair is from untreated cells but the *right-hand track* in each case is gamma-interferon treated. Strip *a* Probed with pooled normal human serum showing no immunoreactive bands. Strip *b* Probed with serum from a patient without TxCAD showing some immunoreactivity (9/20 patients), but not towards the 56–58 kDa doublet. Strips *c* and *d* showing typical immunoreactivity in TxCAD positive sera with recognition of the 56–58 kDa proteins. Fifteen out of twenty-one TxCAD$^+$ patients in this previous study (Dunn et al. 1992) exhibited this pattern of immunoreactivity. Gamma interferon did not increase the amount of immunoreactive proteins in any of the sera tested. Serum samples were obtained 2 years after transplantation. The migration position of molecular weight standards is indicated on the *left* of the figure

stricted to the large coronary vessels. This would explain the localisation of TxCAD to the epicardial vessels and larger myocardial capillaries (Dunn et al. 1992; Dunn and Rose 1993). The 60–62 kDa (later redefined as 56–58 kDa; Crisp et al. 1994) antigens have now been characterised using two-dimensional PAGE, Western immunoblotting, protein microsequencing and antibody pre-adsorbtion studies (Wheeler et al. 1995). The 56–58 kDa proteins were identified as the cytoskeletal protein vimentin and its breakdown products and this has enabled specific measurement of anti-vimentin antibodies in sera from cardiac transplant patients using a dotblot immunoassay (Fig. 2). The reaction of serum antibodies to purified bovine vimentin spotted onto nitrocellulose

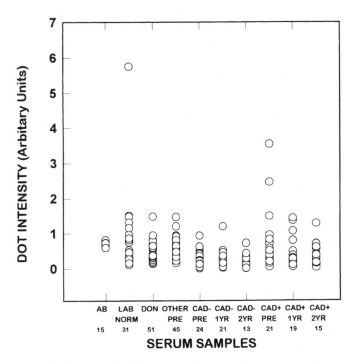

Fig. 2a,b. The titre of IgG (a) and IgM (b) anti-vimentin antibodies in sera from pre- and post-transplant patients, blood donors (*DON*), normal laboratory individuals (*LAB NORM*), and pooled AB serum (*AB*). Data from transplant patients (age and sex matched) is divided into pretransplant (*OTHER PRE*), and post-transplant sera. For patients for whom posttransplant sera were available data are divided into pretransplant samples and their corresponding sera collected 1 (*1YR*) and 2 (*2YR*) years after transplantation. The data are also divided into those who developed TxCAD (*CAD$^+$*) between 1 and 2 years after transplantation and those who did not develop the disease (*CAD$^-$*) during this period (assessed angiographically). Sample numbers are marked below each dataset. Sera from patients were collected prior to transplantation and at annual assessment post-transplant. For dotblot immunoassay, 1-μl aliquots of bovine vimentin (Cymbus, U.K.) dissolved in 6 M urea (1 μg μl^{-1}) were spotted onto nitrocellulose and air dried. Western immunoblotting was then performed (method after Dunn et al. 1992) and spots quantified by enhanced chemiluminesence detection and laser densitometry. A positive (TxCAD$^+$ serum) and negative (AB serum) control were run in parallel with each experimental group and all data were normalised against the positive control sample

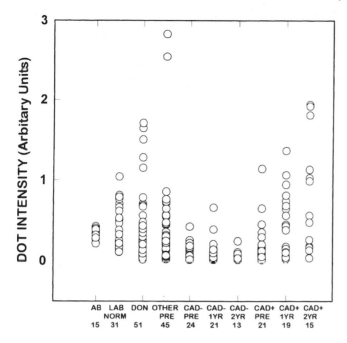

SERUM SAMPLES

Fig. 2b

was determined quantitatively by enhanced chemiluminescence detection combined with laser densitometry (A. Collins et al. in preparation). The titre of IgG and IgM anti-vimentin antibodies was collated with the incidence and timing of the development of TxCAD in these patients (Fig. 2). For IgG antibodies there was no correlation between the titre of antibodies and the development of coronary artery disease (Fig. 2a). Strong IgG reactivity was found in only 2 out of 21 patients in the TxCAD$^+$ group, but there were no significant differences between IgG titres in any of the groups measured.

In patients who did not develop TxCAD, IgM titres 1 and 2 years after transplantation did not differ significantly from their pretransplant samples. However, those patients who developed TxCAD 1–2 years after transplantation exhibited an increase in IgM anti-vimentin titres in their post-transplant sera compared with their pretransplant sera (Fig. 2b). Pretransplant titres from both groups of patients and postransplant TxCAD negative samples did not differ significantly from those in pooled AB serum. However, posttransplant titres in the TxCAD positive group were significantly higher than the AB serum, suggesting that monitoring anti-vimentin IgM titres could be used to assess the presence of TxCAD after transplantation. Interestingly, anti-vimentin IgM titres in normal laboratory individuals, blood donors and other pretransplant patients apparently exhibited a much higher range of titres than either of the transplant study groups. Sera from these individuals were therefore screened against endothelial proteins using Western immunoblotting. Only 1 out of 31 laboratory individuals exhibited weak reactivity towards vimentin, while in the donor and other pretransplant sera, there was a correlation between dotblot intensity and reactivity towards vimentin bands on Western blots. These data showing that normal individuals can have elevated titres of anti-vimentin antibodies suggest that a specific titre of anti-vimentin IgM antibodies will not prove a reliable means of assessing the presence of TxCAD. Nonetheless, individual TxCAD positive patients invariably exhibit an increase in such titres during progression of the disease (A. Collins, unpublished observations) and therefore routine measurement of these antibodies could be used to monitor TxCAD on an individual basis.

The role of anti-vimentin antibodies in the pathogenesis of TxCAD is uncertain. Two questions are fundamental to our understanding of the role of anti-vimentin antibodies in the development of TxCAD. First, how are the auto-antibodies generated and, second, do they exert an effect on the heart? Anti-vimentin antibodies could arise due to direct recognition of vimentin as an alloantigen. Some cytoskeletal proteins such as alpha tubulin exist in many isoforms and may thus be recognised as alloantigens and lead to antibody formation. Vimentin can also exist in different forms in some species (Glasgow et al. 1994) and in humans incompatibility between isoforms in the donor and recipient could lead to allorecognition. Alternatively vimentin may simply cross-react with antibodies which have been raised in response to "foreign" proteins such as those derived from viruses. Vimentin is the major type III intermediate filament protein found in mesenchymal cells (endothelial cells and fibroblasts). In smooth muscle cells the type III intermediate filaments are normally in the form of desmin, but during migration and proliferation, desmin and vimentin are coexpressed. The expression of vimentin in the intima of coronary arteries from transplant recipients is increased (Collins et al. in preparation). Since endothelial cells can present antigens, increased vimentin expression could raise the levels of peptides presented at the cell surface as part of MHC class I antigens which could lead to immune mediated damage to the endothelium. In addition, it is possible that the donor heart presents different peptides of vimentin to those presented by the recipient because they have different allo-MHC class II molecules and thus could represent an alternative form of allorecognition (Crisp 1995). It is likely that vimentin is released also from cells as a result of damage to cardiac tissues due to ischaemia, or lysis by T-cells. Antibodies might thus be raised due to the isoform incompatibility or because the increased levels of protein may simply exceed a threshold of antigenicity. Auto-antibodies towards heart proteins are not uncommon after myocardial infarction and it seems likely that a general release of cell proteins during tissue damage may be a major contributing factor to their formation.

Studies on diseased and normal hearts show that anti-vimentin antibodies only stain within cells, but do not stain the extracellular matrix (Speiser et al. 1992). In addition, commercially available polyclonal and monoclonal antibodies to vimentin do not stain the surface of endothelial cells (P. Taylor, NHLI, UK, personal communication). Intermediate filament antibodies including those against vimentin can occur in autoimmune diseases (Kurki and

Virtanen 1984) and during ageing. In addition, anti-endothelial antibodies are common in autoimmune diseases of the vasculature (Pearson 1994). Anti-vimentin antibodies have been described in patients with normal athero-sclerosis (Nikkari et al. 1993), but the incidence (12%) was much lower than in the present study. Although the appearance of IgM antibodies which recognise epitopes on vimentin is correlated with the incidence of TxCAD it is possible that the antibodies were raised in response to other antigens. A number of antibodies do cross-react with vimentin. Such antibodies could arise due to foreign antigens, but could also be due to histocompatibility antigens. For example, a monoclonal antibody which reacts with the Rhesus D antigen on red blood cells also recognises vimentin (Thorpe 1990). Rhesus incompatibility has been suggested as a possible risk factor in the development of TxCAD (Fyfe et al. 1992) and the possibility that our patients were mismatched for some of the minor Rhesus antigens is currently under investigation. The CD23 antigen is also recognised by monoclonal antibodies towards vimentin. Anti-vimentin antibodies may also be formed in response to infection with Epstein-Barr virus which is thought to be the result of polyclonal stimulation of B cells (Kataaha et al. 1985). In a similar way, the presence of these antibodies in transplant recipients could indicate polyclonal stimulation via the allograft and/or con-comitant viral infection. The M1 protein derived from Group A Streptococci, which causes glomerulonephritis, also shares epitopes with vimentin and desmin (Birkholz et al. 1990).

Do anti-vimentin antibodies play a role in the pathogenesis of TxCAD? Vimentin cross reactive antibodies can be cytotoxic on embryonic spinal cord cells in vitro (Le et al. 1993), but in our own studies (A. Danskine and A. Collins, unpublished observations) transplant patient's sera was not cytotoxic and did not elicit antibody dependent cell mediated cytotoxicity. The possi-bility that anti-vimentin antibodies can activate endothelial cells without da-maging them, as has been shown to occur with alloantibodies (Pidwell et al. 1995), is currently under investigation. The high levels of IgG anti-vimentin antibodies present in sera which were not correlated with TxCAD, suggest that these antibodies are not involved in TxCAD pathogenesis. However it is pos-sible that the dotblot immunoassay used in this work cannot distinguish be-tween specific idiotypes which could be important in pathogenesis against a high background of anti-vimentin IgG titre. IgG could play a protective role in removing antigens liberated due to tissue damage.

It would be expected that antibodies would need to react with cell surface constituents in order to effect disease pathogenesis and there is no evidence to show that anti-vimentin antibodies do so. However, antibodies in TxCAD$^+$ sera do bind to the coronary endothelial cells (Dunn et al. 1992) and can be shown by flow cytometry to bind to the cell surface of various endothelial cell lines (B. Ferry, John Radcliffe Hospital, Oxford, U.K., personal communication). They could therefore exert an effect in activating such cells. It is unclear whether IgM antibodies play any role in the pathogenesis of TxCAD, they may simply be a measure of endothelial or vessel wall damage. Nevertheless their detection could form the basis for a simple quantitative test for the presence and pro-gression of TxCAD. We are presently developing an enzyme linked immunoassay to measure the titre of such antibodies which will allow more rapid and convenient screening of patient's sera.

Summary

Formation of lesions during transplant associated coronary artery disease is a complex process which includes lymphocyte adhesion and migration, smooth muscle cell proliferation, extracellular matrix and lipid deposition. Many factors may affect the rate of progression or severity of TxCAD, but most such factors are probably not causative in their own right. The role of anti-endothelial antibodies in the pathogenesis of TxCAD remains uncertain. Nevertheless, the presence of anti-endothelial antibodies, including anti-vimentin antibodies, is correlated with the appearance of TxCAD in cardiac transplant patients at Harefield Hospital. Characterisation of the antigens responsible for the formation of these antibodies may lead to the development of sensitive and rapid tests for progression of the disease, and contribute to elucidation of the mechanisms of transplant related sclerosis.

Acknowledgements. Original work described in this chapter was supported in part by the British Heart Foundation and Harefield Hospital Trust. We would like to thank Dr Patricia Taylor for her helpful comments and suggestions.

References

Birkholz S, Goroncy-Bermes P, Schonerkark M, Hansch GM, Opferkuch W (1990) Intermediate filaments vimentin and desmin share epitopes with M1 protein of group A Streptococci. Zentralbl Bakt 274: 183–194

Castellot JJ Jr, Wright TC, Karnovsky MJ (1987) Regulation of vascular smooth muscle cell growth by heparin and heparan sulfates. Semin Thromb Haemost 13: 489–503

Cerilli J, Brasile L, Galouzis T, Lempert N, Clarke J (1985) The vascular endothelial cell antigen system. Transplantation 39: 286–289

Clowes AW, Reidy MA, Clowes MM (1983) Kinetics of cellular proliferation after arterial injury. Lab Invest 49: 208–215

Clowes AW, Clowes MM, Fingerle J, Reidy MA (1989a) Kinetics of cellular proliferation after arterial injury V. Role of acute distension in the induction of smooth muscle proliferation. Lab Invest 60: 360–364

Clowes AW, Clowes MM, Fingerle J, Reidy MA (1989b) Regulation of smooth muscle cell growth in injured artery. J Cardiovasc Pharmacol 14 (Suppl 6): S12–S14

Crisp SJ (1995) The role of antiendothelial antibodies in the development of transplantation-associated coronary artery disease. Thesis, University of London, U.K.

Crisp SJ, Dunn MJ, Rose ML, Barbir M, Yacoub MH (1994) Antiendothelial antibodies after heart transplantation: the accelerating factor in transplant-associated coronary artery disease? J Heart Lung Transplant 12: 81–92

Dressler FA, Miller LW (1992) Necropsy versus angiography: how accurate is angiography? J Heart Lung Transplant 11: 556–559

Dunn MJ, Rose ML (1993) Antibody mediated rejection following cardiac transplantation. In: Rose ML, Yacoub MH (eds) Immunology of heart and lung transplantation. Arnold, London, pp 200–215

Dunn MJ, Crisp S, Rose ML, Taylor PM, Yacoub MH (1992) Detection of anti-endothelial antibodies by Western blotting – positive correlation with coronary artery disease after cardiac transplantation. Lancet 339: 1566–1570

Emeson EE, Robertson AL (1988) T lymphocytes in aortic and coronary intimas. Their potential role in atherogenesis. Am J Pathol 130: 369–376

Fish RD, Nabel EG, Selwyn AP, Ludmer PL, Mudge GH, Kirshenbaum JM, Schoen FJ, Alexander RW (1988) Responses of coronary arteries of cardiac transplant patients to acetylcholine. J Clin Invest 81: 21–31

Fyfe AI, Brownfield ED, Kobashigawa JA, Drinkwater DC, Laks H (1992) Rh incompatible cardiac transplantation is associated with increased early rejection and transplant atherosclerosis. Circulation 86 (Suppl 1): 628

Gao S-Z, Hunt SA, Schroeder JS, Alderman EL, Hill I, Stinson EB (1988) Retransplantation for severe accelerated coronary artery disease in the heart transplant recipients. Am J Cardiol 62: 876–881

Gao S-Z, Schroeder JS, Alderman EL, Hunt SA, Valantine HA, Wiederhold V, Stinson EB (1989) Prevalence of accelerated coronary artery disease in heart transplant survivors: comparison of cyclosporine and azathioprine regimens. Circulation 80 (Suppl 3): 100–105

Gao S-Z, Schroeder JS, Hunt SA, Billingham ME, Valantine HA, Stinson EB (1994) Does rapidity of development of transplant coronary artery disease portend a worse prognosis? J Heart Lung Transplant 13: 1119–1124

Gaudin PB, Rayburn BK, Hutchins GM, Kasper EM, Baughman KL, Goodman SN, Leeks LE, Baumgartner WA, Hruban RH (1994) Peritransplant injury to the myocardium associated with the development of accelerated arteriosclerosis in heart transplant recipients. Am J Pathol 18: 338–346

Glagov S, Weinsenberg E, Zarins CK, Stankunavicius R, Kolettis GJ (1987) Compensatory enlargement of human atherosclerotic coronary arteries. N Engl J Med 316: 1371–1375

Glasgow E, Druger RF, Fuchs C, Levine EM, Giordano S, Schecter N (1994) Cloning of multiple forms of goldfish vimentin: Differential expression in CNS. J Neurochem 63: 470–481

Hammond EH, Yowell RL, Nunoda S, Menlove RL, Renlund DG, Bristow MR, Gay WA Jr, Jones KW, O'Connell JB (1989) Vascular (humoral) rejection in heart transplantation: pathologic observations and clinical implications. J Heart Transplant 8: 430–433

Hosenpud JD, Shipley GD, Wagner CR (1992) Cardiac allograft vasculopathy: Current concepts, recent developments, and future directions. J Heart Lung Transplant 11: 9–23

Hruban RH, Beschorner WE, Baumgartner WA (1990) Accelerated arteriosclerosis in heart transplant recipients is associated with a T-lymphocyte-mediated endothelialitis. Am J Pathol 137: 872–882

Johnson DE, Alderman EL, Schroeder JS, Gao S-Z, Hunt S, DeCampli WM, Stinson E, Billingham M (1991) J Am Coll Cardiol 17: 449–457

Kataaha PK, Mortazavi-Milani SM, Russel G, Holborow EJ (1985) Anti-intermediate filament antibodies, antikeratin antibody, and antiperinuclear factor in rheumatoid artheritis and infection mononucleosis. Ann Rheum Dis 44: 446–449

Khaghani A, Yacoub M, McCloskey D, Awad J, Burden M, Fitzgerald M, Hawes R, Holmes J, Smith J, Banner N et al. (1989) The influence of HLA matching, donor/recipient sex, and incidence of acute rejection on survival in cardiac allograft recipients receiving cyclosporine and azathioprine. Transplant Proc 21: 799–800

Koo EWY, Gottlieb AI (1989) Endothelial stimulation of intimal cell proliferation in a porcine aortic organ culture. Am J Pathol 134: 497–503

Kriett JM, Kaye MP (1990) The registry of the International Society for Heart Transplantation; Seventh official report – 1990. J Heart Transplant 9: 323–330

Kurki P, Virtanen I (1984) The detection of antibodies against cytoskeletal components. J Immunol Methods 67: 209–223

Kushwaha S, Maseri A, Mitchell A, Yacoub M (1991) Coronary reactivity in ergonovine: possible relationship to accelerated coronary arterial disease in cardiac transplant recipients. Eur Heart J 12: 524–525

Laden AMK (1972) The effects of treatment on the arterial lesions of rat and rabbit cardiac allografts. Transplantation 13: 281–290

Le WD, Xie WJ, Glenn Smith R, Appel SH (1993) Vimentin cross reactive antibodies induce cell death in primary cultures of embryonic spinal cord. J Neuroimmunol 42: 15–22

Minick CR, Murphy GE (1973) Experimental induction of atheroarteriosclerosis by the synergy of allergic injury to arteries and lipid-rich diet. Am J Pathol 73: 265–292

Nikkari ST, Solakivi T, Sisto T, Jaakola O (1993) Antibodies to cytoskeletal protein in sera of patients with angiographically assessed coronary artery disease. Atherosclerosis 98: 11–16

Oni AA, Ray JA, Norman DJ, Hershberger RA, Wagner Cr, Hovaguimian H, Cobanoglu A, Hosenpud JD (1991) Cardiac allograft venopathy: a correlate to "accelerated transplant atherosclerosis". J Heart Lung Transplant 10: 190 (abstract)

Page C, Rose M, Yacoub M, Pigott R (1992) Antigenic heterogeneity of vascular endothelium. Am J Pathol 141: 673–683

Pearson JD (1994) Autoantibodies to endothelial cells. In: Catravas JD (ed) Vascular endothelium. Plenum, New York

Pfeffer PF, Foerster A, Froysaker T, Simonsen S, Thorsby E (1988) HLA-DR mismatch and histologically evaluated rejection episodes in cardiac transplants can be correlated. Transplant Proc 20: 367–368

Pidwell DJ, Heller MJ, Gabler D, Orosz CG (1995) In vitro stimulation of human endothelial cells by sera from a subpopulation of high-percentage panel-reactive antibody patients. Transplantation 60: 563–569

Pinto FJ, Chenzbraun A, Gao S-Z, St Goar FG, Fischell T, Alderman EL (1993) Serial quantitative angiography and intracoronary ultrasound: do angiographic measurements match morphology? J Am Coll Cardiol 19: A192

Rose ML (1996) Role of antibody and indirect antigen presentation in transplant associated coronary artery vasculopathy. J Heart Lung Transplant 15: 342–349

Rose ML, Dunn MJ (1993) What causes accelerated coronary artery disease after cardiac transplantation? Prim Cardiol 19: 34–39

Rose ML, Coles MI, Griffin RJ, Pomerance A, Yacoub MH (1986) Expression of class I and class II major histocompatibility antigens in normal and transplanted heart. Transplantation 41: 776

Rose EA, Pepino P, Barr ML, Smith CR, Ratner AJ, Ho E, Berger C et al. (1992) Relation of HLA antibodies and graft atherosclerosis in human cardiac allograft recipients. J Heart Transplant 11: S120–123

Ross R (1986) The pathogenesis of atherosclerosis - an update. N Engl J Med 314: 488–500

Ross R, Glomset JA (1976) The pathogenesis of atherosclerosis. N Engl J Med 295: 369–377

Russell PS, Chase CM, Winn HJ, Colvin RB (1994) Coronary atherosclerosis in transplanted mouse hearts II. Importance of humoral immunity. J Immunol 154: 5135–5141

Salomon RN, Hughes CCW, Schoen FJ, Payne DD, Pober JS, Libby P (1991) Human coronary transplantation-associated arteriosclerosis: evidence of a chronic immune reaction to activated graft endothelial cells. Am J Pathol 138: 791–798

Schoen FJ, Libby P (1991) Cardiac transplant graft arteriosclerosis. Trends Cardiovasc Med 1: 216–223

Schook LB, Wood N, Mohanakumar T (1987) Identification of human vascular endothelial cell/monocyte antigenic system using monoclonal antibodies. Transplantation 44: 412–416

Schroeder JS, Gao S-Z (1995) Accelerated graft coronary artery disease in heart-transplant recipients. Coron Artery Dis 6: 226–233

Shirotani M, Yui Y, Kawai C (1993) Restenosis after coronary angioplasty: pathogenesis of neointimal thickening initiated by endothelial loss. Endothelium 1: 5–22

Speiser B, Weihrauch D, Reiss CF, Schaper J (1992) The extracellular matrix in human cardiac tissue. Part II: Vimentin, laminin, and fibronectin. Cardioscience 3: 41–49

St Goar FG, Pinto FJ, Alderman EL, Valantine HA, Schroeder JS, Gao S, Stinson EB, Popp RL (1992) Intracoronary ultrasound in cardiac transplant recipients. In vivo evidence of "angiographically silent" intimal thickening. Circulation 85: 979–987

Taylor PM, Rose ML, Yacoub MH (1993) Coronary artery immunogenicity: a comparison between explanted recipient or donor hearts and transplanted hearts. Transpl Immunol 1: 294–301

Taylor PM, Rose ML, Yacoub MH, Pigott R (1992) Induction of vascular adhesion molecules during rejection of human cardiac allografts. Transplantation 54: 451–457

Thorpe SJ (1990) Reactivity of a human monoclonal antibody against Rh D with intermediate filament protein vimentin. Br J Haematol 76: 116–120

Uretsky BF, Murali S, Reddy PS, Rabin B, Lee A, Griffith BP, Hardesty R, Trento A, Bahnson HT (1987) Development of coronary artery disease in cardiac transplant patients receiving immunosuppressive therapy with cyclosporine and prednisone. Circulation 76: 827–834

Wheeler CH, Collins A, Dunn MJ, Crisp SJ, Yacoub MH, Rose ML (1995) Characterization of endothelial antigens associated with transplant associated coronary artery disease. J Heart Lung Transplant 14: S188–S197

Wick G, Schett G, Amberger A, Kleindienst R, Xu Q (1995) Is atherosclerosis an immunologically mediated disease? Immunol Today 16: 27–33

Willems CH, Astyaldi GCB, De Groot G, Janssen MC, Gonsalvez MD, Zeijlemaker WP, Van Mourik JA, Van Aken WG (1982) Media conditioned by cultured human vascular endothelial cells inhibit the growth of vascular smooth muscle cells. Exp Cell Res 139: 191–197

Xu Q, Oberhuber G, Gruschwitz M, Wick G (1990) Immunology of atherosclerosis: cellular composition and major histocompatibility complex class II antigen presentation in aortic intima, fatty streaks, and atherosclerotic plaques in young and aged human specimens. Clin Immunol Immunopathol 56: 344–359

Xu Q, Dietrich H, Steiner HJ, Gown AM, Schoel B, Mikuz G, Kaufmann SH, Wick G (1992) Induction of arteriosclerosis in normocholesterolemic rabbits by immunization with heat shock protein 65. Arterioscler Thromb 12: 789–799

Xu Q, Willeit J, Marosi M, Kleindienst R, Oberhollenzer G, Kiechl S, Stulnig T, Luef G, Wick G (1993) Association of serum antibodies to heat-shock protein 65 with carotid atherosclerosis. Lancet 341: 255–259

Xu Q, Schett G, Seitz CS, Hu Y, Gupta RS, Wick G (1994) Surface staining and cytotoxic activity of heat-shock protein 60 antibody in stressed aortic endothelial cells. Circ Res 75: 1078–1085

Yacoub M, Rose M (1994) Accelerated coronary artery sclerosis. Ann Cardiac Surg 7: 80–88

Zerbe T, Arena V, Kormos RL, Griffith BP, Hardesty RL, Duquesnoy RJ (1991) Histocompatibility and other risk factors for histological rejection of human cardiac allografts during the first three months following transplantation. Transplantation 52: 485–490

Zerbe T, Uretsky B, Kormos R, Armitage J, Wolyn T, Griffith BP, Hardesty R, DuQuesnoy R (1992) Graft atherosclerosis: Effects of cellular rejection and human lymphocyte antigen. J Heart Lung Transplant 11: 104–110

Role of Ischemia/Reperfusion Injury in Organ Transplantation

H.-A. Lehr[1] and K. Messmer[2]

Introduction

Reperfusion of oxygenated blood into previously ischemic tissue is essential to prevent the progression of cellular injury due to the decreased nutritional blood flow, i.e., the decreased delivery of oxygen and metabolic substrates, as well as the removal of harmful metabolic byproducts. However, it has become obvious that reperfusion also initiates a complex series of pathologic events that contribute to, rather than prevent, further tissue damage. Moreover, a growing body of evidence indicates that ischemia/reperfusion injury is initiated by events that occur at the level of the microcirculation. In the first part of this overview, we will delineate the major components of the microcirculatory manifestations of ischemia reperfusion injury. In the second part, we will focus on a distinct pathophysiological condition in which these microcirculatory manifestations of ischemia/reperfusion injury are operative: the loss of long-term allograft function after organ transplantation.

Microvascular Manifestations of Post-ischemic Tissue Damage:

Ischemia-Induced Cell Swelling and Capillary Perfusion Failure (No-Reflow)

Mammalian cells possess a high intracellular osmotic colloidal pressure due to a higher concentration of protein intracellularly than extracellularly. To balance this, sodium is maintained at a concentration which is lower intracellularly than extracellularly. This cellular homeostasis depends on an energy-dependent sodium/potassium pump. Energy for this and for other cellular functions is provided by adenosine triphosphate (ATP), which is generated by oxidative phosphorylation provided the oxygen tension of the cell is maintained at a sufficiently high level. When blood flow is disrupted and nutritive perfusion of a tissue drops below a critical level, oxygen tension decreases, oxidative

---

[1]Institute of Pathology, Johannes Gutenberg University, Langenbedestr. 1, 55101 Mainz, Germany
[2]Institute for Surgical Research, University of Munich, Marchioninistr. 15, 81377 Munich, Germany

phosphorylation drops, and ATP generation ceases. When the cell loses its ability to maintain the sodium/potassium gradient, sodium accumulates and this is followed by an iso-osmotic influx of water. This results in cell swelling, one of the earliest and most prominent manifestations of ischemic injury.

Cessation of blood flow not only prevents oxygen and nutrients from reaching the tissue, but also prevents the drainage of cellular metabolites. Hence, a second mechanism of cellular swelling in ischemia is the increased intracellular osmotic load, due to the accumulation of catabolites, such as inorganic phosphates, lactate, and purine nucleosides. Finally, there is evidence that cell swelling may also be exacerbated by a sodium–hydrogen exchange process aimed at maintaining a normal intracellular pH [1].

The effects of ischemic cell swelling at the level of the microcirculation are crucially important to the survival of an ischemic tissue, since cellular swelling will further compromise nutritive tissue perfusion, at which point a vicious circle is initiated. Indeed, prolonged ischemia results in the swelling of myo-fibers [2], renal interstitial cells [3], as well as of capillary endothelial cells [3, 4]. In an elegant experimental approach, Mazzoni and coworkers used in-travital microscopy to measure the deformation of red blood cells passing through capillary lumina in skeletal muscle [5]. Using this technique, they found that during hemorrhagic shock, endothelial cells swell and significantly compromise the capillary lumen. Similar observations were later made in striated muscle of hamsters, in which a 4-h ischemia resulted in a significant narrowing of the capillary lumen [6].

The hydraulic resistance to flow in a blood vessel is dependent upon blood viscosity and the inverse of the lumen diameter to the fourth power. Hence, even very small changes in diameter will result in considerably larger changes in resistance to flow. This has a particular impact on capillaries, where the endothelial cell/vessel wall diameter ratio is higher than in any other vessel segment. Within the network of muscle capillaries, blood flow will immediately be shunted from vessel segments with high hydraulic resistance to segments with lower resistance. As a consequence, the heterogeneity of capillary blood perfusion increases [7]. Messmer and coworkers repeatedly demonstrated that as a consequence of prolonged ischemia, roughly 50% of capillaries are thus excluded from the circulation [6–13]. It is important to realise that this ex-clusion of capillaries from the circulation is induced by ischemia and is only minimally affected by reperfusion events. This notion is underscored in studies with the skinfold chamber preparation in hamsters, in which treatment with heparin, superoxide dismutase, or the antioxidant vitamin E almost entirely prevented the reperfusion-induced accumulation and adhesion of leukocytes within the post-ischemic muscle microcirculation, but at the same time had only a limited beneficial effect on the ischemia-induced loss of functional capillary density [7, 8, 10–12].

Reperfusion-Induced Leukocyte Accumulation and Breakdown of Endothelial Barrier Function (Reflow Paradox)

The chemotactic accumulation of circulating leukocytes and their adhesion to the endothelial lining of postcapillary venules have long been recognized as central features of post-ischemic reperfusion injury [9, 14–17]. The mechanisms underlying this leukocyte recruitment into the post-ischemic tissue are well characterized. They include the generation of reactive oxygen species (ROS) and a variety of inflammatory mediators, as well as the up-regulation of adhesion molecules (reviewed in [18]). Through the release of cytotoxic degranulation products, ROS, and inflammatory mediators, leukocytes can directly contribute to tissue damage and to the recruitment of further leukocytes into the post-ischemic tissue. A prominent feature of leukocyte-induced microvascular damage is the breakdown of endothelial cell barrier function, resulting in the leakage of fluid and macromolecules into the interstitial space. Through this mechanism, leukocytes have the potency to contribute to the increase in interstitial pressure and to exacerbate the precarious microvascular perfusion situation. The contribution of leukocytes to post-ischemic tissue damage has been impressively documented in experiments in which tissue damage was significantly attenuated by anti-CD18 antibodies [14] or by leukocyte depletion with Leukopak filters [15]. This finding was confirmed by Klausner et al., who demonstrated that reperfusion-induced increases in skeletal muscle lymph flow and protein concentration were significantly reduced in animals rendered neutropenic by treatment with hydroxyurea or nitrogen mustard [19]. Similarly, Belkin et al. significantly reduced post-ischemic muscle necrosis by radiation-induced neutropenia [20].

The most elegant and conclusive proof for the contribution of leukocytes to reperfusion injury was provided by experiments in which leukocyte adhesion was prevented by monoclonal antibodies directed against leukocyte adhesion molecules. The blocking of CD11b/CD18 adhesion molecules on leukocytes [21–23], or of the intracellular adhesion molecule 1 (ICAM-1) on endothelial cells [23] almost completely prevented leukocyte recruitment into post-ischemic tissue. Consequently, the post-ischemic breakdown of endothelial cell barrier function was blunted and edema formation was significantly reduced. In some tissues, post-ischemic edema may not be too much of a problem or cause for concern. However, in other organs such as liver, brain, and certain muscle groups, which are enclosed in a tight non-expandable compartment, edema may significantly endanger tissue viability by elevating interstitial tissue pressure above a critical point and thus compromising nutritional blood flow. Tissue necrosis, nerve compression, or rhabdomyolysis are the consequences.

The identification of the inflammatory mediators involved in post-ischemic leukocyte chemotaxis and adhesion has resulted in the conduction of a large series of experiments in which post-ischemic tissue damage in a variety of different organ systems was effectively reduced. A variety of pharmacological and dietary approaches have been taken which aimed at blocking the formation and/or action of inflammatory mediators such as complement [24], leukotrienes [17, 19], and platelet-activating factor [25]. In particular, the key role of ROS has been addressed in a series of studies in which reperfusion injury was blocked by scavengers of ROS [7, 8, 10, 11, 15, 27] and by antioxidants [12, 28].

In one recent study, we used intravital fluorescent microscopy to demonstrate that a simple dietary supplementation of animal diets with vitamin E has a significant inhibitory effect on post-ischemic leukocyte adhesion in striated skin muscle [12]. This study is of interest in two respects. Firstly, the maximal inhibitory effect on post-ischemic leukocyte adhesion was already fully expressed at very low vitamin E concentrations. Such concentrations of vitamin E have been added to the diets of laboratory animals by animal food manufacturers for the last few years. Vitamin supplements, which are meant to improve the health of laboratory animals, may have a negative impact on biomedical research since they also prevent the reproduction of pathophysiologically relevant experimental conditions in these animals. As shown in our study, a hamster which is fed with the standard (vitamin E-supplemented) laboratory diet is of no use for the study of ischemia/reperfusion injury. The second interesting point to be made from this study was our observation that inhibition of leukocyte adhesion during the immediate post-reperfusion period by vitamin E did not affect functional capillary density in the first 24 h after reperfusion (as expected from the studies delineated above). However, when we extended the observation period to 1 week, we observed that at days 3–7 after reperfusion, functional capillary density dropped significantly to 20% of baseline values in non-supplemented hamsters, but was maintained in vitamin E-supplemented animals at values that were not statistically significant from baseline values [12]. This suggests that the early inhibition of leukocyte adhesion may exert long-term effects on tissue viability which will most likely be missed in most experimental approaches with only a short-term (hours) observation follow-up period.

Allograft Arteriosclerosis – Rationale for the Use of Antioxidant Vitamins

The transplantation of a solid organ from an organ donor has emerged as a treatment option for many diseases that otherwise lead to death or long-term dependency on life support systems for the patient. The organs are usually obtained from brain-dead donors or from living-related or living-unrelated donors. Despite the shortage of organs for transplantation, careful attention is paid to the fact that only functionally intact, undamaged organs are used for transplantation. However, even with major improvements in the logistics of organ transplantation, surgical technique, preservation techniques, and preservation solutions, every transplantation starts with an inevitable insult on the graft: ischemia and reperfusion.

Prolonged ischemia results in initial non-functioning of the graft after transplantation, which has also been implicated as a clinical risk factor for the long-term loss of organ grafts [29–31]. In the early days of routine renal transplantation it was shown that the duration of warm ischemia had a major influence on long-term allograft function and survival: a 1- min increase in warm ischemia time was statistically correlated with a 1% decrease in the one-year graft survival [32]. Transplantation of organs from living donors (with short ischemia times) has a better long-term outcome compared with cadaveric transplants (with long ischemia times), even in the absence of optimal histocompatibility matching [33]. The most compelling clinical evidence for an impact of ischemia/reperfusion injury on long-term allograft survival has been obtained from a recent study which retrospectively correlated the histomorphological severity of ischemia/ reperfusion injury in early endomyocardial biopsies with long-term graft survival. In this study, the histomorphological degree of peri-transplant myocardial damage (attributed to ischemia/ reperfusion injury) emerged as the strongest predictor of the later development of accelerated transplant atherosclerosis [34].

The microvascular manifestations of ischemia/ reperfusion injury are basically identical in non-transplanted and in transplanted organs. Therefore it is not surprising that the very same therapeutic interventions that have been shown to protect non-transplanted organs from ischemia/ reperfusion injury are also protective in transplanted organs. In light of (i) the central role of leukocyte activation and adhesion in ischemia/ reperfusion injury (see above), and (ii) the demonstration that adhesion molecules are up-regulated in transplanted organs after ischemia and reperfusion (35, 36), blocking monoclonal antibodies against adhesion molecules on leukocytes and/or endothelial cells were tested. They were found to significantly reduce reperfusion injury in renal [37], lung [38], intestinal [39], and heart allografts [40], and also to improve early graft function and survival of the recipients. In an impressive experimental approach, the first ever to successfully use blocking monoclonal antibodies for a therapeutic purpose in humans, Haug and coworkers demonstrated that administration of blocking antibodies against ICAM-1 significantly improved the early function of renal allografts and reduced the incidence of allograft rejection episodes [41].

Inhibition of leukocyte infiltration and adhesion can not only be accomplished by blocking monoclonal antibodies, but also by antioxidants which inhibit the formation and/or action of ROS [7, 8, 16, 27, 42]. ROS are generated during ischemia and reperfusion and account for much of the subsequent microvascular dysfunction (see above). Several studies have demonstrated that pretreatment of animals with ROS scavengers and antioxidants, including the lipid-soluble antioxidant vitamin E, significantly attenuates ischemia/reperfusion damage in transplanted organs and extends allograft and animal survival times [43–49]. These findings have in the meantime been confirmed in clinical organ transplantation. Rabl and coworkers reported that pretreatment of 30 renal allograft recipients with an infusion of several antioxidant vitamins (vs. placebo) significantly blocked lipid peroxidation after transplantation and also significantly improved early allograft function in the vitamin-treated group, as judged from significantly lower creatinine levels, and improved creatinine clearance rates [50]. Although these experimental and clinical studies provide compelling evidence for the impact of ROS and leukocytes on ischemia/reperfusion injury of transplanted organs, they do not help to explain by which mechanism ischemia/ reperfusion injury contributes to long-term allograft failure.

It has been suggested that ischemia and reperfusion up-regulate the expression of major histocompatibility complex (MHC) molecules, particularly class II, thus rendering post-ischemic allografts more immunogenic [51]. Indeed, temporary ischemia was found to significantly up-regulate the expression of MHC class I and class II expression in mouse kidneys compared with the contralateral non-ischemic kidney [52], and also to up-regulate MHC expression in canine lung allografts [53]. Increased expression of MHC antigens leads to a more effective T-cell recognition and the corresponding effector responses [54]. The cytotoxic T-cell response of the recipient against the transplanted organ may be further enhanced by another reperfusion-induced event: the ROS-mediated inactivation of nitric oxide [55]. Nitric oxide has several important roles in the regulation of cardiovascular parameters (reviewed in [56]). Among other important activities it counteracts platelet aggregation and leukocyte adhesion to endothelial cells [57, 58] and also significantly inhibits the development of an allospecific cytotoxic lymphocyte response [59]. Consequently, inhibition of nitric oxide significantly increase the mitogen-induced proliferation of lymphocytes [60].

Taken together, ischemia/reperfusion injury could augment the immunogenicity of transplanted organs by inducing the expression of MHC antigens and/or by enhancing cytotoxic lymphocyte responses. However, a look at the cumulative renal allograft survival curves over the last 15 years indicates that while the improvement of immunosuppression (in particular, the introduction of cyclosporin in the early 1980s) has significantly increased the 1 year allograft survival of transplanted allografts, it has not affected the steady loss of grafts after the first year [30]. This steady loss of allografts (around 6% per year) has been ascribed to chronic rejection. Chronic rejection of transplants has been defined as progressive functional deterioration, occurring months to years after grafting and is associated with characteristic morphologic changes in the vascular tree [61–63]. The vascular histopathology results from infiltration of the intima by mononuclear cells, migration and proliferation of smooth muscle cells and fibroblasts from the media into the intima, and subsequent deposition of extracellular matrix [63].

Despite minor differences in the contribution of individual factors to the generation of "classical" atherosclerosis and the accelerated atherosclerosis occurring in transplanted organs, the basic underlying pathomechanisms are similar. According to the "response to injury" hypothesis of atherogenesis, two important players in atherogenesis are leukocytes (in particular mononuclear cells, which enter the vessel wall and provide the morphological basis for the formation of foam cells) and smooth muscle cells, which migrate and proliferate in response to diverse mediators, cytokines, and growth factors [64]. Indeed, the mediators involved in leukocyte recruitment into the vessel wall during atherogenesis are similar to the mediators involved in leukocyte adhesion during ischemia reperfusion injury. Likewise, the adhesion molecules expressed in early atherosclerotic lesions [65–67] conform largely to the adhesion molecules expressed during ischemia/ reperfusion injury of rat and human allografts [36, 68]. Duijvestijn and coworkers documented the up-regulated expression of ICAM-1 and lymphocyte function associated antigen-1/

CD18 during chronic rejection of rat renal allografts [68]. Besides ROS, which have been shown to directly stimulate smooth muscle cell proliferation [69], several other mediators that have been implicated in smooth muscle proliferation [64, 70] are generated in post-ischemic tissue [71–73]. In agreement with these findings, Yilmaz and coworkers demonstrated that prolonged warm ischemia of rat renal allografts predisposes to allograft loss due to chronic atherosclerosis and vascular obliteration [74]. Similar observations were made in rat renal isografts subjected to temporary ischemia [75]. Later, Wanders and coworkers observed in an aortic transplantation model in rats that the duration of transplant ischemia significantly correlated with the severity of transplant arteriosclerosis [76].

Compelling clinical confirmation of the concept that ischemia/reperfusion injury affects long-term allograft function has been provided by Land and coworkers. They found a significant improvement in renal allograft survival at 4 years after transplantation in patients who had received a single injection of superoxide dismutase immediately prior to reperfusion of the transplanted kidney [77]. These results are of particular importance in that no significant improvement by superoxide dismutase treatment had been observed in these same patients during the first year of clinical follow-up [78]. Although no histological confirmation was presented (no routine renal biopsy protocol), the authors speculate that superoxide dismutase treatment reduced the severity of ischemia/ reperfusion injury and thus disrupted one or several of the mechanisms by which ischemia/ reperfusion injury predisposes to accelerated transplant atherosclerosis [77].

The generation and action of ROS during ischemia and reperfusion of transplanted organs can not only be blocked pharmacologically (for example by superoxide dismutase, catalase, or other scavenging or antioxidant molecules), but can also be counteracted effectively by simple dietary supplementation with antioxidant vitamins, such as the water-soluble vitamin C (ascorbic acid) and the lipid-soluble vitamin E (alpha-tocopherol). As mentioned above, antioxidant vitamins have been used both in experimental models and in clinical renal transplantation to effectively inhibit the severity of reperfusion injury and to improve short-term allograft function and survival [43–50]. Unfortunately, not a single study has focused on the long-term outcome of allograft transplantation in the investigation of the potential impact of antioxidant vitamins on allograft atherosclerosis. It is known from experimental models as well as from data obtained from human allograft recipients that antioxidant vitamins are consumed during reperfusion injury of transplanted grafts [46, 48, 79–81], and that the lipid peroxidation observed after reperfusion can be effectively prevented with antioxidant vitamins, both in animal models [46] and in patients [50]. Furthermore it is known from animal studies that antioxidant vitamins significantly improve early allograft function and both graft and animal survival [44–46, 49]. Yet, far too little attention is paid to the antioxidant status in patients undergoing organ transplantation or who are on a waiting list for organ transplantation. This is dramatically emphasized in a recent report on antioxidant vitamin levels in liver allograft recipients. Even before transplantation, the circulating levels of the antioxidant vitamins A and E, and of carotene and lycopene were significantly lower in these patients than in normal controls. In some patients, carotene and lycopene levels were so low that they could not be measured [81]. As a consequence of the lack of adequate antioxidant protection, levels of thiobarbituric-acid-reactive substances were significantly elevated even before transplantation as evidenced by the increased lipid peroxidation products formed in the circulation of these patients [81]. As previously described in animal models, antioxidant vitamin blood levels dropped even further in human renal and liver allograft recipients [81, 82]. These data are particularly disturbing in light of our knowledge (see above) that (i) antioxidant vitamins have the ability to protect the allograft from damage during ischemia/ reperfusion injury at the time of transplantation, that (ii) the most prominent reason for late allograft loss is the development of atherosclerosis within the organ, and that (iii) blood levels of antioxidant vitamins correlate significantly with the development of atherosclerosis in large epidemiological surveys [83–85]. We believe that clinical studies are warranted to thoroughly test the impact of antioxidant vitamin supplementation in patients on the waiting list for allograft transplantation on parameters of short-term and long-term function and survival after clinical organ transplantation.

Summary

We have delineated the microcirculatory manifestations of ischemia/ reperfusion injury in this review. Microcirculatory injury is characterized by (i) a reduction in functional capillary density (due to ischemia-induced cell swelling), and (ii) the accumulation and adhesion of circulating leukocytes, and the subsequent breakdown of the endothelial cell barrier function at the level of postcapillary venules (reperfusion-associated events). We have demonstrated that the severity of ischemia/reperfusion injury can be effectively attenuated by blocking adhesion molecules and/or inflammatory mediators, including ROS. In particular, the beneficial role of antioxidant vitamins was emphasized. In the second part, we have discussed a clinical condition in which the mechanisms of ischemia/ reperfusion injury are operative: the transplantation of solid organs. We have presented arguments for the concept that ischemia/ reperfusion injury contributes not only to the early non-function and loss of allografts in organ transplantation, but also to the late loss of allografts due to the development of accelerated graft atherosclerosis. Finally, we have discussed a rationale for the prophylactic/therapeutic use of antioxidant vitamins in experimental and clinical transplantation, aimed at improving both short-term and long-term allograft function and viability.

References

1. Cala PM, Anderson SE, Cragoe EJ (1988) Na/H exchange-dependent cell volume and pH regulation and disturbances. Comp Biochem Physiol Physiol 90A: 551–555
2. Nakayama S, Kramer GC, Carlsen RC, Holcroft JW (1985) Infusion of very hypertonic saline to bled rats: membrane potentials and fluid shifts. J Surg Res 38: 180–186
3. Flores J, DiBona DR, Beck CH, Leaf A (1972) The role of cell swelling in ischemic renal damage and the protective effect of hypertonic solute. J Clin Invest 51: 118–126
4. Gidlöf A, Lewis DH, Hammersen F (1987) The effect of prolonged total ischemia on the ultrastructure of human skeletal muscle capillaries. A morphometric analysis. Int J Microcirc Clin Exp 7: 67–86
5. Mazzoni MC, Borgstrom P, Intaglietta M, Arfors KE (1989) Lumenal narrowing and endothelial cell swelling in skeletal muscle capillaries during hemorrhagic shock. Circ Shock 29: 27–29
6. Nolte D, Bayer M, Lehr HA, Becker M, Krombach F, Kreimeier U, Messmer K (1992) Attenuation of post-ischemic microvascular disturbances in striated muscle by hyperosmolar saline dextran. Am J Physiol 263: H1411–H1416
7. Menger MD, Steiner D, Messmer K (1992) Microvascular ischemia-reperfusion injury in striated muscle: significance of "no-reflow". Am J Physiol 263: H1892–H1900
8. Messmer K, Sack FU, Menger MD, Bartlett R, Barker JH, Hammersen F (1988) White cell-endothelium interaction during postischemic reperfusion of skin skeletal muscle. Adv Exp Med Biol 242: 95–98
9. Lehr HA, Hübner C, Nolte D, Kohlschütter A, Messmer K (1991) Dietary fish oil blocks the microcirculatory manifestations of ischemia-reperfusion injury in striated muscle in hamsters. Proc Natl Acad Sci USA 88: 6726–6730
10. Menger MD, Pelikan S, Steiner D, Messmer K (1992) Microvascular ischemia-reperfusion injury in striated muscle: significance of "reflow paradox". Am J Physiol 263: H1901–H1906
11. Becker M, Menger MD, Lehr HA (1994) Heparin-released superoxide dismutase inhibits post-ischemic leukocyte adhesion to venular endothelium. Am J Physiol 267: H925–H930
12. Willy C, Thiery J, Menger MD, Messmer K, Arfors KE, Lehr HA (1995) Impact of vitamin E supplement in standard laboratory animal diet on microvascular manifestation of ischemia/reperfusion injury. Free Radic Biol Med 19: 919–926
13. Nolte D, Menger MD, Messmer K (1995) Microcirculatory models of ischaemia-reperfusion in skin and striated muscle. Int J Microcirc Clin Exp 15 (Suppl): 9–16
14. Hernandez LA, Grisham MB, Twohig B, Arfors KE, Harlan JM, Granger DN (1987) Role of neutrophils in ischemia-reperfusion-induced microvascular injury. Am J Physiol 253: H699–H703
15. Korthuis RJ, Grisham MB, Granger DN (1988) Leukocyte depletion attenuates vascular injury in post-ischemic skeletal muscle. Am J Physiol 254: H823–H827
16. Granger DN, Benoit JN, Suzuki M, Grisham MB (1989) Leukocyte adherence to venular endothelium during ischemia-reperfusion. Am J Physiol 257: G683–G688
17. Lehr HA, Guhlmann A, Nolte D, Keppler D, Messmer K (1991) Leukotrienes as mediators in ischemia-reperfusion injury in a microcirculation model in the hamster. J Clin Invest 87: 2036–2041
18. Granger DN, Kubes P (1994) The microcirculation and inflammation: modulation of leukocyte/endothelial cell adhesion. J Leukoc Biol 55: 662–675
19. Klausner JM, Paterson IS, Valeri CR, Shepri D, Hechtman HB (1988) Limb ischemia-induced increase in permeability is mediated by leukocytes and leukotrienes. Ann Surg 208: 755–760
20. Belkin M, LaMorte ML, Wright JG, Hobson RW (1989) The role of leukocytes in the pathophysiology of skeletal muscle ischemic injury. J Vasc Surg 10: 14–17
21. Carden DL, Smith JK, Korthuis RJ (1990) Neutrophil-mediated microvascular dysfunction in post-ischemic canine skeletal muscle. Role of granulocyte adherence. Circ Res 66: 1436–1444
22. Jerome SN, Akimitsu T, Korthuis RJ (1994) Leukocyte adhesion, edema, and development of post-ischemic capillary no-reflow. Am J Physiol 267: H1329–H1336

23. Nolte D, Hecht R, Schmid P, Botzlar A, Menger MD, Neumüller C, Sinowatz F, Vestweber D, Messmer K (1994) Role of Mac-1 and ICAM-1 in ischemia-reperfusion injury in a microcirculation model of BALB/C mice. Am J Physiol 267: H1320–H1328

24. Maroko RP, Carpenter CB, Chiariello M, Fishbein MC, Radvany P, Knostman JD, Hale SL (1978) Reduction of cobra venom factor of myocardial necrosis after coronary artery occlusion. J Clin Invest 61: 661–670

25. Kubes P, Ibbotson G, Russell J, Wallace JL, Granger DN (1990) Role of platelet-activating factor in ischemia/reperfusion-induced leukocyte adherence. Am J Physiol 259: G300–G305

26. Korthuis RJ, Granger DN, Townsley MI, Taylor AE (1985) The role of oxygen free radicals in ischemia-induced increases in canine skeletal muscle vascular permeability. Circ Res 57: 599–609

27. Suzuki M, Inauen W, Kvietys RP, Grisham MB, Meininger C, Schelling ME, Granger HJ, Granger DN (1989) Superoxide mediates reperfusion-induced leukocyte–endothelial cell interactions. Am J Physiol 257: H1740–H1745

28. Takenaka M, Tatsukawa Y, Dohi K, Ezaki H, Matsukawa K, Kawasaki T (1981) Protective effects of alpha-tocopherol and coenzyme Q10 on warm ischemic damages in the rat kidney. Transplantation 32: 137–141

29. Cho YW, Terasaki PI, Graver B (1989) Fifteen-year kidney graft survival. In: Terasaki P (ed) Clinical Transplants 1989. Los Angeles UCLA Tissue Typing Laboratory, pp 325–331

30. Foster MC, Wenham PW, Rowe PA, Burden RP, Morgan AG, Cotton RE, Blamey RW (1989) The late results of renal transplantation and the importance of chronic rejection as a cause of graft loss. Ann R Coll Surg Engl 71: 44–47

31. Halloran P, Aprile MA, Farewell V, Ludwin D, Smith EK, Tsai SY, Bear RA, Cole EH, Fenton SS, Cattran DC (1988) Factors influencing early renal function in cadaver kidney transplants. Transplantation 45: 122–127

32. Van Es A, Hermans J, Van Bockel JH, Persijn GG, van Hooff JP, de Graeff J (1983) Effect of warm ischemia time and HLA (A and B) matching on renal cadaveric graft survival and rejection episodes. Transplantation 36: 255–258

33. Matas A, Gillingham KJ, Sutherland DER (1993) Half-life and risk factors for kidney transplant outcome – importance of death with function. Transplantation 55: 757–761

34. Gaudin PB, Rayburn BK, Hutchins GM, Kasper EK, Baugham KL, Goodman SN, Lecks LE, Baumgartner WA, Hruban RH (1994) Peritransplant injury to the myocardium associated with the development of acccelerated arteriosclerosis in heart transplant recipients. Am J Surg Pathol 18: 338–346

35. Scoazec JY, Durnad F, Degott C, Delautier D, Bernuau J, Belghiti J, Benhamou JP, Feldmann G (1994) Expression of cyclosporine-dependent adhesion molecules in post-reperfusion biopsy specimens of liver antigens. Gastroenterology 107: 1094–1102

36. Briscoe DM, Yeung AC, Schoen FJ, Allred EN, Stavrakis G, Ganz P, Cotran RS, Pober JS, Schoen EL (1995) Predictive value of inducible endothelial cell adhesion molecule expression for acute rejection of human cardiac allografts. Transplantation 59: 204–211

37. Cosimi AB, Conti D, Delmonico FL, Preffer FI, Wee SL, Rothlein R, Faanes R, Colvin RB (1990) In vivo effects of monoclonal antibody to ICAM-1 (CD54) in nonhuman primates with renal allografts. J Immunol 144: 4604–4612

38. Imaizumi T (1994) Effect of antibodies against neutrophil and endothelial adhesion molecules on reperfusion injury after pulmonary ischemia. Transplant Proc 26: 1851–1854

39. Slocum MM, Granger DN (1993) Early mucosal and microvascular changes in feline intestinal transplants. Gastroenterology 105: 1761–1768

40. Isobe M, Yagita H, Okumura K, Ihara A (1993) Specific acceptance of cardiac allograft after treatment with antibodies to ICAM-1 and LFA-1. Science 255: 1125–1127

41. Haug CE, Colvin RB, Delmonico FL, Auchincloss H, Tolkoff-Rubin N, Preffer FI, Rothlein R, Norris S, Scharschmidt L, Cosimi AB (1993) A phase I trial on immunosuppression with anti-ICAM-1 (CD54) mAb in renal allograft recipients. Transplantation 55: 766–773

42. Marzi I, Knee J, Buhren V, Menger M, Trentz O (1992) Reduction by superoxide dismutase of leukocyte-endothelial cell adherence after liver transplantation. Surgery 111: 90–97

43. Toledo-Pereyra LH, Simmons RL, Najarian JS (1975) Protection of the ischemic liver by donor pre-treatment before transplantation. J Surg Res 129: 513–517

44. Demirbas A, Bozoklu S, Özdemir A, Bilgin N, Haberal M (1993) Effect of alpha tocopherol on the prevention of reperfusion injury caused by free oxygen radicals in the canine kidney autotransplantation model. Transplant Proc 25: 2274
45. Tanemoto K, Sakagami K, Orita K (1993) Beneficial effect of EPC-K1 on the survival of warm ischemic damaged graft in rat cardiac transplantation. Acta Med Okayama 47: 121–127
46. Ikeda M, Sumimoto K, Urushihara T, Fukuda Y, Dohi K, Kawasaki T (1994) Prevention of ischemic damage in rat pancreatic transplantation by pretreatment with alpha tocopherol. Transplant Proc 26: 561–562
47. Rao PN, Walsh TR, Makowka L, Liu T, Demitris AJ, Rubin RS, Snyder JT, Mischinger HJ, Starzl TE (1990) Inhibition of free radical generation and improved survival by protection of the hepatic microvascular endothelium by targeted erythrocytes in orthotopic liver transplantation. Transplantation 49: 1055–1059
48. Oda T, Nakai I, Mituo M, Yamagashi H, Oka T, Yoshikawa Y (1992) Role of oxygen radicals and synergistic effect of superoxide dismutase and catalase on ischemia-reperfusion injury of the rat pancreas. Transplant Proc 24: 797–798
49. Slakey D, Roza A, Pieper G, Johnson C, Adams M (1993) Ascorbic acid and alpha tocopherol prolong rat cardiac allograft survival. Transplant Proc 25: 610–611
50. Rabl H, Khoschsorur G, Colombo T, Petritsch P, Rauchenwald M, Költringer P, Tatzber F, Esterbauer H (1993) A multivitamin infusion prevents lipid peroxidation and improves transplantation performance. Kidney Int 43: 912–917
51. Shackleton CR, Ettinger SL, McLoughlin MC, Scudamore CH, Miller RR, Keown PA (1990) Effect of recovery from ischemia injury on class I and class II MHC antigen expression. Transplantation 49: 641–644
52. Shoskes DA, Parfrey NA, Halloran PF (1990) Increased major histocompatibility complex antigen expression in unilateral ischemia acute tubular necrosis in the mouse. Transplantation 49: 201–207
53. Adoumie R, Serrick C, Giaid A, Shennib H (1992) Early cellular events in the lung allograft. Ann Thorac Surg 54: 1071–1076
54. Bishop GA, Waugh JA, Hall BM (1988) Expression of HLA antigens on renal tubular cells in culture: II. Effect of increased HLA antigen expression on tubular cell stimulation of lymphocyte activation and on their vulnerability to cell-mediated lysis. Transplantation 46: 303–310
55. Beckman JS, Beckman TW, Chen J, Marshall PA, Freeman BA (1990) Apparent hydroxyl radical production by peroxynitrite: implications for endothelial injury from nitric oxide and superoxide. Proc Natl Acad Sci USA 87: 1620–1624
56. Dusting GJ (1995) Nitric oxide in cardiovascular disorders. J Vasc Res 32: 143–161
57. Kubes P, Kanwar S, Niu XF, Gaboury J (1993) Nitric oxide synthesis inhibition induces leukocyte adhesion via superoxide and mast cells. FASEB J 7: 1293–1299
58. Langher JM, Hoffman R, Lancaster JR, Simmons R (1993) Nitric oxide – a new endogenous immunomodulator. Transplantation 55: 1205–1212
59. Langher JM, Dull KE, Ochoa J, Billiar T, Ildstad S, Schaut W, Simmons R, Hoffman R (1992) Evidence that nitric oxide production in in vivo allosensitized cells inhibits the development of allospecific CTL. Transplantation 53: 632–640
60. Mills GD (1991) Molecular basis of "suppressor" macrophages. Arginine metabolism via the nitric oxide synthase pathway. J Immunol 146: 2719–2723
61. Häyry P, Isoniemi H, Yilmaz S, Mennander A, Lernstrom K, Räisänen-Sokolowski A, Koskinen P, Ustinov J, Lautenschlager I, Taskinen E (1993) Chronic allograft rejection Immunol Rev 134: 33–81
62. Azuma H, Tilney NL (1994) Chronic graft rejection. Curr Opin Immunol 6: 770–776
63. Fellström (1995) Vascular mechanisms in the development of chronic rejection. Prog Appl Microcirc 21: 92–99
64. Ross R (1993) Atherosclerosis: a defense mechanism gone awry. Am J Pathol 143: 987–1002
65. Poston RN, Haskard DO, Coucher JR, Gall NP, Johnson-Tidey RR (1992) Expression of intracellular adhesion molecule-1 in atherosclerotic plaques. Am J Pathol 140: 665–673

66. Azuma H, Heemann UW, Tillius SG, Tilney NL (1994) Cytokines and adhesion molecules in chronic rejection. Clin Transplant 8: 168–180
67. Gimbrone MA (1995) Vascular endothelium: an integrator of pathophysiologic stimuli in atherosclerosis. Am J Cardiol 75: 67B–70B
68. Duijvestijn A, Kok M, Miyasaka M, Vriesman PV (1993) ICAM-1 and LFA-1/CD18 expression in chronic renal allograft rejection. Transplant Proc 25: 2867–2868
69. Rao GN, Berk BC (1992) Active oxygen species stimulate vascular smooth muscle cell growth and proto-oncogene expression. Circ Res 70: 593–599
70. Häyry P, Alatalo S, Myllärniemi M, Räisänen-Sokolowski A, Lernström K (1995) Cellular and Molecular Biology of chronic rejection. Transplant Proc 27: 71–74
71. Vender RL, Clemmons DR, Kwock L, Friedman M (1987) Reduced oxygen tension induces pulmonary endothelium to release pulmonary smooth muscle cell mitogen(s). Am Rev Respir Dis 135: 622–627
72. Hassoun PM, Pasricha PJ, Teufel E, Lee SL, Fanburg BL (1989) Hypoxia stimulates the release by bovine pulmonary artery endothelial cells of an inhibitor of pulmonary artery smooth muscle cell growth. Am J Respir Cell Mol Biol 1: 377–384
73. Michiels C, De Leener F, Arnould T, Dieu M, Remacle J (1994) Hypoxia stimulates human endothelial cells to release smooth muscle cell mitogens: role of prostaglandins and bFGF. Exp Cell Res 213: 43–54
74. Yilmaz S, Paavonen T, Häyry P (1992) Chronic rejection of rat kidney allografts. II. The impact of prolonged ischemia on transplant histology. Transplantation 53: 823–827
75. Tullius SG, Heemann U, Hancock WW, Azuma H, Tilney NL (1994) Long-term kidney isografts develop functional and morphologic changes that mimic those of chronic allograft rejection. Ann Surg 220: 425–435
76. Wanders A, Akyürek MI, Waltenberger J, Ren ZP, Stafberg C, Funa K, Larsson E, Fellström B (1995) Ischemia-induced transplant arteriosclerosis in the rat. Arterioscler Thromb Vasc Biol 15: 145–155
77. Land W, Schneeberger H, Schleibner S, Illner WD, Abendroth D, Rutili G, Arfors KE, Messmer K (1994) The beneficial effect of human recombinant superoxide dismutase on acute and chronic rejection events in recipients of cadaveric renal transplants. Transplantation 57: 211–217
78. Schneeberger H, Illner WD, Abendroth D, Bulkley G, Rutili F, Williams M, Thiel M, Land W (1989) First clinical experience with superoxide dismutase in kidney transplantation: results of a double-blind randomized study. Transplant Proc 121: 1245–1246
79. Marubayashi S, Dohi K, Sunimoto K, Oku J, Ochi K, Kawasaki T (1989) Changes in activity of oxygen free radical scavengers and in levels of endogenous antioxidants during hepatic ischemia and subsequent reperfusion. Transplant Proc 21: 1317–1318
80. Serino F, Citterio F, Lippa S, Oradei A, Agnes S, Nanni G, Pozzetto A, Littarru G, Castagneto M (1990) Coenzyme Q, alpha tocopherol and delayed function in human kidney transplantation. Transplant Proc 22: 1375–1378
81. Goode HF, Webster NR, Howdle PD, Leek JP, Lodge JPA, Sadek SA, Walker BE (1994) Reperfusion injury, antioxidants and hemodynamics during orthotopic liver transplantation. Hepatology 19: 354–359
82. Princemail J, Defraigne JO, Franssen C, Bonnet P, Deby-Dupont G, Pirenne J, Deby C, Lamy M, Limet M, Meurisse M (1993) Evidence for free radical formation during human kidney transplantation. Free Radic Biol Med 15: 343–348
83. Riemersma RA, Wood DA, Macintyre CCA, Elton RA, Gey KF, Oliver MF (1991) Risk of angina pectoris and plasma concentrations of vitamins A, C, and E and carotene. Lancet 337: 1–5
84. Enstrom JE, Kanim LE, Klein MA (1992) Vitamin C intake and mortality among a sample of the United States population. Epidemiology 3: 194–202
85. Gey KF, Moser UK, Jordan P, Stählin HB, Eichholzer M, Lüdin E (1993) Increased risk of cardiovascular disease at suboptimal plasma concentrations of essential antioxidants: an epidemiologic update with special attention to carotene and vitamin C. Am J Clin Nutr 57 (Suppl): 787S–797S

The Role of NO Synthases in Immunological Diseases: Importance for Left Ventricular Function

M. Kelm[1] and B. Yilmaz[2]

Introduction

Considering the biological effects of nitric oxide (NO) in the heart and thus its pathophysiological significance in cardiac diseases four major compartments have to be discerned: the blood within the coronary circulation, endocardial and coronary endothelial cells, coronary smooth muscle cells, and cardiomyocytes (see Fig. 1). In contrast, cardiac fibroblasts do not appear to synthesize NO [1]. Under baseline conditions nitric oxide is continuously synthesized from L-arginine within the vascular endothelium. It is released to the luminal side where it inhibits the adhesion of platelets, monocytes and neutrophils, all of which play a key role in the development of an atherosclerotic lesion [2–6]. In addition, NO is also released to the abluminal side where it exerts short-term and long-term effects on coronary vasculature and thus represents an important modulator of coronary vascular tone [7, 8]. Furthermore, NO is capable of modulating cardiac contractility, not only by its effects on coronary flow, but also via direct effects on cardiomyocytes [9, 10]. In addition, preliminary data suggest that NO modulates the release of norepinephrine from cardiac neurons, thus affecting cardiac contractility [2, 11].

Formation of NO by NO Synthases

NO formed within the heart can be synthesized by two different isoforms of NO synthase, the constitutively expressed cNOS and the inducible iNOS [11]. The cNOS, first described in vascular endothelium, continuously produces NO from L-arginine in the low nanomolar range. Basal levels can be increased rapidly and severalfold by stimuli such as acetylcholine, bradykinin, and most importantly by shear stress. In contrast, the inducible enzyme iNOS is only expressed after immunological stimuli, such as lipopolysaccharides and cytokines. Most importantly, the amounts of NO produced by iNOS are a hundred- to a thousandfold higher than those produced by the cNOS. Within the heart, the

---
[1]Department of Medicine, Division of Cardiology, Pneumology, Angiology, Heinrich Heine University, Moorenstr. 5, 40225 Düsseldorf, Germany
[2]Department of Pharmacology, Ege University, 53100 Bornova, Izmir, Turkey

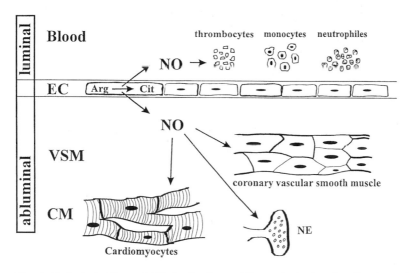

Fig. 1. Biological effects of NO in the heart. NO synthesized at baseline by cNOS and in response to inflammatory stimuli by the iNOS modulates endothelial adhesiveness, coronary blood flow, contractility of cardiomyocytes and cardiac sympathetic activity. *EC*, endothelial cell; *VSM*, vascular smooth muscle cell, *CM*, cardiomyocytes; *NE*, norepinephrine (released from synapses)

cNOS is found in vascular endothelium and most likely also in cardiomyocytes, although the latter is still a matter of debate [12, 13]. iNOS can be expressed in all four major compartments: in macrophages, coronary endothelial and smooth muscle cells, and in cardiomyocytes. Thus, the cardiac effects of NO depend critically on the site and type of stimulated NO synthase.

Metabolism of NO

Apart from its rate of formation, the localized effects of NO within the heart are also dictated by its metabolism [14]. For instance, the dilatory action of NO can be blunted by a disturbed diffusion due to increased wall thickness, a selective resistance of vascular smooth muscle or an enhanced inactivation of NO by, for example, oxyhemoglobin and oxygen-derived radicals [15]. Thus, an exact knowledge of the metabolism of NO is mandatory in order to understand the regulation of its biological effects.

In aqueous solutions, the half-life of NO critically depends on the oxygen tension and ranges from 4–7 s [16]. During single passage through the coronary circulation of isolated saline perfused hearts, NO is also degraded to nitrite, but with a considerably shorter half-life (< 1 s [8, 17]. This indicates that within the heart a mechanism exists which inactivates NO extremely rapidly. In blood, NO is first converted to nitrite, but this unstable intermediate is rapidly further converted to nitrate within the erythrocytes [18, 19]. Thus, within the heart, NO appears to act more as an autocrine than as a paracrine or endocrine messenger. It is exactly this rapid metabolism which hampers quantification of the *L*-arginine–NO–pathway in humans.

Physiological Significance of NO for Left Ventricular Function

NO modulates left ventricular function either via the regulation of coronary blood flow or directly via a reduction in cardiomyocyte contractility. The effects of exogenously applied NO on coronary flow (CF) and left ventricular pressure (LVP) in isolated constant pressure perfused hearts are depicted in Fig. 2. In the range of 1 n*M*–1µ*M*, NO increased coronary flow in a dose-dependent manner, whereas LVP remained unaffected. Only slightly higher concentrations of NO decreased LVP. In the concentration range from 3 to 100 µ*M*, NO significantly decreased LVP. Thus, exogenous NO depresses cardiac contractility at concentrations which potentially can be reached by both iso-

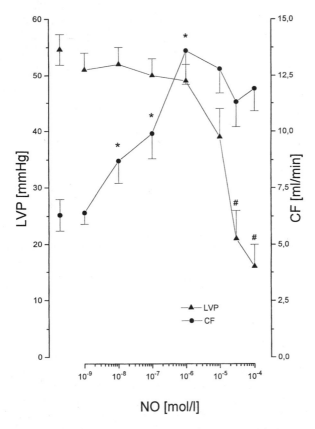

Fig. 2. Effect of NO on coronary flow (*CF*) and left ventricular pressure (*LVP*) in isolated constant-pressure-perfused guinea pig hearts; *n* = 7; mean ± SEM. *, significant difference from control for CF; #, significant difference from control for CVP

forms of NO synthase. Concomitantly, CF decreased, a surprising and as yet unexplained finding. Nevertheless, the decrease in LVP cannot be explained by a critical coronary vasoconstriction as CF at the highest NO concentration is still well above control levels. NO probably exerts its negative inotropic effects directly since neither nitrite nor nitrate influences coronary flow of LVP. No significant decrease in oxygen tension or pH were observed during intracoronary infusion of NO.

Mechanism of NO-Induced Negative Inotropic Effects

Based on experiments performed with isolated cardiomyocytes [20, 21] it was postulated that the negative inotropic effect of NO is mediated, at least in part, by the stimulation of guanylyl cyclase which is the principal target enzyme for NO in many biological systems. In the vasodilatory effective range of NO (as depicted in Fig. 2) we indeed found a concentration-dependent increase in cGMP release: from 360 ± 76 to 1602 ± 312 fmol/min. We cannot discern which proportion of this cGMP is derived from coronary endothelium, smooth muscle or cardiomyocytes, all of which contain guanylyl cyclase. However, at high and negative inotropic concentrations of NO no correlation between cGMP release and decrease in LVP was observed: cGMP release remained constant despite a decreasing contractility. Furthermore, there was a dissociation in the kinetics between NO effects and cGMP release. After cessation of NO infusion, LVP reached control levels within 5 s, whereas cGMP release remained elevated for more than 5 min. These findings argue against a role for cGMP in mediating the negative effects of NO on contractility of cardiomyocytes, at least in our preparation.

Since some data in the literature indicate that NO might modulate norepinephrine release from peripheral nerves [22], we tested the hypothesis that the negative effect of NO on cardiac contractility is mediated by an altered release of norepinephrine. Spillover of norepinephrine into the coronary circulation was measured as a crude index for cardiac formation and release of norepinephrine. However, no significant changes in cardiac release of norepinephrine were observed during infusion of NO. Thus, the negative inotropic effect of NO did not appear to be mediated by an altered metabolism of catecholamines within the heart.

Formation of adenosine represents a sensitive and reliable marker of myocardial energy levels [23–25]. We observed that NO leads to a huge increase in cardiac release of adenosine only at those concentrations which exert negative inotropic effects. The amount of adenosine released equaled that obtained during reactive hyperemia following ischemia in the same preparation. Furthermore, another characteristic feature was that the increase in adenosine release was reversed as rapidly as the decrease in contractility following offset of NO infusion. Thus, a possible explanation for the negative inotropic effect of NO could be that NO or a short-lived NO-derived radical such as peroxynitrite interferes with mitochondrial electron transport in cardiomyocytes. This is in agreement with the very recent observations made by

Radi and Brown, demonstrating that either NO or peroxynitrite inhibits mitochondrial electron transport [26, 27].

Pathophysiological Significance of NO for Left Ventricular Function

Given these essential effects of NO within the heart, it is tempting to speculate that either cNOS or iNOS is involved in various cardiac diseases affecting the coronary circulation and/or the cardiomyocytes (see Table 1). There is increasing evidence in the literature which suggests that dysfunction of the L-arginine–NO pathway is involved in the development of coronary artery disease associated with hypercholesterolemia and arterial hypertension, and that NO modulates cardiac function during myocardial infarction and reperfusion (reviewed in [2]). Furthermore, NO is most likely responsible for the depression of myocardial function in sepsis (reviewed in [10]). Based on rather preliminary data it has also been hypothesized that NO is involved in the pathogenesis of myocarditis, dilated cardiomyopathy and in some types of cardiac dysfunction in transplanted hearts [28].

In 1989, it was first demonstrated that following infusion of endotoxin from *E. coli* into young healthy volunteers, cardiac index and heart rate rose to compensate for the as yet unexplained drop in mean arterial blood pressure, and vascular resistance [29]. The initial increase in stroke volume was followed by a significant drop in myocardial contractility in the time course of septic patients, which further deteriorated circulatory parameters. It has been postulated that some of these hemodynamic responses in septic patients are mediated by pro-inflammatory cytokines which are increased in plasma. Furthermore, it is well known that pro-inflammatory cytokines induce expression of iNOS in various tissues within hours. Thus it was tempting to speculate that increased NOS activity within cardiac myocytes contribute to the depressed cardiac contractility observed in endotoxic shock. Finkel and co-workers were the first to demonstrate that application of the cytokines TNF-alpha, and interleukin-2 and -6 to papillary muscles isolated from hamsters decreased cardiac contractility [30]. The negative inotropic effect was most

Table 1. Significance of NO in the pathogenesis of cardiac diseases[1]

	Coronary arteries	Cardiomyocytes
1. Hypertensive heart disease	+	(+)
2. Hypercholesterolemia	+	–
3. Myocardial infarction and reperfusion	+	(+)
4. Sepsis	+	+
5. DCM	–	(+)
6. Myocarditis	(+)	(+)
7. Transplanted heart	+	+

+, significant role; (+), possible role; –, non-significant role.
[1]As evidenced from experimental and clinical studies.

probably due to enhanced NO formation, since N^G-monomethyl-L-arginine (L-NMMA), the stereospecific inhibitor of NO synthase, entirely blocked these effects of cytokines. In parallel, Poole-Wilson's [20] group demonstrated that iNOS is expressed in isolated cardiomyocytes from endotoxin-treated guinea pigs and that the NO formed within the cardiomyocytes significantly decreased contractility. The negative inotropic effect of bacterial LPS (lipopolysaccharide from *E.coli*)-induced NO formation was reversed by a stereospecific inhibitor of NO synthase, L-NAME (nitro-L-arginine methylester) and was completely prevented by pretreatment with corticoids (dexamethasone, 4 mg kg/BM), which inhibit the expression of iNOS. These experimental findings obtained in isolated tissue and cardiomyocytes from rodents may have important implications for the clinical situation of septic patients with life-threatening infections.

However, in clinical settings the use of corticoids or NO synthase inhibitors in septic patients have been disappointing so far. Nevertheless, metabolites of NO in human blood may represent a valuable diagnostic tool for patients with severely infectious syndromes. Nissel and coworkers demonstrated that in postoperative patients the severity of hemodynamic changes estimated by the Acute Physiology and Chronic Health Evaluation (APACHE) score is directly related to the serum level of nitrate which is the stable end product of NO in human blood [31]. They conclude that serum nitrate, as an indirect index of NO production in vivo, may be useful as a predictive parameter for morbity and mortality of high-risk ICU patients. In this context further randomized studies are needed in which the outcome of ICU septic patients treated with either corticoids or inhibitors of NO synthases is compared with the degree of hemodynamic changes and the rate of NO formation in vivo. At present, the determination of an appropriate dose of NOS inhibitors for septic patients represents a major problem in this field. A possible solution might be the simultaneous administration of NOS inhibitors along with low-dose infusion of NO donors such as sodium nitroprusside. The rationale for this therapeutic concept is to inhibit NOS-inhibitor-induced vasoconstriction without loss of the beneficial effects of NOS inhibitors on cardiomyocytes and macrophages. In summary, experimental and clinical data support the view that NO, which is formed at enhanced rates after stimulation of iNOS by pro-inflammatory cytokines, mediates, at least in part, depression of cardiac contractility and the catecholamine-resistant relaxation of vascular smooth muscle cells. Whether this represents a uniform concept which also holds true for other inflammatory cardiac diseases such as dilative cardiomyopathy, myocarditis, and heart transplantation requires further investigation.

This hypothesis is supported by recent studies using animal models of these cardiac diseases [10]. In a murine model of viral myocarditis, macrophages express iNOS only within inflammatory foci of hearts from infected mice, and NO reduces viral toxicity by inhibiting viral replication. Similarly, it was hypothesized from murine models of allograft rejection [32] that the increased expression of iNOS observed in macrophages, microvascular endothelium, and cardiomyocytes is responsible for cardiac contractile dysfunction and fatal rejection. de Belder and coworkers were the first to report that iNOS activity in ventricular cardiomyocytes was increased in patients suffering from dilated cardiomyopathy (DCM) compared with cardiomyocytes of atrial myocardium obtained from patients with coronary artery disease who underwent coronary artery bypass graft surgery, but with normal LV function [33]. In a further study the same group reported an increased iNOS activity in a small number of patients with inflammatory and non-inflammatory DCM and in post partum DCM [28]. However, the significance of the increased iNOS expression, in terms of a cause-and-effect relationship, for the impaired LV function in patients with DCM remains to be established.

In summary, NO is produced within the heart by the constitutive and inducible isoforms of NO synthase. At baseline, NO is formed by the cNOS within the coronary endothelium and modulates endothelial adhesiveness and coronary vascular tone via short- and long-term effects. This basal NO formation can be increased severalfold by the cNOS and in response to pro-inflammatory cytokines by the iNOS. These high amounts of NO directly affect cardiomyocyte function in addition to the coronary vasculature. Thus, the biological effects of NO on coronary endothelium and smooth muscle and as well as on cardiomyocytes represent a fundamental and principal part of cardiac function, which has to be considered in various cardiac diseases. Although the role of NO in the regulation of cardiac function under physiological and pathophysiological conditions has convincingly been proven in various experimental models, more clinical studies are warranted to establish its clinical significance in cardiac immunological diseases. In particular, further studies are needed to establish a pathophysiological role of NO in cases in which the link between time-dependent and quantitative changes in iNOS expression and subsequent NO formation and hemodynamic alterations is clearly demonstrated.

References

1. Shindo T, Ikeda U, Ohkawa F, Takahashi M, Funayama H, Nishinaga M, Kawahara Y, Yokoyama M, Kasahara T, Shimada K (1994) Nitric oxide synthesis in rat cardiac myocytes and fibroblasts. Life Sci 55: 1101–1108
2. Moncada S, Higgs A (1993) The L-arginine-nitric oxide pathway. N Engl J Med 329: 2002–2012
3. Dzau VJ, Gibbons GH, Morishita R, Pratt RE (1994) New perspectives in hypertension research: Potentials of vascular biology. Hypertension 23: 1132–1139
4. Ross R (1986) The pathogenesis of atherosclerosis – an update. N Engl J Med 324 (8): 488–500
5. Radomski MW, Moncada S (1993) Regulation of vascular homeostasis by nitric oxide. Thromb Haemost 70: 36–41
6. Snyder SH, Bredt DS (1992) Biological roles of nitric oxide. Sci Am 266 (5): 68–77
7. Furchgott RF, Vanhoutte PM (1989) Endothelium-derived relaxing and contracting factors. FASEB J 3: 2007–2018
8. Kelm M, Schrader J (1990) Control of coronary vascular tone by nitric oxide. Circ Res 66: 1561–1575
9. de Belder AJ, Radomski MW, Martin JF, Moncada S (1995) Nitric oxide and the pathogenesis of heart muscle disease. Eur J Clin Invest 25: 1–8
10. Ungureanu-Longrois D, Balligand JL, Kelly RA, Smith TW (1995) Myocardial contractile dysfunction in the systemic inflammatory response syndrome: Role of a cytokine-inducible nitric oxide synthase in cardiac myocytes. J Mol Cell Cardiol 27: 155–167

11. Knowles RG, Moncada S (1994) Nitric oxide synthases in mammals. Biochem J 298: 249–258
12. Schulz R, Nava E, Moncada S (1992) Induction and potential biological relevance of a Ca^{2+}-independent nitric oxide synthase in the myocardium. Br J Pharmacol 105: 575–580
13. Schulz R, Panas DL, Catena R, Moncada S, Olley PM, Lopaschuk GD (1995) The role of nitric oxide in cardiac depression induced by interleukin-1β and tumour necrosis factor-α. Br J Pharmacol 114: 27–34
14. Lancaster Jr. JR (1994) Simulation of the diffusion and reaction of endogenously produced nitric oxide. Proc Natl Acad Sci USA 91: 8137–8141
15. Kelm M, Feelisch M, Krebber T, Deussen A, Motz W, Strauer BE (1995) The role of nitric oxide (NO) in the regulation of coronary vascular tone in hearts from hypertensive rats: maintenance of NO forming capacity and increased basal production of NO. Hypertension 25: 186–193
16. Kelm M, Feelisch M, Spahr R, Piper H, Noack E, Schrader J (1988) Quantitative and kinetic characterization of nitric oxide and EDRF released from cultured endothelial cells. Biochem Biophys Res Commun 154: 236–244
17. Kelm M, Feelisch M, Deussen A, Schrader J, Strauer BE (1991) The role of nitric oxide in the control of coronary vascular tone in relation to partial oxygen pressure, perfusion pressure and flow. J Cardiovasc Pharmacol 17 (Suppl III): 95–99
18. Kelm M, Feelisch M, Grube R, Motz W, Strauer BE (1992) Metabolism of endothelium-derived nitric oxide in human blood. In: Moncada S (ed) The biology of nitric oxide. Portland, Colchester, pp 319–322
19. Kelm M, Yoshida K (1996) Metabolic fate of nitric oxide in vitro and in vivo. In: Feelisch M, Stamler J (eds) Methods in nitric oxide research. Wiley, Chichester pp 46–58
20. Brady AJB, Poole-Wison PA, Harding SE, Warren JB (1992) Nitric oxide production within cardiac myocytes reduces their contractility in endotoxemia. Am J Physiol 1963–1966
21. Balligand JL, Kelly RA, Marsden PA, Smith TW, Michel T (1993) Control of cardiac muscle cell function by an endogenous nitric oxide signaling system. Proc Natl Acad Sci USA 90: 347–351
22. Snyder SH (1994) Nitric oxide: More jobs for that molecule. Nature 372: 504–505
23. Schrader J (1990) Adenosine a homeostatic metabolite in cardiac energy metabolism. Circulation 81: 389–391
24. Deussen A, Schrader J (1991) Cardiac adenosine production is linked to myocardial pO2. J Mol Cell Cardiol 23: 495–504
25. Kammermeier H (1993) Meaning of energetic parameters. Basic Res Cardiol 88: 380–384
26. Radi R, Rodriguez M, Castro L, Telleri R (1994) Inhibition of mitochondrial electron transport by peroxynitrite. Arch Biochem Biophys 308: 89–95
27. Brown GC (1995) Nitric oxide regulates mitochondrial respiration and cell functions by inhibiting cytochrome oxidase. FEBS Lett 369: 136–139
28. de Belder AJ, Radomski MW, Why HJ, Richardson PJ, Martin JF (1995) Myocardial calcium-independent nitric oxide synthase activity is present in dilated cardiomyopathy, myocarditis, and postpartum cardiomyopathy but not in ischaemic or valvar heart disease. Br Heart J 74: 426–430
29. Suffredini AF, Fromm RE, Parker MM, Brenner M, Kovacs JA, Wesley RA, Parrillo JE (1989) The cardiovascular response of normal humans to the administration of endotoxin. N Engl J Med 321: 280–287
30. Finkel MS, Oddis CV, Jacobs TD, Watkins SC, Hattler BG, Simmons RL (1992) Negative inotropic effects of cytokines on the heart mediated by nitric oxide. Science 257: 387–389
31. van Dissel JT, Groeneveld PHP, Maes B, van Furth R, Frolich M, Feuth HDM (1994) Nitric oxide: a predictor of morbidity in postoperative patients? Lancet 343: 1579–1580
32. Yang X, Chowdhury N, Brett J, Marboe C, Sciacca RR, Michler RE, Cai B, Cannon PJ (1994) Induction of myocardial nitric oxide synthase by cardiac allograft rejection. J Clin Invest 94: 714–721
33. de Belder AJ, Radomski MW, Why HJF, Richardson PJ, Bucknall CA, Salas E, Martin JF, Moncada S (1993) Nitric oxide synthase activities in human myocardium. Lancet 341: 84–85

The Role of the Endothelium in Atherosclerosis

J.P. Cooke

Atherosclerosis: An Overview

The most common cause of morbidity and mortality in Western civilization is atherosclerosis. Atherosclerosis is a complex process that is facilitated by hypertension, diabetes mellitus, tobacco use, and hypercholesterolemia. Elevated levels of low density lipoprotein (LDL) cholesterol (particularly oxidized LDL) perturb the cell membrane, alter permeability and secretion, and are associated with the expression of intercellular adhesion molecules, cytokines, and growth factors. Recent evidence suggests that specific glycoprotein adhesion molecules e.g. vascular cell adhesion molecule (VCAM) and chemokines e.g. monocyte chemotactic protein (MCP) elaborated by endothelial cells participate in monocyte adhesion and infiltration in vessels exposed to high levels of serum cholesterol. The expression of these adhesion molecules and chemokines may explain the observation that within several days of a high cholesterol diet, monocytes adhere to the endothelium, particularly at intercellular junctions.

The monocytes migrate into the subendothelium, where they begin to accumulate lipid and become foam cells. This is the earliest event in the formation of the fatty streak. These activated monocytes (macrophages) release mitogens and chemoattractants that recruit additional macrophages as well as vascular smooth muscle cells into the lesion. The smooth muscle cells migrating into the lesion change their phenotype from a "contractile" type to a "secretory" type and elaborate extracellular matrix (i.e. elastin), which transforms the lesion into a fibrous plaque. The smooth muscle cells also become engorged with lipid to form foam cells. The lesion grows with the recruitment of more cells, the elaboration of extracellular matrix, and the accumulation of lipid until it is transformed from a fibrous plaque to a complicated plaque. Platelets also play a role in atherogenesis; injury to or dysfunction of the endothelium permits platelets to adhere to the vessel wall, releasing epidermal growth factor, platelet-derived growth factor, and other mitogens and cytokines that contribute to smooth muscle migration and proliferation.

Myocardial infarctions and stroke are most often precipitated by rupture of this complex plaque. Rupture of the complex plaque exposes the flowing blood

Section of Vascular Medicine, Falk Cardiovascular Research Center, Stanford University School of Medicine, 300 Passteur Drive, Stanford, CA 94305-5246, USA

to the highly thrombogenic constituents of the plaque (such as foam cells, which produce tissue factor). Recent evidence indicates that plaque rupture occurs after the fibrous cap is weakened by collagenases secreted by macrophages. These macrophages typically infiltrate the shoulder region of the plaque, explaining why this area of the plaque is more prone to be the point of rupture.

Endothelial Alterations in Atherosclerosis

Hypercholesterolemia alters vascular reactivity in animal models and in man; vasoconstriction is enhanced, and vasodilation is reduced. This appears to be due in large part to a reduced release or activity of endothelium-derived nitric oxide (NO) and prostacyclin. NO is the most potent endogenous vasodilator and is now known to be derived from L-arginine. The reduced release of NO and prostacyclin may play a role in the initiation of atherogenesis. Since NO and prostacyclin also inhibit platelet adherence and aggregation, and suppress vascular smooth muscle cell proliferation in vitro, a deficiency of these factors would enhance vasoconstriction, promote platelet–vessel wall interactions, and disrupt the balance between growth-inhibiting and growth-promoting influences on the vascular smooth muscle. All of these events would tend to promote atherogenesis.

Another endothelial alteration that may contribute to atherogenesis is oxidative stress. Under the influence of hypercholesterolemia or diabetes mellitus, the endothelium begins to generate superoxide anion. Superoxide anion is a highly reactive oxygen-derived free radical, which can damage cell membranes by lipid peroxidation. In addition, superoxide anion can affect gene expression, adhesion molecules, and chemokines. Certain transcriptional proteins such as nuclear factor κB (NF-κB) are activated by superoxide anion. Normally, NF-κB (a heterodimeric protein) is bound to its intracellular inhibitor IκBα. When the cell is under oxidative stress IκBα become phosphorylated and dissociates from NF-κB. This leaves NF-κB free to translocate to the nucleus, and interact with its binding sequence on the promoter region of several genes (vascular cell adhesion molecule, VCAM-1, MCP-1, and monocyte colony stimulating factor (MCSF)), to enhance their expression. The expression of these genes increases endothelial adhesiveness for monocytes.

NO and Oxidant-Responsive Transcription

The existence of oxidant-responsive transcriptional pathways invokes regulatory molecules which control them. Recent evidence indicates that nitric oxide inhibits NF-κB-mediated transcription. This appears to be due to an effect of NO to reduce endothelial generation of superoxide anion.

In preliminary studies we tested the hypothesis that NO regulates an oxidant sensitive transcriptional pathway regulating the expression of MCP-1. This 76-amino acid chemokine has been implicated as a major culprit in the enticement of monocytes and T lymphocytes into the vessel wall [1, 2]. The expression of MCP-1 is induced by lipopolysaccharides (LPS), cytokines (tumor necrosis factor-α (TNF-α) interleukins-1 and -4), or minimally modified low-density lipoprotein (mmLDL) [3]. Human aortic endothelial and smooth muscle cells exposed to mmLDL express MCP-1; this protein accounts for virtually all of the chemotactic activity produced under these conditions [1]. MCP-1 may also activate or increase the expression of adhesion molecules to facilitate monocyte adhesion [4–6]. The role of this chemokine in human disease has been implicated by immunohistochemical studies of atherosclerotic plaques [7]. The weight of the available evidence indicates that MCP-1 is one of the key factors initiating the inflammatory process of atherogenesis. To determine if vascular NO regulates the expression of this chemokine, we have recently performed a series of in vitro and in vivo studies investigating the effects of NO on MCP-1 expression.

We designed the studies to determine if NO suppresses the expression of MCP-1. In addition, we tested the hypothesis that NO exerts its effect by suppressing redox-sensitive transcriptional pathways regulating MCP-1 expression. Finally, we extended our in vitro observations regarding the interaction of NO and MCP-1 into an animal model of atherogenesis.

Smooth muscle cells (SMC) were isolated from normal rabbit aortae by the explant method. Cells were then exposed to LPS, native LDL or oxidized LDL, for 6 h. We found that the expression of MCP-1 in SMC was induced by LPS or by oxidized LDL, but not native LDL. The induction of MCP-1 by cytokines or oxidized lipoproteins was associated with an increased generation of superoxide anion by the SMC as assessed by lucigenin chemiluminescence. This increase in oxidative stress was associated with the activation of NF-κB. Specifically, electromobility shift assays detected an increased availability of the transcriptional protein NF-κB. Exposure of the cells to an NO donor suppressed this oxidant-sensitive transcriptional pathway. Specifically, the induced expression of MCP-1 and activation of NF-κB was reduced by previous exposure of the SMC to the NO donor DETA-NONOate. To determine if NO exerted its effect at a transcriptional level, SMC were transfected with a 400 bp fragment of the MCP-1 promoter. Promoter activity was enhanced by oxLDL and LPS; DETA-NO suppressed promoter activity induced by oxidized lipoprotein or cytokines.

In subsequent studies we investigated the role of endogenous NO in the regulation of MCP-1 in vivo. NZW rabbits were fed normal chow, normal chow plus nitro-L-arginine (13.5 mg/kg per day, to reduce vascular NO synthesis), high cholesterol diet (Chol), or high cholesterol diet supplemented with L-arginine (to enhance vascular NO synthesis). After 2 weeks, thoracic aortae were harvested and total RNA was isolated. Thoracic aortae harvested from animals treated with L-nitroarginine elaborated about 50% less NO in vitro. By contrast, thoracic aortae of hypercholesterolemic animals treated with L-arginine elaborated significantly more NO (as measured by chemiluminescence of conditioned medium). Northern analysis revealed that MCP-1 expression was increased in thoracic aortae from hypercholesterolemic animals, and was further increased in thoracic aortae from animals treated with L-nitroarginine.

By contrast, MCP-1 expression was reduced in those animals treated with the NO precursor L-arginine.

NO: An Endogenous Anti-atherogenic Molecule

These studies provided insight into the mechanism by which endogenous NO may act to inhibit atherogenesis. Previous observations by our group and others have revealed that modulation of vascular NO activity can significantly influence the course of lesion formation in experimental hypercholesterolemia [8–11]. Hypercholesterolemia reduces the influence of endothelium-derived NO due to its degradation and/or reduced production [12–14]. NO activity can be restored by administration of the NO precursor, L-arginine, in hypercholesterolemic animals and humans [15–17]. In New Zealand white rabbits, hind limb blood flow increases in response to intra-arterial acetylcholine. This increase in flow is believed to be due in part to endothelium-dependent NO mediated vasodilation. This vasodilation is inhibited by hypercholesterolemia and is restored by intravenous infusion of L-arginine. Similarly, in vitro studies using organ chamber technique reveal that endothelium-dependent vasorelaxation is reduced in vascular rings derived from the thoracic aortae of hypercholesterolemic animals. This abnormality can be reversed by an intravenous infusion of L-arginine. A similar phenomenon has been observed in humans. In young hypercholesterolemic humans, forearm vasodilation, in response to intra-arterial acetylcholine, is reduced. Intravenous infusion of L-arginine restores forearm blood flow response to normal levels.

Chronic oral administration of L-arginine to hypercholesterolemic rabbits partially restores endothelium-dependent vasodilation of the thoracic aorta. Direct measurement of NO elaboration (by chemiluminescence) reveals that vascular tissue from arginine treated animals synthesized significantly greater amounts of NO. The chronic enhancement of vascular NO is associated with a striking reduction of intimal lesions in the thoracic aortae and coronary arteries of the treated hypercholesterolemic animals (Fig. 1).

Using a functional binding assay, we have examined the effects of vascular NO upon endothelial adhesiveness for monocytes. The thoracic aorta is harvested from normal or hypercholesterolemic animals treated with L-arginine (to enhance NO synthesis), or L-nitroarginine (to inhibit NO synthesis). The aortae are bisected and pinned flat in a petri dish filled with oxygenated physiologic buffer. Mononuclear cells derived from normal animals, or cells from a monocytoid line are added to the buffer and the preparation is gently rocked for 15 min. Subsequently, non-adherent cells are washed off and adherent cells counted by videomicroscopy. As expected, more cells adhere to the aortae from hypercholesterolemic animals in comparison to aortae from animals on a normal chow diet. Intriguingly, cell adhesion is reduced in aortae harvested from hypercholesterolemic animals that had received L-arginine supplementation (Fig. 2a). By contrast, vessels from normocholesterolemic animals treated with nitro-arginine had greater affinity for monocytes, even more so than aortae from hypercholesterolemic animals (Fig. 2b).

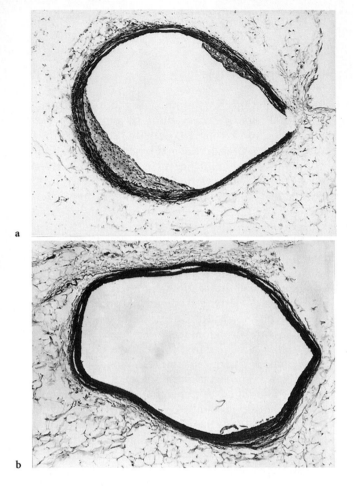

a

b

Fig. 1a,b. Photomicrographs of representative cross sections from the left main coronary arteries of rabbits treated with vehicle (**a**) or supplemental arginine (**b**) after 10 weeks on a 1% cholesterol diet. There is a striking absence of intimal lesions in the coronary arteries of the rabbits given supplemental arginine. (From [18]) × 100

These studies suggested that modulation of vascular NO activity affects endothelial-adhesiveness for monocytes. Indeed, our recent studies and those of other investigators indicate that NO regulates adhesion molecules and chemokines involved in endothelial-monocyte interaction.

Accumulating evidence supports the hypothesis that NO exerts its effect on monocyte adherence and accumulation in part by modulating the activity of redox-responsive transcriptional pathways [19–21]. One way that NO may act is by reducing intracellular oxidative stress. NO can scavenge superoxide anion, although the product of this reaction, peroxynitrate anion, is itself a highly reactive free radical [22]. However, it is possible that peroxynitrate anion could

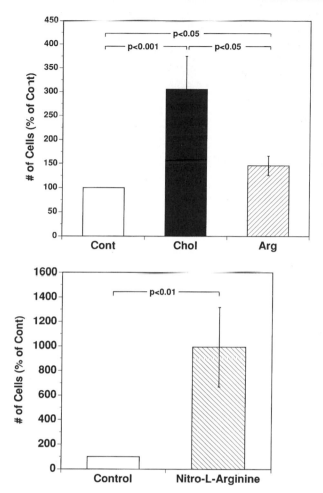

Fig. 2. a Quantification of monocytoid cell binding to rabbit aortic endothelium per high-power field in the ex vivo adhesion assay. Segments of thoracic aortae from control (*Cont*) animals (*n*=7), those fed a high-cholesterol diet (*Chol*; *n*=7), and those fed a high-cholesterol diet supplemented with L-arginine (*Arg*; *n*=7) were harvested and functional binding assays performed as described in the text. On each of seven experimental days, binding assays were performed in parallel with thoracic segments from *Cont*, *Chol*, and *Arg* groups. The number of adherent cells was quantified using epifluorescent microscopy; 30 high-power fields per aortic segment were counted and averaged to give one average value per segment. All values were expressed as a percentage of that of the *Cont* animal. There was a threefold increase in the number of monocytoid cells bound to the thoracic aortae from *Chol* animals. Arginine treatment significantly reduced endothelial adhesiveness. **b** Quantification of monocytoid cell binding to thoracic aortae from normocholesterolemic animals receiving vehicle (*Cont*) or nitro- L-arginine (13.5 mg/kg per day) as described in the text. Chronic oral administration of nitro- L-arginine markedly enhanced cell adhesion to the endothelium ex vivo. (From [10])

subsequently nitrosylate sulfhydryl groups to form S-nitrosothiols. This class of molecules is known to induce vasodilation, inhibit platelet aggregation, and interfere with leukocyte adherence to the vessel wall [23, 24].

Another mechanism by which NO may ameliorate oxidative stress is by terminating the autocatalytic chain of lipid peroxidation that is initiated by oxidized LDL or intracellular generation of oxygen-derived free radicals. Indeed, exogenous NO inhibits copper-induced oxidation of LDL cholesterol, causing a lag in the formation of conjugated dienes [25]. Finally, NO may directly suppress the generation of oxygen-derived free radicals by nitrosylating, and thereby inactivating oxidative enzymes. This hypothesis is supported by the observation that the generation of superoxide anion by stimulated neutrophils is reduced by their exposure to exogenous NO [26]. This is due to the inactivation of NADPH oxidase, a multimeric enzyme, with cytosolic and particulate components. The particulate component is vulnerable to nitrosylation by NO (either at its heme moiety or sulfhydryl group), which prevents its association with the cytosolic component, and reconstitution of the active enzyme. A similar phenomenon may occur in endothelial cells. This would explain the observation of Niu and colleagues, who reported that antagonism of endogenous NO production increases oxidative stress in human umbilical vein endothelial cells (HUVECs), as demonstrated using redox-sensitive fluorophores [27]. Furthermore, Pagano and colleagues [28] have shown that exogenous NO donors inhibit the generation of superoxide anion by the endothelium of rabbit thoracic aortae treated ex vivo with antagonists of superoxide dismutase.

It is well established that hypercholesterolemia reduces the activity of endothelium-derived NO [12]. In parallel, the endothelium begins to generate superoxide anion [14]. This alteration in endothelial redox state triggers a transcriptional cascade that results in the activation of genes encoding molecules that regulate endothelial adhesiveness [20, 29]. Cytokines or oxidized lipoprotein induce the expression by HUVECs of VCAM-1, an endothelial immunoglobulin implicated in monocyte adhesion and atherogenesis [30]. This expression is regulated by an NF-κB-mediated transcriptional pathway that is blocked by exposure of the cells to the antioxidant pyrrolidine dithiocarbamate [20] or aspirin [29].

The cytokine-induced activation of VCAM-1 in human saphenous vein endothelial cells is suppressed by NO donors [20]. This effect of NO appears to be secondary to stabilization and/or increased expression of IκBa, which complexes with NF-κB to inhibit its transcriptional activity [21].

Our data is consistent with this model of an oxidant-responsive NF-κB-mediated pathway that is modulated by NO. Recently, Zeiher and colleagues have also provided evidence that NO inhibits MCP-1 expression in cytokine-stimulated HUVECs, in a cGMP-independent fashion [31].

Hemodynamic Determinants of Atherogenesis: Role of NO

The distribution of atherosclerotic lesions throughout the vascular tree is non-uniform. As early as the nineteenth century, the great pathologists Rokitansky and Virchow independently speculated that this nonuniformity was due to local alterations in hemodynamic forces impinging upon the vascular tree [32, 33]. Indeed, at sites vulnerable to plaque formation – bends, branches and bifurcations – unidirectional laminar flow is disturbed, with areas of re-circulation characterized by low and fluctuating shear stress [34–38]. In these regions of low shear stress, the vulnerability to plaque formation may be due to enhanced monocyte binding. Adhesive interactions between leukocytes in the vessel wall are less likely to be disrupted under conditions of low shear stress. Furthermore, experimental reductions of blood flow enhance endothelial ad-hesiveness for monocytes [39–40]. This may be in part due to the fact that low shear regions exhibit enhanced permeability to macromolecules including LDL [41, 42]. Accumulation and modification of LDL in the vessel wall could trigger a cascade of events leading to changes in the chemotactic and adhesive properties of the endothelium [41, 42].

Tractive forces of fluid flow also modulate the gene expression of en-dothelial adhesion molecules and cytokines that participate in monocyte binding. In the New Zealand White rabbit, an adhesion molecule homologous to the human VCAM-1, is up-regulated by hypercholesterolemia and is ex-pressed at sites of early lesion formation [30, 43]. The expression of VCAM-1 in a murine endothelial cell line is reduced by 75% after 24 h of exposure to laminar fluid flow [44]. The expression of VCAM-1 is regulated in part by oxidant-responsive transcriptional activation. Oxidized LDL and cytokines induce the expression of VCAM-1 via a transcriptional pathway modulated by NF-κB; this NF-κB mediated gene expression can be abrogated by anti-oxidants [20].

Flow is also a potent stimulus for endothelial elaboration of NO [45–47]. Accordingly, we proposed that flow inhibits VCAM-1 expression by triggering the release of endothelium-derived NO and thereby inhibiting oxidant-re-sponsive transcriptional activation.

To test this hypothesis, confluent monolayers of human aortic endothelial cells were exposed to static conditions or to fluid flow using a cone-plate viscometer. After 4 h, the cells were incubated for an additional 4 h with native LDL, oxidized LDL, or LPS plus TNF-α. Whereas native LDL had little effect, incubation with either oxLDL or LPS/TNFα significantly increased endothelial adhesiveness for monocytes, endothelial production of superoxide anion, and expression of VCAM-1. Analysis of nuclear proteins demonstrated that NF-κB activity was increased by the oxidized lipoprotein or cytokines. Previous ex-posure to fluid flow inhibited all of these sequelae of cytokine or lipoprotein stimulation. The effect of fluid flow was most likely due to shear-induced release of NO since coincubation with L-nitroarginine abolished, whereas NO donor mimicked, the effect of flow. These studies suggested that endothelium-derived NO may play a critical role in hemodynamic effects upon the ex-pression of endothelial adhesion molecules. Flow-mediated NO dependent regulation of oxidant responsive transcription may be a critical determinant of the site of a lesion.

To summarize, atherosclerosis is a complex process that is initiated by monocyte adherence to the endothelium. Monocyte interaction with the vessel wall is facilitated by the expression of endothelial adhesion molecules and chemokines. The genes encoding these proteins are regulated in part by an oxidant-sensitive transcriptional protein, NF-κB. The existence of oxidant-sensitive transcriptional pathways invokes the probability of counter-regulatory mechanisms. Endothelium-derived NO appears to be an autocrine modulator of this transcriptional pathway. By suppressing NF-κB-mediated induction of MCP-1 and VCAM-1, NO inhibits monocyte adherence to the endothelium and opposes intimal lesion formation in the vessel wall.

References

1. Navab M, Imes SS, Hama SY, Hough GP, Ross LA, Bork RW, Valente AJ, Berliner JA, Drinkwater DC, Laks H, Fogelman AM (1991) Monocyte transmigration induced by modification of low density lipoprotein in co-cultures of human aortic wall cells is due to induction of monocyte chemotactic protein 1 synthesis and is abolished by high density lipoprotein. J Clin Invest 88: 2939–2046
2. Taub DD, Proost P, Murphy WJ, Anver M, Longo DL, Van Damme J, Oppenheim JJ (1995) Monocyte chemotactic protein-1 (MCP-1), -2, and -3 are chemotactic for human T lymphocytes. J Clin Invest 95: 1370–1376
3. Cushing SD, Berliner JA, Valente AJ, Territo MC, Navab M, Parhami F, Gerrity R, Schwartz CJ, Fogelman AM (1990) Minimally modified LDL induces monocyte chemotactic protein 1 in human endothelial and smooth muscle cells. Proc Natl Acad Sci USA 87: 5134–5138
4. Jiang Y, Beller DI, Frendl G, Graves DT (1992) Monocyte chemoattractant protein-1 regulates adhesion molecule expression and cytokine production in human monocytes. J Immunol 148: 2423–22428
5. Jiang Y, Zhu JF, Luscinskas FW, Graves DT (1992) MCP-1 stimulated monocyte attachment to laminin is mediated by beta-2-integrins. Am J Physiol 267: C1112–C1118
6. Ban K, Kieda U, Takahashi M, Kanbe T, Kasahara T, Shimada K (1994) Expression of intercellular adhesion molecule-1 on rat cardiac myocytes by monocyte chemoattractant protein-1. Cardiovasc Res 28: 1258–1262
7. Yla-Herttuala S, Lipton BA, Rosenfeld ME, Sarkioja T, Yoshimura T, Leonard EJ, Witztum JL, Steinberg D (1991) Expression of monocyte chemoattractant protein 1 in macrophage rich areas of human and rabbit atherosclerotic lesions. Proc Natl Acad Sci USA, 88: 5252–5256
8. Cayette AJ, Palacino JJ, Horten K, Cohen RA (1994) Chronic inhibition of nitric oxide production accelerates neointima formation and impairs endothelial function in hypercholesterolemic rabbits. Arterioscler Thromb 14: 753–759
9. Naruse K, Shimizu K, Muramatsu M, Toki Y, Miyazaki Y, Okumura K, Hashimoto H, Ito T (1994) Long-term inhibition of NO synthesis promotes atherosclerosis in the hypercholesterolemic rabbit thoracic aorta. PGH2 does not contribute to impaired endothelium-dependent relaxation. Arterioscler Thromb 14: 746–752
10. Tsao P, McEvoy LM, Drexler H, Butcher EC, Cooke JP (1994) Enhanced endothelial adhesiveness in hypercholesterolemia is attenuated by L-arginine. Circulation 89: 2176–2182
11. Cooke JP, Singer AH, Tsao PS, Zera P, Rowan RA, Billingham ME (1992) Anti-atherogenic effects of L-arginine in the hypercholesteroemic rabbit. J Clin Invest 90: 1168–1172
12. Heistad DD, Armstrong MLI, Marcus ML, Piegors DJ, Mark AL (1984) Augmented responses to vasoconstrictor stimuli in hypercholesterolemic and atherosclerotic monkeys. Circ Res 43: 711–718

13. McLenahan JM, William JK, Fish RD, Ganz P, Selwyn AP (1991) Loss of flow-mediated endothelium-dependent dilation occurs early in the development of atherosclerosis. Circulation 84: 1273–1278
14. Ohara Y, Petersen TE, Harrison DG (1993) Hypercholesterolemia increases endothelial superoxide anion production. J Clin Invest 91: 2546–2551
15. Creager MA, Gallagher SJ, Girerd XJ, Coleman SM, Dzau VJ, Cooke JP (1992) L-arginine improves endothelium-dependent vasodilation in hypercholesterolemic humans. J Clin Invest 90: 1248–1253
16. Dubois-Rande JL, Zelinsky R, Chabrier PE, Castaigne A, Geschwind H, Adnot S (1992) L-arginine improves endothelium-dependent relaxation of conductance and resistance coronary arteries in coronary artery disease. J Cardiovasc Pharmacol 20 (Suppl 12): S211–S213
17. Rossitch E Jr, Alexander E 3d, Black PM, Cooke JP (1991) L-arginine normalizes endothelial function in cerebral vessels from hypercholesterolemic rabbits. J Clin Invest 87: 1295–1299
18. Wang B, Singer A, Tsao P, Drexler H, Kosek J, Cooke JP (1994) Dietary arginine prevents atherogenesis in the coronary artery of the hypercholesterolemic rabbit. J Am Coll Cardiol 23: 452–458
19. Garg UC, Hassid A (1990) Nitric oxide-generating vasodilators inhibit mitogenesis and proliferation of BALB/C 3T3 fibroblasts by a cyclic GMP-independent mechanism. Biochem Biophys Res Commun 171: 474–479
20. Marui N, Offerman MK, Swerlick R, Kunsch C, Rosen CA, Ahmad M, Alexander RW, Medford RM (1993) Vascular cell adhesion molecule-1 (VCAM-1) gene transcription and expression are regulated through an antioxidant-sensitive mechanism in human vascular endothelial cells. J Clin Invest 92: 1866–1874
21. DeCaterina R, Libby P, Peng H-B, Thannickal VJ, Rajavashisth TB, Gimbrone MA Jr., Shin WS, Liao JK (1995) Nitric oxide decreases cytokine-induced endothelial activation. J Clin Invest 96: 60–68
22. Radi R, Beckman JS, Bush KM, Freeman BA (1991) Peroxynitrite oxidation of sulfhydryls. The cytotoxic potential of superoxide and nitric oxide. J Biol Chem 266: 4244–4250
23. Stamler JS, Simon DI, Osborne JA, Mullins ME, Jaraki O, Michel T, Singel DJ, Loscalzo J (1992) S-nitrosylation of proteins with nitric oxide: Synthesis and characterization of biologically active compounds. Proc Natl Acad Sci USA 89: 444–448
24. Stamler JS, Mendelsohn ME, Amarante P, Smick D, Andon N, Davies PF, Cooke JP, Loscalzo J (1989) N-acetylcysteine potentiates platelet inhibition by endothelium-derived relaxing factor. Circ Res 65: 789–795
25. Hogg N, Kalyanaramer B, Joseph J, Struck A, Parthasarathy S (1993) Inhibition of low-density lipoprotein oxidation by nitric oxide. Potential role in atherogenesis. FEBS Lett 334: 170–174
26. Clancy RM, Leszczynska P, Piziak J, Abramson SB (1992) Nitric oxide, an endothelial cell relaxation factor, inhibits neutrophil superoxide anion production via a direct action on NADPH oxidase. J Clin Invest 90: 1116–1121
27. Niu X-F, Smith CW, Kubes P (1994) Intracellular oxidative stress induced by nitric oxide synthesis inhibition increases endothelial cell adhesion to neutrophils. Circ Res 74: 1133–1140
28. Pagano PJ, Tornheim K, Cohen RA (1993) Superoxide anion production by rabbit thoracic aorta: effect of endothelium-derived nitric oxide. Am J Physiol 265: H707–H712
29. Weber C, Erl W, Pietsch A, Strobel M, Ziegler-Heitbrock HWL, Weber PC (1994) Antioxidants inhibit monocyte adhesion by suppressing nuclear factor-κB mobilization and induction of vascular cell adhesion molecule-1 in endothelial cells stimulated to generate radicals. Arterioscler Thromb 14: 1665–1673
30. Cybulsky MI, Gimbrone MA Jr (1991) Endothelial expression of a mononuclear leukocyte adhesion molecule during atherogenesis. Science 251: 788–791
31. Zeiher AM, Fisslthaler B, Schray-Utz B, Busse R (1995) Nitric oxide modulates the expression of monocyte chemoattractant protein 1 in cultured human endothelial cells. Circ Res 76: 980–986

32. Rokitansky C (1952) The pathological anatomy of the organs of respiration and circulation. A manual of pathological anatomy, vol 4. Sydenham Society, London. (Translated from German by GE Day)
33. Virchow R (1860) Cellular pathology as based upon physiological and pathological histology. Churchill, London (Translated from German by F Clance)
34. Montenegro MR, Eggen DA (1968) Topography of atherosclerosis in the coronary arteries. Lab Invest 18: 586–593
35. Sinzinger H, Siberbauer K, Auerswald W (1980) Quantitative investigation of sudanophilic lesions around the aortic ostia of human fetuses, newborns and children. Blood Vessels 17: 44–52
36. Cornhill JF, Barrett WA, Herderick EE, Mahley RW, Fry DF (1985) Topographic study of sudanophilic lesions in cholesterol-fed minipigs by image analysis. Arteriosclerosis 5: 415–426
37. Glagov S, Zarins C, Giddens DP, Ku DN (1988) Hemodynamics and atherosclerosis. Insights and perspectives gained from studies of human arteries. Arch Pathol Lab Med 112: 1018–1031
38. Asakura T, Karino T (1990) Flow patterns and spatial distribution of atherosclerotic lesions in human coronary arteries. Circ Res 66: 1045–1066
39. Walpola PL, Gotlieb AI, Langille BL (1993) Monocyte adhesion and changes in endothelial cell number, morphology, and F-actin distribution elicited by low shear stress *in vivo*. Am J Pathol 142(5): 1392–1400
40. Walpola PL, Gotlieb AI, Cybulsky MI, Langille BL (1995) Expression of ICAM-1 and VCAM-1 and monocyte adherence in arteries exposed to altered shear stress. Arterioscler Thromb 15(1): 2–10
41. Schwenke DE, Carew TE (1988) Quantification *in vivo* of increased LDL content and rate of LDL degradation in normal rabbit aorta occurring at sites susceptible to early atherosclerotic lesions. Circ Res 62: 699–710
42. Berliner JA, Navab M, Fogelman AM, Frank JS, Demer LL, Edwards PA, Watson AD, Lusis AJ (1995) Atherosclerosis: basic mechanisms. Oxidation, inflammation, and genetics. Circulation 91(9): 2488–2496
43. Li H, Cybulsky MI, Gimbrone MA Jr, Libby P (1993) An atherogenic diet rapidly induces VCAM-1, a cytokine-regulatable mononuclear leukocyte adhesion molecule, in rabbit aortic endothelium. Arterioscler Thromb 13(2): 197–204
44. Ohtsuka A, Ando J, Korenaga R, Kamiya A, Toyama-Sorimachi N, Miyasaka M (1993) The effect of flow on the expression of vascular adhesion molecule-1 by cultured mouse endothelial cells. Biochem Biophys Res Commun 193(1): 303–310
45. Pohl V, Holtz J, Busse R, Bassenge E (1986) Crucial role of the endothelium in the vasodilator response to increase flow in vivo. Hypertension 8: 37–44
46. Cooke JP, Stamler JS, Andon N, Davies PR, Loscalzo J (1990) Flow stimulates endothelial cells to release a nitrovasodilator that is potentiated by reduced thiol. Am J Physiol 28: H804–H812
47. Cooke JP, Rossitch E, Andon N, Loscalzo J, Dzau VJ (1991) Flow activates an endothelial potassium channel to release an endogenous nitrovasodilator. J Clin Invest 88: 1663–1671

Immune and Inflammatory Responses in the Human Atherosclerotic Plaque

A.C. van der Wal, O.J. de Boer, and A.E. Becker

Introduction

Atherosclerotic plaques are the underlying cause of most cardiovascular diseases, with myocardial infarction as a major consequence. The development of arterial lesions starts in childhood, and they progress slowly and become clinically manifest only after an event-free interval of many decades. The sudden onset of symptoms is usually initiated by complications in an advanced plaque, such as plaque disruption and superimposed thrombosis [1].

A current concept of the development of lesions is that they result from a fibroproliferative inflammatory response to some form of chronic injury [2]. This concept, which extends the original "response to injury" hypothesis formulated by Ross and Glomset 20 years earlier [3], emphasizes inflammation as an important mechanism in the ongoing process of injury and repair.

The recent view of atherosclerosis as a chronic inflammatory process emerged from cellular and molecular biological studies of human and experimental lesions which characterized the various cellular constituents and their secretory products more precisely. Macrophages, which for a long time were considered to be solely lipid scavengers and processors, are capable of secreting many proinflammatory molecules in the micromilieu of the intimal plaque. Moreover, substantial amounts of T lymphocytes have now been detected in the lesions of atherosclerosis.

The presence of these immunocompetent cells raises two questions with respect to the pathogenesis of atherosclerosis. First, are specific immune responses involved which may initiate and/or sustain chronic inflammation in the plaque? Second, are inflammatory cells and their secretory products involved in modulating plaque morphology which could underlie the variability in morphology of advanced lesions?

In Situ Immune Responses in Atherosclerotic Lesions

Immunocytochemical studies of human intimal lesions have demonstrated variable but substantial amounts of T lymphocytes in virtually every stage of

Department of Cardiovascular Pathology, Academic Medical Center,
University of Amsterdam, Meibergdreef 9, 1105 AZ Amsterdam, The Netherlands

lesion development, such as in fatty streaks, in the fibrous caps of early fibrofatty lesions, and in advanced plaques. B lymphocytes or plasma cells are scarce or absent in all of these stages.

Advanced plaques obtained at autopsy or from carotid endarterectomy specimens contained a dominant subpopulation of CD4+ cells [4]. On the other hand, in early or precursor lesions, CD8+ lymphocytes are more frequently encountered [5–7]. The reason for this phenotypic shift as the disease progresses is still unclear. However, it is of interest that CD8+ lymphocytes also slightly predominate in the intima adjacent to fully developed lesions which themselves contain a majority of CD4+ cells in their fibrous cap [4]. Therefore, CD8+ cells may have a regulatory role in localizing the inflammatory response, and thus contribute to the focal nature of lesions which is one of the hallmarks of atherosclerosis.

By using immunodouble stains it can be seen that T cells virtually always colocalize with macrophages within the plaque tissue, and that both cell types express MHC class II molecules (HLA-DR) on their cell surfaces, indicating a state of activation [7]. The presence of clustered and activated immunocompetent cells both in early and advanced lesions is suggestive of an ongoing cell-mediated immune response during the development of atherosclerosis.

There is indeed more evidence for the activation of T cells in the plaques. Using FACscan flow cytometry on isolated T cells, Stemme and co-workers showed that the population of T cells in carotid plaques is phenotypically different from T cells in the peripheral blood of the same patients. In their study, 64% of plaque T cells were CD45RO+ memory cells (versus 49% in the blood), and 31% expressed the very late activation antigen VLA-1 (versus only 1% in the blood), which suggests that they are in a late stage (more than 2–3 weeks) of activation. A smaller population of 5%–15% (albeit still significantly more than in the blood) exhibited a state of recent activation, indicated by HLA-DR and CD26 expression [8]. Moreover, a small number of T cells express receptors for the autocrine growth factor interleukin-2 [7–9] and the proliferating-cell nuclear antigen [10], which indicates that a small number is involved in local proliferation following antigenic stimulation. Similar numbers of recently activated T cells are found when the expression of co-stimulatory molecules is studied. Co-stimulatory molecules are sets of receptors and ligands on lymphocytes and antigen-presenting cells that provide accessory signals during antigen-specific activation. Their interaction leads to clonal expansion and cytokine production [11]. The expression of these molecules on a subset of T cells and on most macrophages, in particular B7-1 and CD28 on T cells and B7-1,2 and CD70 on macrophages, implies that the microenvironment of the plaque provides sufficient signals for antigen-specific stimulation [12].

Thus it appears that there are two main subpopulations present: a small population of recently stimulated cells that participate in active inflammation, and a large population of resting or late activated cells which may function as bystander cells. Indeed, in most cell-mediated immune responses only a small proportion of the local T cells are antigen specific, and it is of major interest, therefore, to know which antigens are involved in atherosclerosis.

Recently it has been shown that about 10% of T-cell clones generated from populations of isolated human plaque T cells are able to recognize antigenic determinants of oxidized low density lipoproteins (ox-LDL). The recognition is HLA-DR restricted and the cells respond by proliferating and producing cytokines [13]. Although it is not excluded that there are more antigens involved in the plaque immune response, the identification of ox-LDL epitopes as inciting antigens is of importance since it provides a link between inflammation and lipids in the atherosclerotic plaque.

Antibodies against ox-LDL can also be detected in arterial tissue [14] and in the serum of patients with atherosclerosis [15]. Moreover, serum titers increase with the severity of disease in symptomatic patients [15]. As previously noted, the intimal plaques contain no B cells, and it is unclear where the antibodies are raised. Antigenic stimulation of B cells could take place in the locoregional lymphnodes. Perhaps a more likely source are the adventitial infiltrates that surround the vessel wall at sites of extensive intimal plaque formation. In contrast to the intimal plaque these cuff-like infiltrates contain many B cells and plasma cells; ceroid pigment, an endproduct of lipid oxidation, is also frequently found at these sites [16]. It is still unknown whether these auto-antibodies have a protective role or whether they are involved in the progression of the disease. However, they show that epitopes of ox-LDL molecules may have autoantigenic properties.

Another association between lipid constituents and inflammation can be observed with macrophages, which are the most important source of inflammatory mediators in addition to their recognized function as lipid scavengers [17]. Plaque macrophages are derived from monocytes circulating in the blood. Once they have entered the intima and during their migration through the intimal lesion, they endocytose lipids, especially via scavenger receptors which specifically recognize ox-LDL. Unlimited uptake of ox-LDL takes place, leading to the formation of lipid-laden macrophages known as foam cells. At the border of the atheromatous core, foam cells eventually die, and their cytoplasmic lipids are spilled into the extracellular space. This process contributes to the formation and growth of the lipid rich, necrotic atheromatous core [18]. Like T cells, the population of macrophages in the plaque is by no means homogeneous. In the superficial parts of the fibrous cap, they express HLA-DR molecules and co-stimulatory molecules abundantly, but the expression of CD36, a scavenger receptor for lipids, is low or absent [12, 19]. This macrophage phenotype can function as an immunocompetent cell together with activated T cells, and the resulting secretion of cytokines such as tumor necrosis factor (TNF) and interferon -(IFN-) γ has been shown to down-regulate the expression of scavenger receptors [20]. Macrophages near the atheroma, however, most of which have a morphology of foam cells, exhibit a different phenotype. At these sites macrophages express high numbers of CD36 molecules and no co-stimulatory molecules, indicating that they function principally as lipid scavengers. When these differentiation markers are used in immunodouble stains, a gradual phenotypic shift towards the center (atheroma) is seen; this pattern is highly suggestive of a differentiation of macrophages from immunocompetent cells towards lipid scavenging cells. This unique dual role for macrophages in atherosclerosis could be the basis for the characteristic morphology of atherosclerotic plaques.

A large number of proinflammatory cytokines and vascular growth factors have now been identified, and it is presently beyond doubt that complex paracrine regulatory networks are active in the plaque tissue (for a review see [2]). Taken together these factors are capable of influencing all of the important pathologic features of atherosclerosis, including endothelial dysfunction, smooth muscle cell growth, synthesis/breakdown of extracellular matrix components, lipid metabolism, and thrombus formation. It is therefore reasonable to assume that inflammatory mechanisms have a modulating effect on the growth and differentiation of lesions.

Inflammation and Plaque Morphology

Other immune-mediated long-standing inflammatory diseases, such as sarcoidosis and rheumatoid arthritis, have a remodeling effect on the affected soft tissues and organs, inducing either fibrosis or tissue lysis and necrosis. Chronic inflammation may well have similar remodeling effects on the composition of the plaque.

The tissue composition of advanced atherosclerotic plaques is highly variable, and this is considered of prime clinical importance with respect to complications such as plaque fissuring and thrombosis. On this basis it is customary to distinguish between stable and unstable plaques. The stable plaque is almost solely composed of fibrous tissue, whereas unstable plaques are characterized by large pools of extracellular lipid-rich debris (atheromas) and a thin or virtually absent fibrous cap [1]. Immunohistochemical studies on a series of advanced atherosclerotic plaques have shown that particular types of plaque morphology often relate to different patterns of cellular composition [21, 22]. Plaques which are histologically classified as lipid-rich contain almost exclusively macrophages and T lymphocytes in the attenuated fibrous cap. On the other hand, plaques classified as fibrous, in which the atheroma is inconspicuous or absent, are either acellular or dominated by smooth muscle cells. However, the majority of plaques have an intermediate architecture with variably sized atheromas and fibrous caps in which smooth muscle cells intermingle with inflammatory cells either diffusely or focally. In the latter situation, closely packed inflammatory cells occupy distinct and well-demarcated areas in which the amount of collagen and the number of smooth muscle cells are markedly decreased. These observations suggest that plaque morphology depends on interactions between inflammatory cells, smooth muscle cells, and extracellular matrix components.

Several other investigations support this concept. Smooth muscle cells play a reparative role in the plaque by producing extracellular matrix components such as collagens and elastin, and are thus responsible for maintainance of the stability of the fibrous cap. Disappearance of smooth muscle cells, however, indicates a decline in the reparative response and therefore may give rise to vulnerable regions in plaques. Inflammatory products of macrophages and T cells are considered to be involved in these processes.

Of particular importance in this respect is IFN-γ, a T-cell-derived cytokine which was immunolocalized in human atherosclerotic plaques a few years ago [8]. This cytokine activates immunoregulatory functions of macrophages and also affects the plaque smooth muscle cells. In vascular smooth muscle cell cultures, the administration of IFN-γ causes inhibition of proliferation as well as a marked decrease in basal and cytokine-stimulated interstitial collagen synthesis [23, 24]. Moreover, at the same time these IFN-γ stimulated cultured smooth muscle cells exhibit an aberrant expression of HLA-DR antigens; this is only observed with IFN-γ stimulation [25]. In experimental animal studies, this particular cytokine inhibits the vascular wall response to balloon injury, which essentially consists of smooth muscle cell proliferation [26]. These findings are of great interest since in the human plaque HLA-DR antigens are expressed on smooth muscle cells only in the proximity of inflammatory foci [21] and interstitial collagen protein expression is decreased at sites of T-cell accumulation [27]. These features strongly suggest that IFN-γ exerts effects in the human plaque, which are similar to those seen in culture studies and experimental balloon injury.

Apart from having inhibitory effects on matrix synthesis, inflammatory products may also cause active breakdown of the connective tissue matrix. Among the vast repertoire of toxic products and lytic enzymes produced by macrophages, interest is presently focussed on the family of extracellular matrix degrading metalloproteinases (MMPs). Using immunocytochemical and in situ hybridization techniques, members of all three subgroups of MMPs, including collagenases [28], gelatinases [28, 29] and stromelysins [28, 30] have now been detected in atherosclerotic plaque tissue. Their importance is illustrated by the fact that, once activated by cytokines like TNF and IL-1, together they can degrade all the extracellular matrix components of an atherosclerotic plaque. The presence of both the zymogen and the active form of these enzymes at sites of foam-cell (macrophage) accumulations, which can be regarded as vulnerable regions, makes it conceivable that they indeed play an important role in local connective tissue breakdown [28].

Inflammation and Plaque Rupture

The destabilizing effects of active inflammation are strikingly evident when ruptured and thrombosed plaques are studied using the same methodologies. Plaque disruption is the final consequence of a multifactorial process in which plaque composition and biomechanical factors are the most important contributors [31].

Davies et al. [22] showed that plaque morphologies, as alluded to above, indeed enhance the risk of plaque rupture. These authors compared a large series of intact (two morphologic types: fibrous and lipid-rich) and ulcerated (ruptured) aortic plaques and concluded that instability of plaques can be viewed as a function of increasing amounts of extracellular lipids, increasing macrophage contents and diminishing smooth muscle cell contents. The most extreme values were found in the group of ruptured lesions. Other studies have primarily focused on biomechanical or hemodynamic aspects (for a review see [31]). Among these, the distribution of circumferential tensile stress was computed in simulated plaques [32] and ruptured plaques [33] and studied in combination with immunocytochemical detection of macrophages in ruptured plaques. It was found that regions with high circumferential stress correlated with sites of rupture. However, the site of rupture was influenced by variations in mechanical strength of the fibrous cap, due to focal accumulations of macrophages. In other words, although inflammation is by no means the one single mechanism involved, it may set the scene for tensile stresses, vaso-spasms or hemodynamic forces to cause rupture by inducing weak areas in the fibrous cap.

This view is further supported by immunocytochemical investigations on the exact sites of plaque rupture. In an autopsy series of thrombosed coronary plaques obtained from 20 patients who died of acute myocardial infarction, we found that the immediate site of rupture is invariably associated with the occurrence of large numbers of macrophages and T lymphocytes. In-flammatory cells and some smooth muscle cells adjacent to the infiltrate ex-press HLA-DR antigens, indicating cell activation and the secretion of cytokines. Moreover, the number of smooth muscle cells and the total amount of collagen is low at these sites. This is in contrast to the overall cellular composition of the entire plaque which is much more heterogeneous, and it shows that the area of inflammation associated with the site of rupture can indeed be very discrete [34]. More recently, in vivo studies on atherectomy specimens from patients with various ischemic coronary syndromes (stable angina, unstable angina, non-Q-wave myocardial infarction) have confirmed the relation between inflammation and plaque complications. It was shown that the macrophage contents of specimens, planimetrically quantified in im-munostained tissue sections and related to the clinical status of the patient, increased with the severity of the ischemic syndromes [35].

Conclusions

There is ample evidence for the participation of inflammatory responses in the pathogenesis of atherosclerosis, which are at least in part sustained and probably also initiated by T-cell-mediated immune mechanisms. Of pivotal clinical importance is the fact that exaggeration or activation of the in-flammatory response in the advanced lesions of atherosclerosis destroys the structural integrity of the plaque in such a way that ruptures of plaques and thrombotic occlusion of the vessels may occur.

There is a growing awareness that the inflammatory response is related to the presence of lipid constituents, particularly the products of lipid oxidation, in the plaque. This relationship could explain why lipid-lowering strategies result in only a limited angiographic regression of coronary stenoses but a dramatic decrease in the rate of occurrence of acute coronary events. Stabilization of these lesions could be the result of reducing the inflammatory stimuli provided by lipids [36, 37]. Since inflammatory reactions occur constitutively during the development of lesions, as does the infiltration of lipids, these considerations may also have implications for the growth and maturation of lesions at younger ages, before atherosclerosis becomes clinically manifest.

References

1. Davies MJ (1990) A macro and micro view of coronary vascular insult in ischemic heart disease. Circulation 82 (Suppl II): 38–46
2. Ross R (1993) The pathogenesis of atherosclerosis: a perspective for the 1990s. Nature 362: 801–809
3. Ross R, Glomset JA (1976) The pathogenesis of atherosclerosis. N Engl J Med 295: 369–377, 420–425
4. Jonasson L, Holm J, Skalli O, Bondjers G, Hansson GK (1986) Regional accumulations of T cells, macrophages and smooth muscle cells in the human atherosclerotic plaque. Arteriosclerosis 6: 131–138
5. Munro JM, van der Walt JD, Munro CS, Chalmers JAC, Cox EL (1987) An immunohistochemical analysis of human aortic fatty streaks. Hum Pathol 18: 375–380
6. Emeson EE, Robertson AL (1988) T lymphocytes in aortic and coronary intimas. Their potential role in atherogenesis. Am J Pathol 130: 369–376
7. van der Wal AC, Das PK, Bentz van de Berg DB, van der Loos CM, Becker AE (1989) Atherosclerotic lesions in humans. In situ immunophenotypic analysis suggesting an immune mediated response. Lab Invest 61: 166–170
8. Hansson GK, Holm J, Jonasson L (1989) Detection of activated T lymphocytes in the human atherosclerotic plaque. Am J Pathol 135: 169–175
9. Stemme S, Holm J, Hansson GK (1991) T lymphocytes in human atherosclerotic plaques are memory cells expressing CD 45RO and the integrin VLA-1. Arterioscler Thromb 12: 206–211
10. Rekhter MD, Gordon D (1995) Active proliferation of different cell types, including lymphocytes, in the human atherosclerotic plaque. Am J Pathol 147: 668–677
11. Mondino A, Jenkins MK (1994) Surface proteins involved in T-cell stimulation. J Leukoc Biol 55: 805–815
12. de Boer OJ, Hirsch F, van der Wal AC, Das PK, Becker AE (1995) T-cell activation in human atherosclerotic plaques: in situ expression of costimulatory molecules. Atherosclerosis 115 (Suppl): S26
13. Stemme S, Faber, Holm J, Wiklund O, Witztum JL, Hansson GK (1995) T-lymphocytes from human atherosclerotic plaques recognize oxidized low density lipoprotein. Proc Natl Acad Sci U S A 92: 3893–3897
14. Parums DV, Brown DL, Mitchinson MJ (1990) Serum antibodies to oxidized LDL and ceroid in chronic priaortitis. Arch Pathol Lab Med 114: 383–387
15. Solonen JT, Yla-Herttuala S, Yamamoto R (1992) Autoantibody against oxidized LDL and progression of carotid atherosclerosis. Lancet 339: 883–887
16. Ramshaw AL, Parums DV (1990) Immunohistochemical characterization of inflammatory cells associated with advanced atherosclerosis. Histopathology 17: 543–552
17. Mitchinson (1987) Macrophages and atherogenesis Lancet ii: 146–148
18. Witzum JL (1994) The oxidation hypothesis of atherosclerosis Lancet 344; 793–795
19. van der Wal AC, Das PK, Tigges AJ, Becker AE (1992) Macrophage differentiation in atherosclerosis. An immunohistochemical analysis in humans. Am J Pathol 141: 161–168
20. Geng YJ, Hansson GK (1992) Interferon gamma inhibits scavenger receptor expression and foam cell formation in human monocyte derived macrophages. J Clin Invest 89: 1322–1330
21. van der Wal AC, Becker AE, van der Loos CM, Tigges AJ, Das PK (1994) Fibrous and lipid rich atherosclerotic plaques are part of interchangeable morphologies related to inflammation: a concept. Coron Artery Dis 5: 463–469

22. Davies MJ, Richardson PD, Woolf N, Katz DR, Mann J (1993) Risk of thrombus in human atherosclerotic plaques: role of extracellular lipid, macrophage and smooth muscle cell content. Br Heart J 69: 377–381
23. Hansson GK, Jonasson L, Holm J, Clowes M, Clowes AW (1988) Gamma interferon regulates vascular smooth muscle proliferation and Ia antigen expression in vivo and in vitro. Circ Res 63: 712–719
24. Amento EP, Ehsain N, Palmer H, Libby P (1991) Cytokines and growth factors positively and negatively regulate interstitial collagene expression in human vascular smooth muscle cells. Arterioscler Thromb 11: 1223–1230
25. Warner SJC, Friedman GB, Libby P (1989) Regulation of major histocompatibility gene expression in cultured human vascular smooth muscle cells. Arteriosclerosis 9: 279–288
26. Hansson GK, Holm J, Holm S, Fotev Z, Hedrich HJ, Fingerle J (1991) T lymphocytes inhibit the vascular response to injury. Proc Natl Acad Sci U S A 88: 10530–10534
27. Rekhter MD, Zhanb K, Narayanan AS, Phan S, Schork MA, Gordon D (1993) Type I collagen gene expression in human atherosclerosis. Localization to specific plaque regions. Am J Pathol 143: 1634–1648
28. Galis Z, Sukhova GK, Lark MW, Libby P (1994) Increased expression of matrix-metalloproteinases and matrix degrading activity in vulnerable regions of human atherosclerotic plaques. J Clin Invest 94: 2493–2503
29. Brown DL, Hibbs MS, Kearney M, Loushin C, Isner JM (1995) Identification of 92-kD gelatinase in human coronary atherosclerotic lesions: association of active enzyme synthesis with unstable angina. Circulation 91: 2125–2131
30. Henney AM, Wakely, Davies MJ, Foster K, Hembry R, Murphy G, Humphries S (1991) Localization of stromelysin gene expression in atherosclerotic plaques by in situ hybridization. Proc Natl Acad Sci U S A 88: 8154–8158
31. Falk E, Shah PK, Fuster V (1995) Coronary plaque disruption. Circulation 92: 657–671
32. Richardson PD, Born GVR, Davies MJ (1989) Influence of plaque configuration and stress distribution on fissuring of coronary atherosclerotic plaques. Lancet ii: 941–944
33. Cheng GC, Loree HM, Kamm RD, Fishbein MC, Lee RT (1993) Distribution of circumferential stress in ruptured and stable atherosclerotic lesions: a structural analysis with histopathological correlation. Circulation 87: 1179–1187
34. van der Wal AC, Becker AE, van der Loos CM, Das PK (1994) Site of intimal rupture or erosion of thrombosed coronary atherosclerotic plaques is characterized by an inflammatory process irrespective of the dominant plaque morphology. Circulation 89: 36–44
35. Moreno PR, Falk E, Palacios IF, Newell JB, Fuster V, Fallon J (1994) Macrophage infiltration in acute coronary syndromes: implications for plaque rupture. Circulation 90: 775–778
36. Alexander RW (1994) Inflammation and coronary artery disease. N Engl J Med 331: 468–469
37. Libby P (1995) Molecular bases of the acute coronary syndromes. Circulation 91: 2844–2850

Inflammation in Acute Coronary Syndromes

P.R. Moreno[1] and J.T. Fallon[2]

Introduction

Coronary atherosclerosis without acute thrombosis is generally a benign disease that is asymptomatic or presents as chronic stable angina. The great majority of patients can be treated pharmacologically. For those with intractable angina, percutaneous and surgical revascularization are available with high initial success and good long-term prognosis. Acute manifestations of coronary atherosclerosis either unstable angina, acute myocardial infarction, or sudden cardiac death share a common pathophysiologic phenomenon: acute coronary thrombosis. This life threatening complication occurs usually at the site of plaque fissure or rupture. Several studies have shown that plaque rupture plays a key role in the pathophysiology of acute coronary syndromes [1, 2].

This chapter reviews the potential inflammatory related determinants of plaque rupture and its consequences. An initial section reviews plaque composition, vulnerability, and the role of inflammation in plaque rupture. The subsequent section discusses the relations between inflammation and coronary thrombosis emphasizing the role of macrophages and tissue factor (TF) as the predominant thrombogenic substrate in patients with acute coronary syndromes.

Plaque Rupture

Plaque Composition

Atherosclerosis is an intimal disease characterized by two main components: atheromatous 'gruel' and sclerotic tissue. The former is rich in extracellular lipid and is 'soft', while the latter is rich in collagen and 'hard', i.e., non-compliant. Extracellular lipid is predominantly blood derived, insudated from

[1]Cardiac Catherization Laboratories, Massachusetts General Hospital, 32 Fruit Street, Boston, MA 02114, USA
[2]Mount Sinai Medical Center, The Cardiovascular Institute, Department of Medicine & Pathology, Box 1194, One Gustave, L. Levy Place, New York, NY 10029, USA

the lumen and deposited directly due to trapping and matrix binding or indirectly due to necrosis of lipid-filled foam cells, the majority of which are macrophages. In patients with ischemic heart disease, the coronary arteries are diffusely involved with confluent 'plaquing', and the composition of coronary plaques varies greatly without any obvious relation to coronary risk factors [3]. Regarding size, the sclerotic component usually dominates, while the atheromatous component is much less impressive, constituting less than 20% of the average stenotic coronary plaque. The sclerotic plaque component limits coronary flow and gives rise to chronic angina pectoris, but it may, in fact, stabilize the plaque. On the contrary, the atheromatous component is dangerous, because it softens and destabilizes plaques making them vulnerable, i.e., prone to rupture, a process that is frequently complicated by thrombosis.

Vulnerability to Rupture

A vulnerable plaque typically consists of a central core of soft atheromatous gruel separated from the vascular lumen by a cap of fibrous tissue (Fig. 1). The mechanical properties of plaques and particularly the size and consistency of the atheromatous component are critical in determining the distribution of

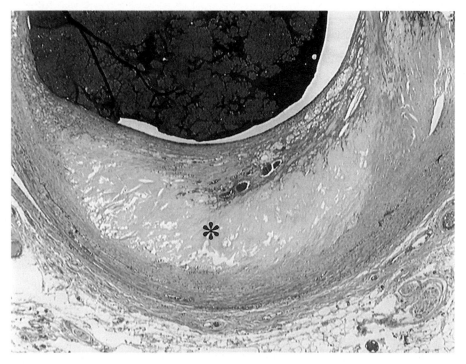

Fig. 1. Photomicrograph of typical vulnerable atherosclerotic plaque with lipid-rich core (∗) separated from lumen by a fibrous cap

stresses that may precipitate plaque rupture [4–6]. Post-mortem studies of human aortic atherosclerotic plaques show that plaques undergoing thrombosis contain larger atheromatous cores than intact plaques [7]. Gertz and Roberts reported the composition of infarct-related coronary plaques and found much larger atheromatous cores in the 39 segments with plaque disruption than in the 339 segments with intact surfaces (32% and 5%–12% of plaque area respectively) [8]. The atheromatous core contains water, cholesterol crystals, cholesterol esters (oils), phospholipids, collagen remnants and cellular degradation products. The ratio of liquid (oily) cholesterol esters to free (crystalline) cholesterol monohydrate determines the stiffness of the plaque. In vitro combinations of atheromatous components have demonstrated that increasing the cholesterol monohydrate concentration up to 50% increases the stiffness of the plaque by 4.5 times compared with plaques containing less cholesterol monohydrate and more phospholipid and triglyceride [9]. This later concept of 'stiffening' of the lipid pool may be one of the mechanisms of enhanced plaque stability responsible for the observed reduction of acute coronary events associated with lipid-lowering therapy [10].

The atheromatous gruel is separated from the vascular lumen by a fibrous cap which may be very thin and is often heavily infiltrated with foam cells of macrophage origin. This structure is the "Achilles tendon" of the atherosclerotic plaque and must bear all the biomechanical forces that tend to rupture the plaque. The maximum circumferential stress in the plaque is inversely related to the thickness of the fibrous cap and directly related to the size of the lipid pool. That is, the thinner the cap, the more vulnerable the plaque is to rupture [11]. The fibrous cap is usually thinnest and probably weakest at its junctions with the nearby intima, also known as the shoulder regions [12]. These areas contain less collagen with resultant reduced tensile strength.

Cellularity and calcification play a significant role considering that calcified plaques are stiffer than cellular or hypocellular ones [13–15]. Rupture of the fibrous cap occurs at the region of maximum circumferential stress in 58% of patients with fatal coronary thrombosis. This suggests that the concentration of circumferential stress in a plaque plays an important role in plaque rupture. However, rupture does not always occur in this region, implying that local compositional variations in the plaque in combination with fibrous cap characteristics are also determinants of plaque rupture [16].

Role of Inflammation in Plaque Rupture

Considering atherosclerosis as an inflammatory disease has provided for new insights into the pathogenesis of acute coronary syndromes [17]. These life-threatening events may reflect acute exacerbation or activation of a chronic inflammatory response in the fibrous cap with subsequent rupture and exposure of thrombogenic materials to the flowing blood leading to coronary thrombosis [18, 19]. Systemic markers of inflammation, such as neutrophil elastase-derived fibrinopeptide and cytokines, are elevated in patients with unstable angina and acute myocardial infarction [20]. The identification of sensitive and specific markers for acute coronary syndromes might facilitate the diagnosis of atherosclerosis and help stratify high risk patients. Furthermore, it could provide a potential therapeutic end point for the activity of the disease. Liuzzo et al., documented that the acute-phase reactants C-reactive protein and amyloid A protein are elevated in the serum of patients with unstable angina and acute myocardial infarction with a high sensitivity and specificity for predicting cardiac death, myocardial infarction, or the urgent need of coronary revascularization [21]. However, it is not clear why these acute-phase proteins are elevated.

Local leukocyte-vessel wall interactions are mediated through integrin receptors and endothelial cell receptors known as intercellular adhesion molecules, including ICAM-1 and ICAM-2 and vascular cell adhesion molecule VCAM-1 [22]. Mazzone et al., demonstrated a transcoronary increase in the membrane expression of the integrin receptor CD11b/CD18 on coronary sinus monocytes and granulocytes from patients with unstable angina when compared with simultaneous control samples drawn from the aortic blood. This suggests an association of acute inflammation and unstable angina [23]. Normally, integrin receptors on circulating monocytes are in an inactive or low avidity state. The mechanism by which monocytes undergo activation has not yet been completely clarified. Endothelial-derived chemoattractant proteins like monocyte chemoattractant protein 1 (MCP-1) [24–28], tumor necrosis factor (TNF) [29, 30], interleukin (IL-1) [30, 31], and monocyte colony-stimulating factor (M-CSF) [32, 33] appear to be increased in atherosclerotic lesions in both humans and experimental animals. However, it is not clear that endothelial cells are the source of all of these factors in vivo. Rather, it appears to be the expression of these factors by smooth muscle cells and monocyte/macrophages already resident within the developing lesions that further attract monocytes into the plaque [34]. Other factors like shear stress, thrombin and lysophosphatidylcholine, a component of oxidized low density lipoproteins (LDL) that is increased in the plasma of hypercholesterolemic patients, are also monocyte chemoattractive and induce VCAM-1 and ICAM-1 expression by arterial endothelial cells in vitro [35–37].

Newly immigrated monocytes develop functional competence, as well as undergo further divisions, after they enter the subendothelial space [38]. The transformation into tissue macrophages is presumably a response to colony-stimulating factors [39]. Monocytes spontaneously undergo programmed cell death (apoptosis) unless they are stimulated by M-CSF or inflammatory cytokines [40]. However, as monocytes differentiate into mature macrophages, this requirement is lost, and tissue macrophages are resistant to apoptotic stimuli such as ionizing radiation [41]. Sensitivity to activation-induced apoptosis appears to be determined in part by previous exposure to particular cytokines.

Macrophages taken from sites of active inflammation have increased properties for endocytosis, digestion, secretion of proteins, cytokines and growth factors that may be involved in coronary plaque rupture as well as in the subsequent intravascular thrombotic response [34, 42]. Interestingly, macrophages in their terminal stage of maturation exhibit a 20- to 30-fold increase in production of oxygen free radicals and a down regulation of c-fms, the M-CSF receptor [43]. Because M-CSF appears to be required for the survival of macrophages and is thought to act by suppressing apoptosis [44, 45], either terminal differentiation or a failure in the local production of M-CSF could lead to an increase in oxygen free radicals with a decrease in macrophage survival. The subsequent accumulation of necrosis debris from macrophages increases the size of the atheromatous core and may augment the vulnerability of a coronary plaque to rupture.

Studies of macrophages in human atherosclerosis have been limited to postmortem aortic experiments and coronary autopsy analyses [7, 8, 12 18, 46]. Lendon et al., measured the total density of macrophages and the maximum stress (force per unit area) in human aortic plaques, and found that ulcerated plaques showed a significant increase in macrophage density and a decreased maximum stress at fracture sites when compared with intact plaques [15]. Davies et al. quantified the percentage of the total plaque area occupied by lipid pool, macrophages and smooth muscle cells in three different groups of human aortic specimens: intact plaques from aortas without thrombosis, intact plaques from aortas with plaques undergoing thrombosis, and thrombosed plaques. Aortic thrombosed plaques contained larger lipid pools and macrophage infiltration areas with a smaller volume of smooth muscle cells, suggesting that atherosclerotic plaque rupture is preceded by a shift in cell population as lipid pool increases, with increased numbers of macrophages and loss of smooth muscle cells in the fibrous cap [7]. Richardson et al. documented lipid-filled foam cells at fibrous cap rupture areas, and van der Wal et al., identified activated macrophages as the dominant cell at the site of superficial erosion or rupture of the fibrous cap in patients with fatal coronary thrombosis [12, 18].

The retrieval of plaque material during percutaneous directional coronary atherectomy has created new possibilities for the study of coronary artery disease in living patients. We tested the hypothesis that macrophage rich areas were increased in coronary plaque tissue from patients with unstable rest angina and non-Q wave myocardial infarction in comparison with coronary plaque tissue from patients with stable angina using directional coronary atherectomy samples [46]. Human macrophage antibody staining was performed with an antihuman pan-macrophage antibody to CD68. The percentage of the total plaque area occupied by macrophages was significantly larger in plaque tissue from patients with unstable angina (13.3% ± 5.6%) and non-Q wave myocardial infarction (14.6% ± 4.6%) than in plaque tissue from patients with stable angina (3.14% ± 1%).

Matrix Degrading Metalloproteinases

The secretion of matrix degrading metalloproteinases by macrophages with subsequent degradation of the fibrous cap may be the principal mechanism of plaque rupture but this hypothesis is still controversial and awaits further studies. Macrophages can influence matrix turnover and plaque rupture by secreting matrix degrading metalloproteinases (MMPs) and plasminogen activators [47]. MMPs are a family of Zn^{2+} and Ca^{2+}-dependent enzymes, which are important in the turnover of extracellular matrix protein in both physiological and pathological states. Twelve MMPs have been identified, cloned, and sequenced, and these are divided into three groups based on substrate preferences [48]. MMPs include the collagenases which degrade structural types I and III collagen, the type IV gelatinases which degrade basement membrane collagen, and the stromelysins which have broad substrate specificity against proteoglycans, laminin, fibronectin, gelatin, and types IV and IX collagen. Stromelysins also plays a major role as collagenase activators [49].

MMPs require activation from proenzyme precursors to attain enzymatic activity. Plasmin is a potent activator of most MMPs, promoting cleavage of the latent propeptides to the active molecule [50, 51]. The roles of urokinase-like plasminogen activator (uPA) and its specific receptor (uPA-r) and their inhibitors (PAI-1 and PAI-2) have been studied in relation to tissue invasion and cell surface proteolysis [52]. uPa and uPA-r are expressed by a variety of cells, including macrophages, and it has been shown that antibodies and inhibitors of uPA prevent matrix degradation [53]. There are similarities between this proteolytic system and the clotting cascade; while plasmin cleaves and therefore activates stromelysin, the resultant active enzyme can activate other proenzymes, forming a positive-feedback loop. When the collagenases are cleaved by stromelysin, there is a five- to eightfold increase in their proteolytic activity. Also, reminiscent of other protease cascades involved in regulation of key biological processes, ubiquitous inhibitors known as tissue inhibitors of metalloproteinases (TIMPs) control the activity of these enzymes. Three members of this family have been identified to date [54, 55]. TIMP 1 is synthesized by human vascular smooth muscle cells as well as macrophages, and forms high-affinity, irreversible complexes with the active forms of collagenases, stromelysin, and gelatinases. It is highly expressed in granulation tissue, and its role is to regulate enzyme activity at the level of activation of MMPs in both latent and catalytic forms [55]. TIMP-2 binds to progelatinase A, stabilizing this inactive form of the enzyme [56]. TIMP-3 is localized specifically to the extracellular matrix, and is involved in the connective tissue remodeling process, as seen in the Sorsby's fundus dystrophy [57]. As a result, the net level of proteinase activity in a given tissue is dependent on a tight balance between these enzymes, their activators, and their inhibitors.

Degradation of Matrix in Human Atherosclerotic Plaques

The expression of MMPs by macrophage-derived foam cells was documented by Galis et al, using a balloon injury model in the hypercholesterolemic rabbit [58]. Such lesion-derived foam cells expressed stromelysin and interstitial collagenase both in situ and in vitro. In contrast, alveolar macrophages from the same animals did not display autonomous expression of these MMPs. More recently, Shah et al. incubated macrophages with human aortic plaque caps to test the hypothesis that human monocyte-derived macrophages may induce fibrous cap collagen degradation [59]. The average hydroxyproline release was increased ninefold in fibrous caps incubated with macrophages in comparison with cell-free incubated tissue. Furthermore, immunostaining for MMP-1 and MMP-2 showed expression by macrophages with zymographic evidence of gelatinolytic activity. Previous experiments have demonstrated diffuse expression of mRNA for MMP-3 (stromelysin) and MMP-9 (92-kDa gelatinase) in human atherosclerotic plaques [60, 61]. Galis et al., also documented immunohistochemical evidence of MMP-1, MMP-2, and MMP-3 expression with gelatinolytic and caseinolytic activity in human carotid endarterectomy specimens. In addition, the use of recombinant TIMP-1 inhibitor reduced this lytic activity, suggesting a mismatch between MMPs and TIMPs in complex atherosclerotic plaques [62]. More recently, Nikkari et al. demonstrated a strong correlation between MMP-1 and the presence of hemorrhage in the atheromatous core from human carotid plaques [63]. Davies has shown an increased immunostaining activity for stromelysin at the edges of the lipid core, suggesting a lytic effect for gruel expansion in the atherosclerotic plaque [64].

Two neutral proteases, tryptase and chymase, are capable of triggering degradation of the extracellular matrix via activation of MMPs [65, 66]. The presence of mast cells which contain these enzymes has been documented by Kovanen et al., who identified an increased percentage of mast cells in areas of erosion or rupture of coronary lesions from patients who died from acute myocardial infarction. The percent of all cells in areas of plaque rupture was 6% for mast cells in comparison to 1% in the adjacent atheromatous area and 0.1% in the unaffected intimal area. In addition, the proportion of these mast cells that were activated, i.e., stimulated to degranulate and release their enzyme content, was 86% in areas of plaque rupture, 63% in the adjacent atheromatous area, and 27% in the unaffected intimal area suggesting an important role for mast cells in the pathophysiology of plaque rupture [67].

Cytokine Regulation of Collagen Breakdown:
The Role of Lymphocytes and Smooth Muscle Cells

A number of cytokines and growth factors are known to induce the synthesis of MMPs, including TNF-α, IL-1, interferon gamma (IFN-γ), and platelet-derived growth factor (PDGF), whereas others, such as transforming growth factor-β (TGF-β), heparin and corticosteroids, have an inhibitory effect [48, 68]. TNF-α, its receptor (sTNF-R1) and IL-1 are increased in the serum of patients with acute myocardial infarction and may reflect myocardial tissue damage with ongoing necrosis [69, 70].

An interesting cycle encompasses collagen metabolism, metalloproteinase regulation and smooth muscle cell homeostasis in the atherosclerotic plaque. Collagen exists in many forms. Principally, the interstitial form of fibrillar collagen concerns us in the context of the plaque's fibrous cap. Triple helical coils derived from specific procollagen precursors make up the types I and III collagen found in the fibrils of the plaque. Vascular smooth muscle cells synthesize and assemble these macromolecules. TGF-β, increases mRNA and protein synthesis of interstitial collagens types I and III by smooth muscle cells, and is considered the most potent stimulus for interstitial collagen expression by these cells [68, 71]. Whereas IFN-γ markedly decreases the expression by human smooth muscle cells of the interstitial collagens not only in the basal, unstimulated state, but also upon exposure to TGF-β.

Among the cells found in human atherosclerotic plaques, only T lymphocytes are known to elaborate the IFN-γ [72]. Van der Wal et al. provides evidence connecting activated T cells to plaque rupture showing that smooth muscle cells and leukocytes express high levels of a transplantation antigen known as HLA-DRα which when expressed suggests a state of "activation" of smooth muscle cells [18]. Previous studies by Warner et al. showed that of a wide variety of cytokines tested, only IFN-γ induced the expression of HLA-DRα in culture smooth muscle cells [73]. Therefore, the finding of cells bearing this marker of activation indicates the presence of IFN-γ at the sites of coronary plaque rupture in humans with fatal myocardial infarction. Moreover, Rekhter et al. found an inverse correlation between the presence of T lymphocytes and the amount of interstitial collagen mRNA and protein in human atherosclerotic lesions, a finding that also supports this concept [74]. Taken together, these results concordantly suggest that chronic immune stimulation within atheroma leads to elaboration of IFN-γ by T cells, inhibiting collagen synthesis in vulnerable regions of the plaque's fibrous cap. In addition to inhibiting collagen gene expression, IFN-γ can inhibit proliferation, induce apoptosis in human vascular smooth muscle cells and activate metalloproteinases that further increase collagen degradation predisposing to plaque rupture [68, 75, 76].

Antigens

The presence of activated T cells and macrophages imply an ongoing immunologic reaction in the atherosclerotic plaque. An immune response normally starts when a T lymphocyte recognizes a foreign antigen. Viral proteins, such as antigens of herpes simplex virus type I and cytomegalovirus (CMV) are present in the arterial wall during atherosclerosis [77, 78]. In experimental models, viral replication can lead to increased leukocyte adherence to endothelium, thrombin generation, and smooth muscle cell proliferation [79–81]. In addition, CMV infection is associated with restenosis after coronary angioplasty [82]. However, the hypothesis that CMV replication is associated with instability of coronary artery plaques was tested by Kol et al., who did not find evidence for CMV cDNA encoding gene in twenty atherectomy specimens from patients with unstable angina [83].

The presence of Chlamydia pneumoniae in coronary atheroma has been documented in several human populations [84–86]. Chlamydia isolates were demonstrated in macrophages and smooth muscle cells of aortic atherosclerotic plaques and in carotid endarterectomy specimens [87]. Furthermore, a sero response to an epitope of chlamydia lipopolysaccharide has been documented in patients with acute myocardial infarction. The presence of elevated antibody titers and immune complexes was a significant independent risk factor for acute myocardial infarction in the Helsinki Heart Study, suggesting a potential role for *C. pneumoniae* during the inflammatory response in coronary tissue from patients with acute myocardial infarction [88].

Antibodies to oxidized LDL (oxLDL-Ab) are common in humans and their titers appear to correlate with the progression of coronary artery disease [89]. Patients with early onset of peripheral vascular disease as well as diabetics have an increased level of oxLDL-Ab [90, 91], but their role in acute coronary syndromes are unclear and remain to be elucidated. Recently, Schumacher et al. quantified oxLDL-Ab in 15 patients with acute myocardial infarction and correlated the levels with CK-MB levels. Ten patients with marked elevation of the MB isoenzyme had significant decreases of oxLDL-Ab during the acute phase suggesting that the decrease of oxLDL-Ab appears to be a marker for the severity of acute myocardial infarction [92].

Finally, heat shock proteins (hsp), intracellular chaperones that stabilize other proteins, are elevated in patients with atherosclerosis [93, 94]. Kleindienst et al., described hsp65 expression at the site of human atherosclerotic lesions and the intensity of expression correlated with lesion severity [95]. Increased titers of circulating hsp65 antibody are a strong independent risk factor for the presence of carotid atherosclerosis [96]. Furthermore, Birnie et al. examined the titers of anti-IgG hsp65 before and at days 3 and 5 after acute myocardial infarction in 11 patients successfully treated with intravenous thrombolysis [97]. Antibodies against hsp65 were present in all samples but their levels were not significantly increased which is presumably related to chronic hsp65 exposure from the underlying atherosclerotic disease.

Coronary Thrombosis

Coronary thrombosis is the result of a dynamic interplay between the arterial wall and the flowing blood. About 75% of thrombi responsible for acute coronary syndromes are precipitated by plaque rupture whereby a thrombogenic substrate is exposed to flowing blood. In this section, we discuss evidence for a role of TF as the predominant thrombogenic substrate in patients with acute coronary syndromes.

Thrombogenic Substrate

Collagen is considered a major thrombogenic substrate in the vessel wall and the platelet-vessel wall interaction was extensively studied under that concept [98]. Badimón et al., have used an ex vivo perfusion chamber to study the thrombogenicity of components of the human atherosclerotic plaques [99, 101]. The pivotal role of fibrous cap rupture in the pathophysiology of acute coronary syndromes emphasized the importance of the atheromatous gruel as the most vulnerable plaque component and suggested that the lipid-rich core together with macrophages could be involved in the subsequent thrombotic reaction [102]. The relative thrombogenicity of atherosclerotic plaque components was elegantly studied by Fernández-Ortiz et al. who found that the lipid core was the most potent substrate for thrombus formation in vitro. However, the substance responsible for this potent reaction was still unclear at that time [19].

TF is the primary initiator of thrombosis in vivo. TF is a specific trans-membrane glycoprotein expressed in circulating monocytes, monocyte-derived macrophages, endothelial cells and smooth muscle cells [103–109]. TF antigen is also present in the atheromatous gruel [110] and has been found in coronary tissue from patients with unstable angina [103, 111]. Therefore, TF is a candidate for the procoagulant activity of ruptured coronary plaques. TF acts by binding with and enhancing the enzymatic activity of factor VIIa towards its substrates, factors IX and X with proteolytic conversion of these zymogens to active enzymes (factors IXa and Xa) followed by the formation of the pro-thrombinase complex, thrombin generation and the subsequent cleavage of fibrinogen to fibrin [106]. Recently, we have developed a novel approach to the localization of TF by specific binding of labeled factors VIIa and X (Fig. 2). TF was clearly shown in the lipid-rich gruel, plaque macrophages and smooth muscle cells, and in the adventitia of atherosclerotic arterial specimens [112]. The functional significance of this finding was further investigated by Toschi et al., who correlated the TF staining intensity with the amount of ^{111}In-platelet deposition on different tissue components of fifty human aortic segments

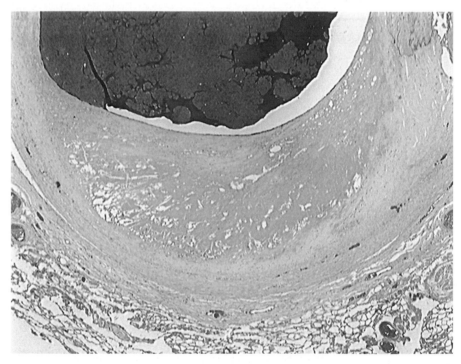

Fig. 2. Photomicrograph of same atherosclerotic plaque shown in Fig. 1 stained for tissue factor using digoxigenin-labelled factor VIIa method

[113]. Thrombogenicity was highest for lipid core followed by normal adventitia and normal tunica media and was directly correlated with TF content.

Tissue factor is not readily available to coagulation factors in the blood unless there is a loss of vascular integrity and requires insertion into membranes containing acidic phospholipids in order to function efficiently as a cofactor [114]. Macrophages and smooth muscle cells are the major cells in atherosclerotic plaques, with scattered lymphocytes and mast cells [115]. To evaluate TF-dependent thrombogenicity in acute coronary syndromes, we performed computerized planimetry of coronary specimens from 50 patients who underwent directional coronary atherectomy for unstable angina [116]. Macrophages, smooth muscle cells and TF were identified with antibodies to CD68, alpha actin and TF, respectively. Multiple stepwise regression analysis showed that macrophages and smooth muscle cells were independent predictors for TF content. Furthermore, colocalization analysis in the atheromatous gruel demonstrated a strong relationship between tissue factor content and macrophages ($r = 0.98$; $P < 0.0001$). The results of this study support the hypothesis that macrophages and smooth muscle cells are re sponsible for coronary plaque TF content. Within the lipid gruel, TF is associated with macrophages and macrophage-derived membranous debris [117], emphasizing the role of macrophages as a predominant contributor to the thrombogenic substrate in patients with acute coronary syndromes. These findings support the hypothesis that TF in the lipid-rich cores of vulnerable plaques is the immediate cause of intra-arterial thrombosis when plaques rupture and the gruel is exposed to flowing blood.

Conclusions

The vulnerability of atherosclerotic plaques to rupture and the degree of the subsequent thrombotic reaction are closely related to the ongoing inflammation in the fibrous cap and the macrophage expression of tissue factor in the soft lipid-rich atheromatous core exposed to the flowing blood. Macrophages produce matrix metalloproteinases that digest the hard structure of the plaque weakening the fibrous cap. These enzymes are regulated by cytokines produced by smooth muscle cells, lymphocytes and mast cells and blocked by specific inhibitors. The net level of proteinase activity is therefore dependent on the balance between active enzymes and their inhibitors. The basic inflammatory reaction that involves the initial stimuli (antigen) is unclear but recent data suggests that autoantibodies against oxidized LDL, and external agents like CMV, *C. pneumoniae* and hsp may play a role.

Finally, coronary thrombosis, the event immediately responsible for acute coronary syndromes is influenced by the degree of plaque thrombogenicity, mostly mediated by TF. Macrophages are not only involved in the process of plaque rupture but also responsible for tissue factor context of lipid-rich plaques, rupture of which underlie the majority of episodes of unstable angina, acute myocardial infarction, and sudden cardiac death.

References

1. Fuster V, Badimon L, Badimon JJ, Chesebro JH (1992) The pathogenesis of coronary artery disease and the acute coronary syndromes: parts 1 and 2. N Engl J Med 326: 242–250, 310–318
2. Falk E, Shah PK, Fuster V (1995) Coronary plaque disruption. Circulation 92: 657–671
3. Kragel AH, Reddy SG, Wittes JT, Roberts WC (1989) Morphometric analysis of the composition of atherosclerotic plaques in the four major epicardial coronary arteries in acute myocardial infarction and in sudden coronary death. Circulation 80: 1747–1756
4. Gertz SD, Roberts WC (1990) Hemodynamic shear force in rupture of coronary arterial atherosclerotic plaques. Am J Cardiol 66: 1368–1372
5. Bostrom K, Watson KE, Horn S, Wortham C, Herman IM, Demmer LL (1993) Bone morphometric protein expression in human atherosclerotic lesions. J Clin Invest 91: 1800–1809
6. Falk E: Coronary thrombosis (1991) Pathogenesis and clinical manifestations. Am J Cardiol 68: 28B–35B
7. Davies MJ, Richardson PD, Woolf N, Katz DR, Mann J (1993) Risk of thrombosis in human atherosclerotic plaques: role of extracellular lipid, macrophage, and smooth muscle cell content. Br Heart J 69: 377–381
8. Gertz SD, Roberts EC (1990) Hemodynamic shear force in rupture of coronary arterial atherosclerotic plaques. Am J Cardiol 66: 1368–1372
9. Loree HM, Tobias BJ, Gibson LJ, Kamm RD, Small DM, Lee RT (1994) Mechanical properties of model atherosclerotic lesion lipid pools. Arterioscler Thromb 14: 230–234
10. Fuster V (1994) Lewis A Conner Memorial Lecture: Mechanisms leading to myocardial infarction: insights from studies of vascular biology. Circulation 90: 2126–2146
11. Loree HM, Kamm RD, Stringfellow RG, Lee RT (1992) Effects of fibrous cap thickness on peak circumferential stress in model atherosclerotic vessels. Circ Res 71: 850–858
12. Richardson PD, Davies MJ, Born GVR (1989) Influence of plaque configuration and stress distribution on fissuring of coronary atherosclerotic plaques. Lancet 2: 941–944
13. Lee RT, Grodzinsky AJ, Frank EH, Kamm RD, Schoen FJ (1991) Structuredependent dynamic mechanical behavior of fibrous caps from human atherosclerotic plaques. Circulation 83: 1764–1770
14. Burleigh MC, Briggs AD, Lendon CL, Davis MJ, Born GVR, Richardson P (1992) Collagen types I and II, collagen content, GAGs and mechanical strength of human atherosclerotic plaque caps: span-wise variations. Atherosclerosis 96: 71–81
15. Lendon CL, Davis MJ, Born GVR, Richardson PD (1991) Atherosclerotic plaque caps are locally weakened when macrophages density is increased. Atherosclerosis 87: 87–90
16. Cheng GC, Loree HM, Kamm RD, Fishbein MC, Lee RT (1993) Distribution of circumferential stress in ruptured and stable atherosclerotic lesions. A structural analysis with histopathological correlation. Circulation 87: 1179–1187
17. Alexander RW (1994) Inflammation and coronary artery disease. N Engl J Med 331: 468–469
18. van der Wal AC, Becker AE, van der Loos CM, Das PK (1994) Site of intimal rupture or erosion of thrombosed coronary atherosclerotic plaques is characterized by an inflammatory process irrespective of the dominant plaque morphology. Circulation 89: 36–44
19. Fernández-Ortiz A, Badimón JJ, Falk E, Fuster V, Meyer B, Mailhac A, Weng D, Shah PK, Badimón L (1994) Characterization of the relative thrombogenicity of atherosclerotic plaque components. J Am Coll Cardiol 23: 1562–1569
20. Dinerman JL, Mehta JL, Saldeen TGP, Emerson S, Davda R, Davinson A (1990) Increased neutrophil elastase release in unstable angina pectoris and acute myocardial infarction. J Am Coll Cardiol 15: 1559–1563
21. Liuzzo G, Biasucci LM, Gallimore R, Grillo R, Rebuzzi A, Pepys MB, Masseri A (1994) The prognostic value of c-reactive protein and serum amyloid A protein in severe unstable angina. New Engl J Med 331: 417-424

22. Davies MJ, Gordon JL, Gearing AJ, Pigott R, Woolf N, Katz D, Kyriakopoulos A (1993) The expression of the adhesion molecules ICAM-1, VCAM-1, PECAM and E-Selectin in human atherosclerosis. Am J Pathol 171: 223–229
23. Mazzone A, De Servi S, Riceuvuti G, Mazzucchrlli I, Pasotti F, Specchia G, Notario A (1993) Increased expression of neutrophil and monocyte adhesion molecules in unstable coronary disease. Circulation 22: 358–363
24. Yla-Herttuala S, Lipton BA, Rosenfeld ME, Sarkioja T, Yoshimura T, Leonard EJ, Witztum JL, Steinberg D (1991) Expression of monocyte chemoattractant protein-1 in macrophage rich areas of human and rabbit atherosclerotic lesions. Proc Natl Acad Sci USA 88: 5252–5256
25. Yu X, Dluz S, Grsves DT, Zhang L, Antoniades HN, Hollander W, Prusty S, Valente AJ, Schwartz CJ, Sonenshein GE (1992) Elevated expression of monocyte chemoattractant protein 1 by vascular smooth muscle cells in hypercholesterolemic primates. Proc Natl Acad Sci USA 89: 6953–6957
26. Takeya M, Yoshimura T, Leonard EJ, Takahashi K (1993) Detection of monocyte chemoattractant protein-1 monoclonal antibody. Hum Pathol 24: 534–539
27. Koch AE, Kunkel SL, Pearce WH, Shah MR, Parikh D, Evanoff HL, Haines GK, Burdick MD, Strieter RM (1993) Enhanced production of the chemoattractant cytokines interleukin-8 and monocyte chemoattractant protein-1 in human aortic aneurysms. Am J Pathol 142: 1423–1431
28. Nelken NA, Coughlin SR, Gordon D, Wilcox JN (1991) Monocyte chemoattractant protein-1 in human atherosclerotic plaques. J Clin Invest 88: 1121–1127
29. Barath P, Fishbein MC, Cao J, Berenson J, Helfant RH, Forrester JS (1990) Detection and localization of tumor necrosis factor in human atheroma. Am J Cardiol 65: 297–302
30. Tipping PG, Hancock WW (1993) Production of tumor necrosis factor and interleukin-1 by macrophages from human atherosclerotic plaques. Am J Pathol 141: 1721–1728
31. Moyer CF, Sajuthi D, Tulli H, Williams JK (1991) Synthesis of IL-1 alpha and IL-1 beta by arterial atherosclerosis. Am J Pathol 138: 951–960
32. Clinton SK, Underwood R, Hayes L, Sherman ML, Kufe DW, Libby P (1992) Macrophage-colony stimulatin factor gene expression in vascular cells and in experimental and human atherosclerosis. Am J pathol 140: 301–316
33. Rosenfeld ME, Yla-Herttuala S, Lipton BA, Ord VA, Witztum JL, Steinberg D (1992) Macrophage colony-stimulating factor mRNA and protein in atherosclerotic lesions of rabbits and man. Am J Pathol 140: 291–300
34. Raines EW, Rosenfeld ME, Ross R (1996) The role of macrophages. In: Fuster V, Topol E, Ross R (eds) Atherosclerotic and coronary artery disease. Lippincott–Raven. Philadelphia, pp 539–555
35. Emtman ML, Ballantyne CM: Inflammation in acute coronary syndromes (1993) Circulation 22: 800–803
36. Quinn MT, Parthasarathy S, Fong L, Steinberg D (1987) Oxidatively modified low density lipoproteins: A potential role in the recruitment and retention of monocyte/macrophages during atherogenesis. Proc Natl Acad Sci USA 84: 2995–2998
37. Kume N, Cybulsky MI, Gimbrone MA Jr (1992) Lysophosphatidylcholine, a component of atherogenic lipoproteins induces mononuclear leukocyte adhesion molecules in cultured human rabbit endothelial cells. J Clin Invest 90: 1138–1144
38. van Furth R (1989) Origen and turnover of monocytes and macrophages. Curr Top Pathol 79: 125–150
39. Adams DO, Hamilton TA (1984) The cell biology of macrophage activation. Ann Rev Immunol 2: 283–318
40. Magnan DF, Wahl SM (1991) Differential regulation of human monocyte programmed cell death (apoptosis) by chemotactic factors and cytokines. J Immunol 147: 3408–3412
41. van Furth R (1988) Phagocytic cells: Development and distribution of mononuclear phagocytes in normal steady state and inflammation. In: Gallin JI, Goldstein IM, Snyderman R (eds) Inflammation: basic principles and clinical correlates. Raven, New York, pp 218–295

226   P.R. Moreno and J.T. Fallon

42. Elliot DE, Boros DL (1984) Schistosome egg antigen(s) presentation and regulatory activity by macrophages isolated from vigorous or immunomodulated liver granulomas of *Schistosoma mansoni*-infected mice. J Immunol 132: 1506–1510
43. Kreipe H, Radzun HJ, Rudolph P, Barth J, Hansmann ML, Heidorn K, Parawaresch MR. Multinucleated giant cells generated in vivo (1988) Terminally differentiated macrophages with down regulated c-fos expression. Am J Pathol 130: 232–243
44. Munn DH, Beall AC, Song D, Wrenn RW, Throckmorton DC (1995) Activation induced apoptosis in human macrophages: Developmental regulation of a novel cell death pathway by macrophage colony-stimulation factor and interferon gamma. J Exp Med 181: 127–136
45. Williams GT, Smith CA, Spoonser E, Dexter TM, Taylor DR (1990) Haemopoietic colony stimulating factors promote cell survival by suppressing apoptosis. Nature 343: 76–79
46. Moreno PR, Falk E, Palacios IF, Newell JB, Fuster V, Fallon JT (1994) Macrophage infiltration in acute coronary syndromes: implications for plaque rupture. Circulation 90: 775–778
47. Woessner JF (1991) Matrix metalloproteinases and their inhibitors in connective tissue remodeling. FASEB 5: 2145–2154
48. Dollery AM, McEwan JR, Henney AM (1995) Matrix metalloproteinases and cardiovascular disease. Circ Res 77: 863–868
49. Chin JR, Murphy G, Werb Z (1985) Stromelysin, a connective tissue-degrading metalloendopeptidase secreted by stimulated rabbit synovial fibroblasts in parallel with collagenase. J Biol Chem 260: 12367–12376
50. Sperti G, van Leeuwen RTJ, Quax PHA, Maseri A, Kluft C (1992) Cultured rat aortic vascular smooth muscle cells digest naturally produced extracellular matrix: involvement of plasminogen-dependent and plasminogen-independent pathways. Circ Res 71: 385–392
51. Nagase H, Enghild JJ, Suzuki K, Salvesen G (1990) Stepwise activation mechanisms of teh precursor of matrix metalloproteinase 3 (stromelysin) by proteases and (4-aminophenyl) mercuric acetate. Biochem 29: 5783–5789
52. Liotta LA, Steeg PS, Stetler-Stevenson WG (1991) Cancer metastasis and angiogenesis: an imbalance of positive and negative regulation. Cell 64: 327–336
53. Esdtreicher A, Wohlwend A, Berlin D, Schleuning WD, Vassalli JD (1989) Characterization of the cellular binding site for the urokinase-type plasminogen activator. J Biol Chem 264: 1180–1189
54. Murphy G, Reynolds JJ (1993) Extracellular matrix degeneration. In: Royce PM, Steinmann B (eds) Connective tissue and its heritable disorders. Wiley-Liss, New York, pp 287–316
55. Leco KJ, Khokha R, Pavloff N, Hawkes SP, Edwards DR (1994) Tissue inhibitors of metalloproteinases-3 (TIMP-3) is an extracellular matrix associated protein with a distinctive pattern of expression in mouse cells. J Biol Chem 269: 9352–9360
56. Denhardt DT, Feng B, Edwards DR, Cocuzzi ET, Malyankar UM (1993) Tissue inhibitor of metalloproteinases (TIMP aka EPA): structure, control of expression and biological functions. Pharmacol Ther 59: 329–341
57. Weber BHF, Vogt G, Pruett RC, Stöhr H, Felbor U (1994) Mutations in the tissue inhibitor of metalloproteinase-3 (TIMP-3) in patients with Sorsby's fundus dystrophy. Nat Genet 8: 352–355
58. Galis ZS, Sukhova GK, Kranzhöfer R, Clark S, Libby P (1995) Macrophage foam cells from experimental atheroma constitutively produce matrix-degrading proteinases. Proc Natl Acad Sci USA 92: 402–406
59. Shah PK, Falk E, Badimón JJ, Fernández-Ortiz A, Mailhac A, Levy G, Fallon JT, Regnstrom J, Fuster V (1995) Human monocyte-derived macrophage induce collagen breakdown in fibrous cap of atherosclerotic plaques: potential role of matrix degrading metalloproteinasas and implications for plaque rupture. Circulation 92: 1565–1569
60. Henney AM, Wakeley PR, Davies MJ, Foster K, Hembry R, Murphy G, Humphries S (1991) Localization of stromelysin gene expression in atherosclerotic plaques by in situ hybridization. Proc Natl Acad Sci USA 88: 8154–8158

61. Brown DL, Hibbs MS, Kearney M, Topol EJ, Loushin C, Isner JM (1995) Expression and cellular localization of 92 kDa gelatinase in coronary lesions of patients with unstable angina. Circulation 91: 2125–2131
62. Galis ZS, Sukhova GK, Lark MW, Libby P (1994) Increased expression of matrix metalloproteinases and matrix degrading activity in vulnerable regions of human atherosclerotic plaques. J Clin Invest 94: 2493–2503
63. Nikkari ST, O'Brien KO, Ferguson M, Hatsukami T, Welgus HG, Alpers CE, Clowes AW (1995) Interstitial collagenase (MMP-1) expression in human carotid atherosclerosis. Circulation 92: 1393–1398
64. Davies MJ (1995) Stability and Instability: two faces of coronary atherosclerosis. Paul Dudley White International Lecture. Circulation 92: 1–C
65. Saarien J, Kalkkinen N, Welgus HG, Kovanen PT (1994) Activation of human interstitial procollagenase through direct cleavage of the Leu^{83}-Thr^{84} bond by mast cell chymase. J Biol Chem 269: 18134–18140
66. Gruber BL, Marchese MJ, Suzuki K, Schwartz LB, Okada Y, Nagase H, Ramamurthy NS (1989) Synovial procollagenase activation by human mast cell tryptase: dependence upon matrix metalloproteinase 3 activation. J Clin Invest 84: 1657–1662
67. Kovanen PT, Kaartinen M, Paavonen T (1995) Infiltrated of activated mast cells at the site of coronary atheromatous erosion or rupture in myocardial infarction. Circulation 92: 1084–1088
68. Libby P (1995) Molecular bases of the acute coronary syndromes. Circulation 91: 2844–2850
69. Letini R, Bianchi M, Correale E, Dinarello CA, Fantuzzi G, Fresco C, Maggioni AP, Mengozzi M, Romano S, Shapiro L (1994) Cytokines in acute myocardial infarction: selective increase in circulating tumor necrosis factor, its soluble receptor, and interleukin-1 receptor antagonist. J Cardiovasc Pharmacol 23: 1–6
70. Blum A, Sclarovsky S, Rehavia E, Shohat B (1994) Levels of T-lymphocyte subpopulations, interleukin-1 beta, and soluble interleukin 2 receptor in acute myocardial infarction. Am Heart J 127: 1226–1230
71. Amento EP, Ehsani N, Palmer H, Libby P (1991) Cytokines positively and negatively regulate interstitial collagen gene expression in human vascular smooth muscle cells. Arterioscler Thromb 11: 1223–1230
72. Hansson GK, Holm J, Jonasson L (1989) Detection of activated T lymphocytes in the human atherosclerotic plaque. Am J Pathol 135: 169–175
73. Warner SJC, Friedman GB, Libby P (1989) Regulation of major histocompatibility gene expression in cultured human vascular smooth muscle cells. Arteriosclerosis 9: 279–288
74. Rekther M, Zhang K, Narayanan A, Phan S, Schork M, Gordon D (1993) Type I collagen gene expression in human atherosclerotic localization to specific plaque regions. Am J Pathol 143: 1634–1648
75. Hansson GK, Jonasson L, Holm J, Clowes MK, Clowes A (1988) Gamma interferon regulates vascular smooth muscle proliferation and Ia expression in vivo and in vitro. Circ Res 63: 712–719
76. Warner SJC, Friedman GB, Libby P (1989) Immune interferon inhibits proliferation and induces 2'-5'-oligoadenylate synthetase gene expression in human vascular smooth muscle cells. J Clin Invest 83: 1174–1182
77. Benditt EP, Barrett T, McDougall JK (1983) Viruses in the etiology of atherosclerosis. Proc Natl Acad Sci USA 80: 6386–6389
78. Hendrix MGR, Salimans MMM, van Boven CPA, Bruggeman CA (1990) High prevalence of latently present cytomegalovirusin arterial walls of patients suffering from grade III atherosclerosis. Am J Pathol 136: 23–28
79. Sapn AHM, van Boven CPA, Bruggeman CPA (1989) The effect of cytomegalovirus infection in the adherence of polimorphonuclear leukocytes to endothelial cells. Eur J Clin Invest 19: 542–548
80. Visser MR, Tracy PB, Vercellotti GM, Goodman JL, White JG, Jacob HS (1988) Enhanced thrombin generation and platelet binding on herpes simplex virus infected endothelium. Proc Natl Acad Sci USA 85: 8227–8230

81. Lemström KB, Bruning JH, Bruggeman CA, Lautenschlager IT, Häyry PJ (1993) Cytomegalovirus infection enhances smooth muscle cell proliferation and intimal thickening of rat allografts. J Clin Invest 92: 549–558
82. Speir E, Modali R, Huang ES, Leon MB, Shawl F, Finkel T, Epstein SE (1994) Potential role of human cytomegalovirus and p53 interaction in coronary restenosis. Science 265: 391–394
83. Kol A, Sperti G, Shani J, Schulhoff N, van de Greef W, Landini MP, La Placa M, Maseri A, Crea F (1995) Cytomegalovirus replication is not a cause of instability in unstable angina. Circulation 91: 1910–1913
84. Shor A, Kuo C-C, Patton DL (1992) Detection of Chlamydia pneumoniae in coronary arterial fatty streaks and atheromatous plaques. S Afr Med J 82: 158–161
85. Kuo C-C, Shor A, Campbell LA, Fukushi H, Patton DL, Grayston JT (1993) Demonstration of Chlaamydia pneumoniae in atherosclerotic lesions of coronary arteries. J Infect Dis 167: 841–849
86. Campbell LA, O'brien ER, Cappuccio AL, Kuo C-C, Wang S-P, Stewart D, Patton DL, Cummings PK, Grayston JT (1995) Detection of Chlamydia pneumoniae (TWAR) in human atherectomy tissues. J Infect Dis 172: 585–588
87. Grayston JT, Kuo CC, Coulson AS, Campbell LA, Lawrence RD, Lee MJ, Strandness ED, Wang SP (1995) Chlamydia pneumoniae (TWAR) in atherosclerosis of the carotid artery. Circulation 92: 3397–3400
88. Saikku P, Leinonen M, Tenkanen L, Linnanmaki E, Ekman MR, Manninen V, Manttari M, Frick MH, Huttunen JK (1992) Chronic Chlamydia pneumoniae infection as a risk factor for coronary heart disease in the Helsinki Heart Study. Ann Intern Med 116: 273–278
89. Hansson GK, Libby P (1996) The role of lymphocyte In: Fuster V, Topol EJ, Ross R (eds) Atherosclerosis and coronary artery disease. Lippincott-Raven. Philadelphia, New York, pp 557–568
90. Bergmark C, Wu R, de Faire U, Lefvert AK, Swedenborg J (1995) Patients with early-onset peripheral vascular disease have increased levels of autoantibodies to oxidized LDL. Arterioscler Thromb Vasc Biol 15: 441–445
91. Bellomo G, Maggi E, Poli M, Agosta FG, Bollati P, Finardi G (1995) Autoantibodies against oxidatively modified low-density lipoproteins in NIDDM. Diabetes 44: 60–66
92. Schumacher M, Eber B, Tatzber F, Kaufmann P, Halwachs G, Fruhwald FM, Zweiker R, Esterbauer H, Klein W (1995) Transient reduction of autoantibodies against oxidized LDL in acute myocardial infarction. Free Radical Biol Med 18: 1087–1091
93. Xu Q, Willeit J, Waldenberger FR, Weimann S, Wick G (1993) Demonstration of heat shock protein 60 expression and T lymphocytes bearing alpha/beta or gamma/delta receptor in human atherosclerotic lesions. Am J Pathol 142: 1927–1937
94. Wick G, Kleindienst R, Schett G, Amberger A, Xu Q (1995) The role of heat shock protein 65/60 in the pathogenesis of atherosclerosis. Intern Arch Allerg Immunol 107: 130–131
95. Kleindienst R, Xu Q, Willeit J, Waldenberger FR, Weiman S, Wick G (1995) Immunology of atherosclerosis. Demonstration of heat shock protein 60 expression and T lymphocytes bearing alpha/beta or gamma/delta receptor in human atherosclerotic lesions. Am J Pathol 142: 1927–1937
96. Xu Q, Willeit J, Marosi M, Klindienst R, Oberhollenzer F, Kiechl S, Stulnig T, Luef G, Wick G (1993) Association of serum antibodies to heat shock protein 65 with carotid atherosclerosis. Lancet 341: 255–259
97. Birnie DH, Hood S, Holmes E, Hillis W (1994) Anti-heat shock protein 65 titers in acute myocardial infarction. Lancet 344: 1443
98. Badimón L, Badimón JJ, Turitto VT, Vallabhajosula S, Fuster V (1988) Platelet cthrombus formation on collagen type I: A model of deep vessel wall injury – influence of blood rheology, von Willebrant factor, and blood coagulation. Circulation 78: 1431–1442
99. Badimón L, Badimón JJ, Galvez A, Chesebro JT, Fuster V (1986) Influence of arterial damage and wall shear rate on platelet deposition: ex vivo study in a swine model. Arteriosclerosis 6: 312–320

100. Ip JH, Fuster V, Badimón L, Taubman M, Badimón JJ, Chesebro JH (1990) Syndromes of accelerated atherosclerosis: Role of vascular injury and smooth muscle cell proliferation. J Am Coll Cardiol 15: 1667–1687
101. Meyer BJ, Badimón JJ, Mailhac A, Fernández-Ortiz A, Chesebro JT, Fuster V, Badimón L (1994) Inhibition of growth of thrombus on fresh mural thrombus. Targeting optimal therapy. Circulation 90: 2432–2438
102. Falk E (1992) Why does plaque rupture? Circulation 86: III30–42
103. Leathman EW, Bath PM, Tooze JA, Camm AJ (1995) Increased monocyte tissue factor expression in coronary artery disease. Br Heart J 73: 10–13
104. Lo SK, Cheung A, Zheng Q, Silverstein RL (1995) Induction of tissue factor on monocytes by adhesion to endothelial cells. J Immunol 154: 4768–4777
105. Ruf W, Edgington TS (1994) Structural biology of tissue factor, the initiator of thrombogenesis in vivo. FASEB J 8: 385–390
106. Carson SD, Brozna JP (1993) The role of tissue factor in the production of thrombin. Blood Coagul Fibrinol 4: 281–292
107. Edwards RL, Rickles FR (1992) The role of leukocytes in the activation of blood coagulation. Semin Hematol 29: 202–212
108. Drake TA, Ruf W, Morrisey JH, Edgington TS (1989) Functional tissue factor is entirely cell surface expressed on lipopolysaccharide-stimulated human blood monocytes and constitutively tissue factor-producing neoplastic cell line. J Cell Biol 109: 389–395
109. Taubman MB, Marmur JD, Rosenfield C-L, Guha A, Nichtberger S, Nemerson Y (1993) Agonist-mediated tissue factor expression in cultured vascular smooth muscle cells: role of Ca^{2+} mobilization and protein kinase C activation. J Clin Invest 91: 547–552
110. Wilcox JN, Smith KM, Schwartz SM, Gordon D (1989) Localization of tissue factor in the normal vessel wall and in the atherosclerotic plaque. Proc Natl Acad Sci USA 86: 2839–2843
111. Annex BH, Denning SM, Keith MC, Sketch MH, Stack RS, Morrisey JH, Peters KG (1995) Differential expression of tissue factor protein in directional atherectomy specimens from patients with stable and unstable coronary syndromes. Circulation 91: 619–622
112. Thiruvikraman SV, Guha A, Roboz J, Taubman MB, Nemerson Y, Fallon JT (1996) In situ localization of tissue factor in human atherosclerotic plaques by binding of digoxigenin labelled factors VIIa and X. Lab Invest (in press)
113. Toschi V, Fallon JT, Gallo R, Lettino M, Fernández-Ortiz A, Badimón L, Chesebro JT, Nemerson Y, Fuster V, Badimón JJ (1995) Tissue factor predicts thrombogenicity of human atherosclerotic plaque components. Circulation I-112 (abstract)
114. Nemerson Y (1992) The tissue factor pathway of blood coagulation. Semin Hematol 29: 170–176
115. Ross R (1993) The pathogenesis of atherosclerosis: a perspective for the 1990s. Science 362: 801–809
116. Moreno PR, Bernardi VH, López-Cuellar J, Palacios IF, Gold HK, Nemerson Y, Fuster V, Fallon JT (1996) Macrophages, smooth muscle cells and tissue factor in unstable angina: implications for cell mediated thrombogenicity in acute coronary syndromes. Circulation (in press)
117. Ball RY, Stowers EC, Burton JH, Cary NRB, Skepper JN, Mitchinson MJ (1995) Evidence that the death of macrophage foam cells contributes to the lipid core of atheroma. Atherosclerosis 114: 45–54

Immunological Mechanisms in Myocardial Reperfusion Injury

D.J. Lefer

Introduction

Polymorphonuclear leukocytes (PMNs) play a prominent role in the tissue injury associated with ischemia and reperfusion of a number of organs [4]. The adhesion of PMNs to the vascular endothelium is a critical step in PMN-mediated reperfusion injury [4, 5]. Furthermore, recent experimental evidence suggests that a number of adhesion molecules expressed on the surface of the PMNs and the endothelial cell (EC) regulate PMN-EC interactions [1, 17]. PMN-EC interactions occur in a highly orchestrated manner with the expression of distinct families of PMN and EC adhesion molecules at various times during the inflammatory response [17].

The selectin family of adhesion molecules modulates the initial "rolling" of PMNs along the activated endothelium and allows for subsequent PMN-EC interactions [1, 15]. The selectin family of glycoprotein adhesion molecules includes E-selectin, P-selectin, and L-selectin (Fig. 1). P-selectin and E-selectin are "vascular selectins" and are expressed following stimulation of the vascular endothelium with a variety of stimuli [13]. P-selectin is stored in the Weibel Palade bodies of endothelial cells and is rapidly translocated to the endothelial cell surface following activation with thrombin, histamine, and reactive oxygen species [13]. E-selectin is expressed on the endothelium 4–6 h following stimulation with various cytokines [1, 17] including tumor necrosis factor-alpha (TNF-α) and interleukin-1β (IL-1β). In contrast to the other two selectins, L-selectin is basally expressed on the microvillous processes of PMNs and is thought to mediate initial PMN "rolling" prior to PMN activation [16]. It has previously been demonstrated that this "homing receptor" can interact with the vascular selectins and can present carbohydrate ligands such as sialyl Lewis^x (SLe^x) which promotes further PMN-endothelial cell interactions [16]. Furthermore, experimental evidence suggests that SLe^x is a common carbohydrate ligand for all three members of the selectin receptor family [15]. The result of the various carbohydrate-selectin interactions between PMNs and endothelial cells is the tethering of PMNs to the endothelium and ultimately the recruitment of activated PMNs to the sites of inflammation.

Department of Medicine, Cardiology Section, Tulane University School of Medicine, 1430 Tulane Avenue, SL 48, New Orleans, LA 70112, USA

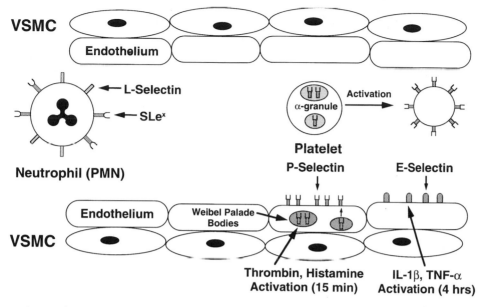

Fig. 1. Selectin interactions within the circulation (*VSMC*, vascular smooth muscle cell; *SLe*ˣ, Sialyl Lewisˣ)

Although the modes and time courses of their expression varies, the involvement of the selectin family of adhesion molecules in PMN-EC interactions in vivo is well-established. P-selectin, is thought to perform a cardinal role in PMN-mediated inflammation and is perhaps the most well-defined of the selectins. Previous experimental investigations [10, 19] have definitively implicated P-selectin in the sequelae of PMN-mediated vascular injury. Furthermore, recent clinical investigations [6, 7, 18] point to a role for P-selectin in the pathogenesis of coronary vascular injury associated with myocardial ischemia in man. Kaikita et al. [7] have demonstrated that the soluble form of P-selectin is released into the coronary circulation in patients following acute coronary artery vasospasm. In addition, another recent report [6] revealed that plasma levels of soluble P-selectin were approximately twofold greater in patients suffering from unstable angina than in patients experiencing stable effort angina or healthy volunteers. Similarly, our laboratory has reported that tissue expression of P-selectin in coronary artery atherectomy specimens from unstable angina patients is dramatically enhanced compared to specimens obtained from stable angina patients. We have also determined [18] that tissue expression of E-selectin was not elevated in the unstable angina patients compared to those with stable angina. This clinical evidence clearly suggests that P-selectin may play a pivotal role in the development of myocardial injury during coronary artery ischemia in man. Additional studies are required to further substantiate the role of the selectin glycoproteins and SLeˣ in coronary vascular injury in humans.

Following selectin-mediated PMN-EC interactions PMNs can undergo firm attachment to the inflamed endothelium and this process is regulated by the PMN β2 integrins and intercellular adhesion molecule-1 (ICAM-1) [17]. The neutrophil β_2 integrins (LFA-1, MAC-1, and p150,95) are largely responsible for firm adhesion of PMNs to ICAM-1 expressed on the endothelium [17]. ICAM-1 is constitutively expressed on the vascular endothelium at moderate levels and can be markedly upregulated 4–24 h following stimulation of endothelial cells with a variety of agonists including TNF-α and ILβ [17].

Transendothelial migration of PMNs can occur following firm adhesion of PMNs to the endothelium and this process is highly regulated by platelet-endothelial cell adhesion molecule-1 (PECAM-1) expressed primarily at the junctions of endothelial cells and by PMNs [14]. In vitro experiments have clearly demonstrated that PECAM-1 is required for PMN extravasation [14]. Interestingly, the PMN-EC involved in PMN emigration is a homophilic interaction since neutrophil PECAM-1 binds endothelial PECAM-1 is required for transendothelial migration.

The Role of Selectins and Sialyl Lewis^x in Myocardial Reperfusion Injury

In the circulation, leukocytes must adhere to the vascular endothelium under conditions of high shear rates and the initial interactions between PMNs and the endothelium are characterized by rolling rates approximately 100 times slower than the velocity of blood flow [9]. It has been well characterized that PMN adhesion to the endothelium is a multistep process whereby the initial PMN-EC interactions are low affinity in nature, are required for firm adhesion, and are regulated by a recently described class of adhesion molecules which includes the selectins (P-, E-, and L-selectin) and the carbohydrate SLe^x [8, 9]. Coincident with these observations was the development of novel agents which blocked the function of the selectins and SLe^x both in vitro and in vivo. Our laboratory and others have utilized selectin-SLe^x inhibitors as tools to examine the precise function of these adhesion receptors in myocardial ischemia-reperfusion injury.

A number of investigators have examined the cardioprotective effects of monoclonal antibodies directed against P-selectin in animal models of myocardial ischemia-reperfusion injury. Weyrich et al. [19] was the first to report profound coronary vascular and myocardial protective actions of a specific monoclonal antibody directed against P-selectin in a feline model of myocardial ischemia-reperfusion. Administration of the anti-P-selectin monoclonal antibody (mAb) PB1.3 10 min prior to reperfusion attenuated myocardial necrosis by 55%, inhibited PMN accumulation in the ischemic-reperfused myocardium, and dramatically preserved coronary endothelial vascular reactivity at 4.5 h of reperfusion. In a subsequent study [10], our laboratory tested PB 1.3 in canine model of coronary artery occlusion and reperfusion in which the left circumflex coronary artery was occluded for 120 min followed by 4 h of reperfusion. We also observed a dramatic reduction in myocardial necrosis (Fig. 2) in conjunction with coronary vascular protection and reduced

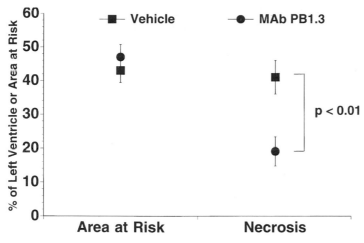

Fig. 2. Myocardial necrosis in dog hearts subjected to 2 h of ischemia and 4 h of reperfusion. Dogs (n=7 per group) received either saline vehicle or the anti-P-selectin monoclonal antibody PB1.3 (1 mg/kg), 5 min prior to reperfusion. PB1.3 treatment significantly reduced myocardial necrosis at 4 h of reperfusion. Area at risk is expressed as a percentage of the left ventricle, and necrosis as a percentage of the area at risk

PMN infiltration. Interestingly, despite the marked protective effects of PB1.3, we failed to observe any significant preservation of postischemic myocardial blood flow or myocardial contractile function. The results of these studies clearly implicate a role for P-selectin in myocardial reperfusion injury.

Monoclonal antibodies directed against L-selectin have also been developed and have previously been studied in animal models of myocardial ischemia-reperfusion injury. Ma et al. [12] studied the effects of DREG-200 in cats subjected to coronary artery ischemia (90 min) and reperfusion (270 min). Administration of DREG-200 10 min before reperfusion reduced myocardial necrosis in the ischemic zone by greater than 50% and also attenuated PMN accumulation in the myocardium. More recently, Buerke et al. [3] employed a humanized form of DREG-200 (HuDREG-200) in a feline model of myocardial ischemia-reperfusion and observed a very similar cardioprotection. Furthermore, Buerke et al. [3] demonstrated that treatment with HuDREG-200 significantly preserved left ventricular function throughout the reperfusion period. In addition, analysis of L-selectin expression on neutrophils obtained from the blood of cats subjected to myocardial ischemia and reperfusion revealed pronounced L-selectin shedding within minutes of reperfusion that persisted for 4 h into reperfusion.

More recently, our laboratory has utilized several selectin inhibitors that are SLe^x mimetics which effectively neutralize all three of the selectin adhesion glycoproteins. Initially, we investigated the effects of selectin inhibition with an SLe^x containing oligosaccharide (SLe^x-OS) in an acute canine model of myocardial reperfusion injury [11] in which the left circumflex coronary artery is occluded for 1.5 h followed by 4.5 h of reflow. Treatment with the SLe^x-OS, CY-

1503, reduced myocardial necrosis by approximately 70% in the risk zone and also markedly reduced the release of creatine kinase (CK) from the ischemic-reperfused myocardium (Fig. 3). We also determined that broad spectrum selectin inhibition with CY-1503 afforded marked coronary vascular protection as evidenced by preservation of coronary vasodilation to acetylcholine and nitroglycerin. The results of our study confirm the earlier results of Buerke et al. [2] utilizing CY-1503 to prevent myocardial reperfusion injury in cats subjected to coronary artery ischemia and reperfusion.

In order to further investigate the role of selectins in myocardial reperfusion injury we performed additional experiments in which dogs were subjected to 1.5 h of myocardial ischemia and 48 h of reperfusion. Animals were randomized to receive either an intravenous (iv) bolus of CY-1503 (35 mg/kg), a bolus of CY-1503 (35 mg/kg) + continuous iv infusion (1.75 mg/kg per hour) for 24 h, or saline. We observed a 56% reduction in myocardial necrosis (Fig. 3), a 55% reduction in myocardial PMN accumulation, and significant preservation of regional myocardial blood flow and myocardial contractility at 48 h in dogs receiving the bolus plus infusion of CY-1503. Treatment with the bolus alone resulted in marked cardioprotection at 4.5 hours of reperfusion, yet failed to significantly reduce the ultimate extent of myocardial injury at 48 h of reperfusion. Thus, the results of these studies clearly demonstrate that selectin inhibition with a soluble form of SLe^x can provide prolonged myocardial protection in the setting of myocardial reperfusion injury.

In additional studies our laboratory has studied the effects of a newly synthesized small molecule selectin antagonist, TBC-1269, in acute myocardial

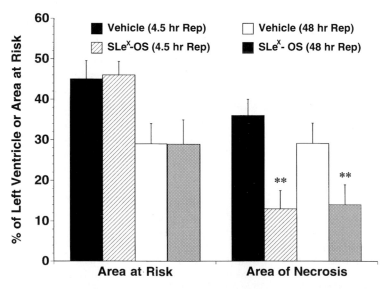

Fig. 3. Myocardial infarct size in dogs subjected to 90 min of ischemia and either 4.5 or 48 h of reperfusion (*Rep*). Treatment with the Sialyl Lewis^x containing carbohydrate (*SLe^x-OS*), dramatically reduce the extent of myocardial infarction at both 4.5 h and 48 h of reperfusion

ischemia and reperfusion in dogs. Interestingly, TBC-1269 treatment reduced myocardial necrosis of the ischemic-reperfused myocardium by 60% and significantly reduced myocardial CK release at 4.5 h following reperfusion (Fig. 4). In isolated, perfused pig hearts subjected to global ischemia and reperfusion TBC-1269 treatment dramatically reduced the extent of postischemic myocardial contractile dysfunction and PMN accumulation. It appears that selectin inhibition with SLe^x containing oligosaccharides or with small molecule selectin inhibitors provide marked protection of the ischemic myocardium from PMN-mediated reperfusion injury.

Summary

The results of these experimental investigations point to a clear role for the SLe^x and P-selectin in the pathophysiology relating to myocardial ischemia-reperfusion injury. Studies conducted in our laboratory conclusively demonstrate that inhibition of P-selectin with a blocking monoclonal antibody drastically reduce the extent of coronary vascular injury and myocardial cell death in the postischemic heart. Furthermore, we have also demonstrated that a SLe^x containing oligosaccharide as well as a small molecule inhibitor can salvage myocardium following ischemia and reperfusion. It is clear that the cardioprotective actions of anti-selectin therapy are not just acute since we observed prolonged myocardial salvage at 48 h following reperfusion with the SLe^x oligosaccharide. Additionally, the inhibition of neutrophil L-selectin function with a monoclonal antibody also results in the avoidance of myo-

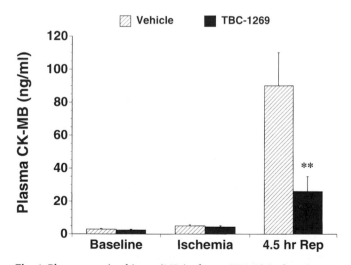

Fig. 4. Plasma creatine kinase (MB isoform; *CK-MB*) in dogs ($n=8$ per group) subjected to 90 min of ischemia and 4.5 h of reperfusion *Rep*). Dogs receiving saline vehicle demonstrated a significant elevation in plasma CK at 4.5 h of reperfusion which was largely inhibited by treatment with the novel, small molecule selectin inhibitor, TBC-1269

cardial reperfusion injury. At present, it is unclear if E-selectin contributes to myocardial cell injury following coronary artery occlusion and reperfusion. Additional studies, utilizing species specific E-selectin monoclonal antibodies are required to elucidate the potential role of E-selectin in this disease process.

Finally, it is also unclear if the selectins contribute to myocardial reperfusion injury in man despite clinical evidence that some of the selectins are expressed on cells in man following episodes of coronary ischemia. Definitive proof for the involvement of the selectins will come when novel selectin inhibitors are employed in the treatment of myocardial reperfusion injury in humans. It will also be important to see if anti-selectin treatment is safe for use in the clinical setting since this anti-inflammatory treatment might potentially interfere with the normal healing process of the myocardium following the development of myocardial infarction.

References

1. Bevilacqua MP, Nelson RM (1993) Selectins. J Clin Invest 91: 379–387
2. Buerke M, Weyrich AS, Zheng Z, Gaeta FCA, Forrest MJ, Lefer AM (1994) Sialyl Lewis[x]-containing oligosaccharide attenuates myocardial reperfusion injury in cats. J Clin Invest 93: 1140–1148
3. Buerke M, Weyrich AS, Murohara T, Queen C, Klingbeil CK, Co MS, Lefer AM (1994) Humanized monoclonal antibody DREG-200 directed against L-selectin protects in feline myocardial reperfusion injury. J Pharmacol Exp Ther 271: 134–142
4. Harlan JM, Winn RK, Vedder NB, Doerschuk CM, Rice CL (1991) In vivo models of leukocyte adherence to endothelium. In: Harlan JM, Liu DY (eds) Adhesion: its role in inflammatory disease. Freeman, New York, pp 117–150
5. Hansen PR (1995) Role of neutrophils in myocardial ischemia and reperfusion. Circulation 91: 1872–1885
6. Ikeda H, Takajo Y, Ichiki K, Ueno T, Maki S, Noda T, Sugi K, Imaizumi T (1995) Increased soluble form of P-selectin in patients with unstable angina. Circulation 92: 1693–1696
7. Kaikita K, Ogawa H, Yasue H, Sakamoto T, Suefuji H, Sumida H, Okumura K (1995) Soluble P-selectin is released into the coronary circulation after coronary spasm. Circulation 92: 1726–1730
8. Lawrence MB, Springer TA (1991) Leukocytes roll on a selectin at physiologic flow rates: distinction from and prerequisite for adhesion through integrins. Cell 65: 859–873
9. Lasky LA (1992) Selectins: interpreters of cell-specific carbohydrate information during inflammation. Science 258: 964–969
10. Lefer DJ, Flynn DM, Buda AJ (1996) Effects of a monoclonal antibody directed against P-selectin after myocardial ischemia and reperfusion. Am J Physiol (Heart and Circ Physiol 39) 270: H88–H98
11. Lefer DJ, Flynn DM, Phillips ML, Ratcliffe M, Buda AJ (1994) A novel sialyl Lewis[x] analog attenuates neutrophil accumulation and myocardial necrosis following ischemia and reperfusion. Circulation 90: 2390–2401
12. Ma X-L, Weyrich AS, Lefer DJ, Buerke M, Albertine KH, Kishimoto TK, Lefer AM (1993) Monoclonal antibody to L-selectin attenuates neutrophil accumulation and protects ischemic reperfused cat myocardium. Circulation 88: 649–658
13. McEver RP (1991) Leukocyte interactions mediated by selectins. Thromb Haemost 66: 80–87
14. Muller WA, Weigel SA, Deng X, Phillips DM (1993) PECAM-1 is required for transendothelial migration of leukocytes. J Exp Med 178: 449–460
15. Paulson JC Selectin/carbohydrate-mediated adhesion of leukocytes. In: Harlan JM, Liu DY (eds) Adhesion: its role in inflammatory disease. Freeman, New York, pp 19–38

16. Picker LJ, Warnock RA, Burns AR, Doerschuk CM, Berg EL, Butcher EC (1991) The neutrophil selectin LECAM-1 presents carbohydrate ligands for the vascular selectins ELAM-1 and GMP-140. Cell 66: 921–933
17. Springer TA (1994) Traffic signals for lymphocyte recirculation and leukocyte emigration: the multistep paradigm. Cell 76: 301–314
18. Tenaglia AN, Buda AJ, Wilkins RG, Barron MK, Jeffords PR, Vo KD, Jordan MO, Kusnick BA, Lefer DJ (1995) Increased expression of P-selectin in coronary atherectomy specimens from patients with unstable angina: evidence for leukocyte-endothelial cell interactions in unstable angina. Circulation 92 [Suppl I]: I-341
19. Weyrich AS, Ma X-L, Lefer DJ, Albertine KH, Lefer AM (1993) In vivo neutralization of P-selectin protects feline heart and endothelium in myocardial ischemia and reperfusion injury. J Clin Invest 91: 2620–2629

Metalloproteinases and Atherosclerotic Plaque Rupture

R.T. Lee and P. Libby

Introduction

Over the past decade, epidemiologic, pathologic, and clinical studies have demonstrated that the abrupt transition of stable vascular syndromes to acute ischemia is not a random, inevitable event in the natural history of the atheroma. Instead, we now realize that not all atherosclerotic lesions are destined to undergo acute plaque rupture and thrombosis, and that understanding the differences between stable and unstable lesions may provide novel strategies for prevention of acute myocardial infarction. In addition, emerging evidence implicates plaque rupture as an important component of acute stroke, peripheral vascular disease, and even in the asymptomatic progression of atherosclerosis [1]. Thus, strategies to prevent plaque rupture may have far reaching benefits beyond prevention of acute myocardial infarction.

The Pathogenesis of Acute Plaque Rupture

In the 1980's, careful pathologic studies by Davies and others established the validity of a concept that had been controversial for decades: that acute plaque rupture is a common precipitant of coronary thrombosis and myocardial infarction [2, 3]. These studies also showed that lesions that rupture and cause acute coronary syndromes are more likely to have large lipid cores and thin overlying fibrous caps when compared to stable lesions, even in the same patients. In addition, we learned that angiographic stenosis severity itself does not correlate well with lesion instability [1]. The failure of angiography, our current standard method of evaluating the extent of coronary artery disease, to predict future myocardial infarction was at first surprising, and emphasized our incomplete understanding of the plaque rupture event. In fact, the average diameter reduction of the coronary artery lumen prior to myocardial infarction is approximately 50%; more severe lesions tend to progress to total occlusion without causing myocardial infarction, probably due to collateral vessel formation.

Vascular Medicine and Atherosclerosis Unit, Cardiovascular Division, Brigham and Women's Hospital and Harvard Medical School, 75 Francis St., Boston, MA 02115, USA

To link these pathologic and clinical observations into a mechanism of plaque rupture, we and others have used a modern engineering technique called finite element analysis to understand why some plaques rupture and others do not [4, 5]. In finite element analysis, a complicated structure is broken down into smaller, simpler sections called "elements". Each element has its own mechanical properties, but different elements can have different properties. Powerful computers are used to solve the interactions between these elements. These studies indicate that a certain type of mechanical stress called circumferential tensile stress is the most likely cause of atherosclerotic plaque rupture. Locations of high calculated circumferential stress colocalize with actual locations of atherosclerotic plaque rupture in patients who died of acute myocardial infarction and plaque rupture [6]. In addition, these studies also explain, in part, why angiographic stenosis severity does not predict future myocardial infarction. In fact, when stenosis severity increases, the computer model predicts a gradual *decrease* in the peak circumferential stress in the lesion. In contrast, fibrous cap thickness is a dominant feature of plaque stability. When fibrous cap thickness is decreased from 250 to 50 microns, peak stress in the fibrous cap of the lesion *increases fivefold* [5]. These data are consistent with pathologic observations, which suggest that a peak fibrous cap thickness of less than 200 microns is a critical parameter characterizing plaques that have ruptured (M. Davies, personal communication).

Inflammation and Plaque Stability

The ability of any tissue to withstand an imposed stress depends not only on the magnitude of the stress, but on the inherent strength of the tissue. Although analyses of plaque structural mechanics implicate high mechanical forces as a major contributor to plaque rupture, several findings emphasize the critical contribution of the inherent strength of the fibrous cap. First, not all plaques with high stress regions undergo rupture. Second, many plaques have two or more high stress regions, and plaques frequently rupture at the second or third highest stress region [6]. Third, local areas of inflammation with macrophage-derived foam cells are commonly found in regions of ruptured fibrous caps [1, 7]. This inflammation may affect metabolism of the extracellular matrix at sites of lethal coronary plaque rupture. This collagenous matrix determines in large part the structural integrity of the plaque's fibrous cap. Thus, acute myocardial infarction may result from several simultaneous pathophysiologic changes, including adverse plaque structure, matrix degradation, and a prothrombotic state (Fig. 1).

Matrix degradative enzymes are broadly classified in three types: serine proteinases (such as plasmin), cysteine proteinases (such as lysosomal protease Cathepsin B), and the matrix metalloproteinases (Table 1). Members of metalloproteinase family of proteinases all have a zinc ion at their active site, as well as sharing sequence similarity [8]. Each of these enzymes is synthesized in a latent form and requires a conformational change often accompanied by partial proteolytic cleavage to attain enzymatic activity. This family of pro-

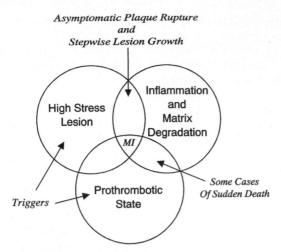

Fig. 1. Schematic diagram of factors that lead to atherosclerotic plaque rupture. Some lesions ("High Stress Lesion") have high lipid content and thin, eccentric fibrous caps; this combination leads to regions of greatly magnified tensile stresses on the plaque. The fibrous cap may also be subjected to inflammation and matrix degradation, such as by matrix metalloproteinases, rendering it more susceptible to rupture. The natural balance of thrombosis and thrombolysis may be altered to form a prothrombotic state which favors thrombosis when the fibrous cap ruptures. "Triggers" such as physical activity may increase mechanical stress on the lesion as well as tilt the balance of thrombosis-thrombolysis toward the prothrombotic state. If a lesion ruptures due to high mechanical stresses and matrix degradation, the artery may not occlude without the prothrombotic state, and the lesion may heal with further reduction of the arterial lumen diameter. Some cases of sudden cardiac death without infarction appear to be due to erosions of the plaque matrix without major fibrous cap rupture, with overlying thrombosis. If all three major factors are present, extensive plaque rupture can lead to complete thrombosis of the lumen, and acute myocardial infarction may develop

teinases, which now includes over ten members, is an attractive therapeutic target, because extracellular activity of metalloproteinases may be inhibited by naturally-occurring or synthetic inhibitors, and overactivity of these enzymes is closely related to many pathologic states, including cancer metastasis, forms of arthritis, and certain acute vascular syndromes. We will briefly review recent evidence that metalloproteinases may play an important role in the patho-

Table 1. Some members of the metalloproteinase family

	Name	Typical matrix substrates
MMP-1	Interstitial collagenase	Collagen types I, II, III, VII, X
MMP-2	72 kDa gelatinase	Gelatin type I, fibronectin, elastin
MMP-3	Stromelysin	Proteoglycans, fibronectin, some collagens
MMP-7	Matrilysin	Gelatins, proteoglycans, fibronectin
MMP-8	Neutrophil collagenase	Collagens I, II, III
MMP-9	92 kDa gelatinase	Gelatins, collagens IV, V

MMP, metalloproteinase

genesis of acute myocardial infarction, as well as some of the complexities of this powerful matrix degradation system.

Metalloproteinases and the Atheroma

The most important load-bearing molecule of the atherosclerotic fibrous cap is fibrillar collagen, predominantly types I and III. Fibrillar collagen degradation is generally initiated at a specific cleavage site by interstitial collagenase (MMP-1) or neutrophil collagenase (MMP-8), with further degradation of the fragments by gelatinolytic enzymes. Human vascular smooth muscle cells constitutively express 72 kDa gelatinase (MMP-2), a gelatinase that is generally secreted by cultured cells [9]. Human smooth muscle cells can also be induced to secrete MMP-1, MMP-3, and MMP-9 when stimulated with cytokines such as interleukin-1 and TNF-α. Thus these cytokines, present in the human atheroma, can lead to the synthesis of a complement of enzymes that can digest all of the major components of the atheroma matrix. In addition, cytokine stimulation leads to only marginal changes in synthesis of the endogenous inhibitors called Tissue Inhibitor of Metalloproteinases (TIMPs) by smooth muscle cells, so that the balance appears to be altered in favor of matrix degradation.

Cultured cells share important differences from cells in vivo, so that several laboratories have studied expression of metalloproteinases in the atheroma itself. Henney et al. have shown evidence for stromelysin mRNA expression in human atheroma [10]. Galis et al. showed that smooth muscle cells, T cells, and macrophages of the human atheroma all expressed MMP-1, MMP-3, and MMP-9 [11]. In addition, Brown et al. found increased MMP-9 immunoreactivity in atheroma specimens from patients with unstable angina compared to patients with stable angina, suggesting that unstable coronary syndromes are associated with elevated levels of gelatinolytic zymogens [12]. These investigations indicate metalloproteinase overexpression in human atheroma, and that in vitro studies of vascular smooth muscle cells exposed to cytokines in vitro parallel the activated in vivo cell with regard to metalloproteinase expression.

Metalloproteinase Activation

An important level of regulation of the metalloproteinase system is control of matrix degradation activity after the zymogen has been secreted into the extracellular milieu. We have already mentioned one potent control mechanism – the endogenous inhibitor TIMPs which can bind reversibly but with high affinity to form an inactive complex with the metalloproteinase. An additional less-understood mechanism is the activation step required to convert the inactive zymogen to the fully active metalloproteinase. In vitro, metalloproteinases can be activated by a variety of agents, including sodium dodecyl sulfate, trypsin, and aminophenylmercuric acetate. The activation step may be achieved by a conformational change that unfolds a highly conserved cysteine residue in the "pro" portion of the precursor that otherwise coordinates with and inhibits the zinc at the active site. This conformational change usually causes proteolytic cleavage of approximately 10kD of the amino terminus of the zymogen. In vivo, activation is probably achieved by autolytic cleavage, by a newly-described class of cell surface-associated metalloproteinases that contain a transmembrane region [13], or by other proteinases (e.g., plasmin).

Currently-available antibodies do not distinguish between the active and inactive enzymes. Therefore, the presence of immunoreactive metalloproteinases in a tissue does not necessarily indicate active matrix degradation. However, the technique of in situ zymography can localize matrix degradation activity [11]. In situ zymography is performed by laying frozen sections of tissue upon suitable substrates (such as casein for MMP-3 activity) and evaluating lysis of the substrate. These studies have indeed demonstrated increased matrix-degradation activity in human atheroma. In addition, this increased degradation activity appeared greatest at the "shoulder" region of the plaque, where the fibrous cap joins the more normal artery wall. This region of the plaque is also a region of high mechanical stress and frequently is the location of lethal plaque rupture.

How is a metalloproteinase such as MMP-1 activated in the atheroma? One possibility is MMP-3, which is frequently co-expressed with MMP-1 and can activate other metalloproteinases. Another possibility alluded to above is plasmin, a serine protease which can not only degrade fibrin but also several components of the extracellular matrix. We have investigated the ability of plasminogen and plasmin in the induction and activation of MMP-1 and MMP-3 in cultured human vascular smooth muscle cells [14]. While cytokines such as TNF-α and IL-1 induce the zymogens of MMP-1 and MMP-3, plasmin can induce and activate these metalloproteinases. Interestingly, TNF-α can inhibit the cleavage of plasminogen to plasmin through the induction of plasminogen activator inhibitor-1, so that metalloproteinase activation by plasminogen is inhibited. Thus, smooth muscle cells may regulate the activation step through modulation of the plasminogen-plasmin system, even after the metalloproteinase zymogens have been secreted into the extracellular space. This may be accomplished by secretion of TIMPs or plasminogen activator inhibitor-1, which will not only downregulate metalloproteinase activation but also inhibit the formation of matrix-degrading plasmin.

The Macrophage and Metalloproteinases

Although smooth muscle cells have the machinery to degrade extracellular matrix and destablize the atheroma, a growing body of evidence indicates that the macrophage plays a critical role in matrix degradation of the fibrous cap. Greater densities of macrophages are found at plaque rupture locations, and macrophage-rich human atherosclerotic tissue is much more prone to fracture at a given stress [15]. One reason may be direct secretion of metalloproteinases by the macrophage [16, 17]; in addition, the macrophage is a potent source of cytokines that may stimulate smooth muscle cells to secrete metalloproteinases. We have investigated the interactions between freshly-isolated human monocytes and vascular smooth muscle cells in culture [18]. Coculture of these two cell types leads to a dramatic induction of MMP-1 and MMP-3 (greater than 20-fold), and conditioned media experiments indicate that the source of this marked increase is the smooth muscle cell, not the monocyte. Recombinant interleukin-1 receptor antagonist, an inhibitory member of the interleukin-1 family, blocked almost all of the synthesis of MMP-1 and MMP-3 by smooth muscle cells that was induced by monocytes, indicating that interleukin-1 is the major cytokine responsible for this induction. Thus, while human monocytes and smooth muscle cells are both potential sources of metalloproteinases, under some circumstances smooth muscle cell synthesis stimulated by monocyte-derived cytokines may be the primary mechanism.

However, in vivo evidence indicates that the macrophage is more than a cytokine source in the matrix degradation cascade. Galis et al. isolated lipid-laden macrophages from rabbit aortic lesions produced by balloon injury and hypercholesterolemia [19]. Freshly isolated foam cells from these lesions contained and released MMP-1 and MMP-3, while alveolar macrophages from the lungs of the same rabbits did not. Both macrophage sources released gelatinolytic activity. Thus, even without further stimulation and in the absence of smooth muscle cells, atheroma macrophage-derived foam cells can produce the metalloproteinases to degrade the atheroma. In addition, human atheromata often have a paucity of smooth muscle cells at the location of fibrous cap rupture, possibly due to cell death (perhaps by apoptosis, a form of programmed cell death) [20]. Although this could prevent adequate repair of the extracellular matrix by smooth muscle cells at sites of high stress (due to reduced cell number), it suggests that smooth muscle cells themselves may not be the principle source of matrix degradation in the final stage of the plaque prior to rupture.

Increased Mechanical Stresses and Metalloproteinases: A Link?

The proposed processes that lead to an increased probability of plaque rupture (see Fig. 1) assume that matrix degradation and the presence of high stress locations in the fibrous cap are independent events. In fact, these processes may be closely associated. Galis et al. [11] and Nikkari et al. [21] noted that metalloproteinases are preferentially overexpressed at the "shoulder" region of the atheroma, where many plaque ruptures occur and computer analyses predict the highest circumferential stresses. We have found that in human coronary atheromata expression of MMP-1 is two to five-fold higher at regions of high circumferential stress compared to low stress regions (unpublished observations). Thus, mechanical stress and matrix-degradation activity do not appear to be independent.

One simple explanation for this association is that the plaque grows near the shoulder region, and metalloproteinases are simply participating in the remodeling process. However, regulation of metalloproteinases also relates to mechanical forces at the cellular level. In monolayers of vascular smooth muscle cells, mechanical wounding of the cell layer leads to metalloproteinase expression [22]. In addition, Werb et al. have demonstrated close links between the commitment of expression of MMP-1 and MMP-3 with deformation of cytoskeletal architecture [23]. This suggests that mechanical stresses may be "sensed" by the cytoskeleton or other mechanotransduction mechanisms and translated into the remodeling activity of metalloproteinase secretion. In most circumstances, this could prove adaptive, promoting tissue remodeling to a configuration with less stress; in the atheroma, it may trigger fibrous cap rupture.

Conclusion

With the recognition that plaque rupture is a major cause of acute vascular syndromes, inhibition of plaque rupture has become a potential therapeutic target for prevention of cardiovascular events. Successful therapies such as cholesterol reduction and aspirin have led to dramatic improvements in both primary and secondary prevention studies, but a significant proportion of acute vascular events are not prevented by these therapies. The matrix metalloproteinase family of enzymes may participate in the pre-thrombus pathogenesis of plaque rupture and myocardial infarction, and, as extracellular enzymes, can be inhibited by a variety of means. It is attractive to propose that orally active metalloproteinase inhibitors could stabilize lesions by preventing degradation of the collagenous fibrous cap, a benefit that may be independent of the mechanisms of cholesterol reduction or platelet inhibition.

However, experience with metalloproteinases in other diseases such as cancer and arthritis tells us to proceed with caution when considering the modulation of vascular metalloproteinases. First, the metalloproteinases have overlapping specificities for matrix molecules; this redundancy reduces the possibilities for specific inhibition strategies. Second, chemical inhibition of one metalloproteinase is rarely specific for that enzyme. Third, the extracellular matrix system, as the critical system for maintaining tissue structure, has regulatory controls (such as metalloproteinase activation) that are incompletely understood. These complexities are some of the reasons that, despite extensive characterization of metalloproteinases and the matrix biology of tumor metastasis and articular cartilage degradation, no clinical advances have emerged from metalloproteinase inhibition to date in these areas.

The most critical obstacle to inhibiting plaque rupture in patients remains our lack of understanding of the natural history of the atheroma, particularly the time course and matrix-degrading implications of episodes of fibrous cap inflammation. Until a representative animal model of this process is well characterized, we will continue to learn from single time point snapshots of matrix degradation in the human atheroma as well as the cell biology and biochemistry of the metalloproteinases. However, it may difficult to bring metalloproteinase inhibition into the clinical arena of cardiovascular disease without strong evidence that this approach is successful in a representative animal model.

Acknowledgement. Supported by grants HL54749 and HL34636 from the National Heart, Lung and Blood Institute.

References

Fuster V (1994) Lewis A. Connor Memorial Lecture. Mechanisms leading to myocardial infarction: insights from studies of vascular biology. Circulation 90: 2126–2146

Davies MJ, Thomas AC (1985) Plaque fissuring: the cause of acute myocardial infarction, sudden ischemic death and crescendo angina. Br Heart J 53: 363–373

Falk E (1985) Unstable angina with fatal outcome: dynamic coronary thrombosis leading to infarction and/or sudden death: autopsy evidence of recurrent mural thrombosis with peripheral embolization culminating in total vascular occlusion. Circulation 71: 699–708

Richardson PD, Davies MJ, Born GVR (1989) Influence of plaque configuration and stress distribution on fissuring of coronary atherosclerotic plaques. Lancet 2: 941–944

Loree HM, Kamm RD, Stringfellow RG, Lee RT (1992) Effects of fibrous cap thickness on peak circumferential stress in model atherosclerotic vessels. Circ Res 71: 850–858

Cheng GC, Loree HM, Kamm RD, Fishbein MC, Lee RT (1993) Distribution of circumferential stress in ruptured and stable atherosclerotic lesions: a structural analysis with histopathologic correlation. Circulation 87: 1179–1187

Moreno PR, Falk E, Palacios IF, Newell JB, Fuster V, Fallon JT (1994) Macrophage infiltration in acute coronary syndromes. Implications for plaque rupture. Circulation 90: 775–778

Mignatti P, Rifkin DB (1993) Biology and biochemistry of proteinases in tumor invasion. Physiol Rev 73: 161–195

Galis ZS, Muszynski M, Sukhova GK, Simon-Morrissey E, Unemori EN, Lark MW, Amento E, Libby P (1994) Cytokine-stimulated vascular smooth muscle cells synthesize a complement of enzymes required for extracellular matrix digestion. Circ Res 75: 181–189

Henney AM, Wakeley PR, Davies MJ, Foster K, Hembry R, Murphy G, Humphries S (1991) Localization of stromelysin gene expression in atherosclerotic plaques by in situ hybridization. Proc Natl Acad Sci U S A 88: 8154–8158

Galis ZS, Sukhova GK, Lark MW, Libby P (1994) Increased expression of matrix metalloproteinases and matrix degrading activity in vulnerable regions of human atherosclerotic plaques. J Clin Invest 94: 2493–2503

Brown DL, Hibbs MS, Kearney M, Loushin C, Isner JM (1995) Identification of 92-kD gelatinase in human coronary atherosclerotic lesions. Circulation 91: 2125–2131

Sato H, Takino T, Okada Y, Cao J, Shinagawa A, Yamamoto E, Seiki M (1994) A matrix metalloproteinase expressed on the surface of invasive tumour cells. Nature 370: 61–65

Lee E, Vaughan DE, Parikh SH, Grodzinsky AJ, Libby P, Lark MW, Lee RT (1996) Regulation of matrix metalloproteinase and plasminogen activator inhibitor-1 synthesis by plasminogen in cultured human vascular smooth muscle cells. Circ Res 1996 (in press)

Lendon CL, Davies MJ, Born GVR, Richardson PD (1991) Atherosclerotic plaque caps are locally weakened when macrophages density is increased. Atherosclerosis 87: 87–90

Werb Z, Banda MJ, Jones PA (1980) Degradation of connective tissue matrices by macrophages. I. Proteolysis of elastin, glycoproteins, and collagen by proteinases isolated from macrophages. J Exp Med 152: 1340–1357

Welgus HG, Campbell EJ, Cury JD, Eisen AZ, Senior RM, Wilhelm SM, Goldberg GI (1990) Neutral metalloproteinases produced by human mononuclear phagocytes. Enzyme profile, regulation, and expression during cellular development. J Clin Invest 86: 1496–1502

Lee E, Grodzinsky AJ, Libby P, Clinton SK, Lark MW, Lee RT (1995) Human vascular smooth muscle cells -monocyte interactions and metalloproteinase secretion in culture. Arterioscler Thromb Vasc Biol 15: 2284–2289

Galiz ZS, Sukhova GK, Kranzhofer R, Clark S, Libby P (1995) Macrophage foam cells from experimental atheroma constitutively produce matrix-degrading proteinases. Proc Natl Acad Sci U S A 92: 402–406

Geng YJ, Libby P (1995) Evidence for apoptosis in advanced human atheroma. Colocalization with interleukin-1 beta-converting enzyme. Am J Pathol 147: 251–266

Nikkari ST, O'Brien KD, Ferguson BS, Hatsukami T, Welgus HG, Alpers CE, Clowes AW (1995) Intersititial collagenase (MMP-1) expression in human carotid atherosclerosis.
Circulation 92: 1393–98
James TW, Wagner R, White LA, Zwolak RM, Brinckerhoff CE (1993) Induction of collagenase and stromelysin gene expression by mechanical injury in a vascular smooth muscle-derived cell line. J Cell Physiol 157: 426–437
Werb Z, Hembry RM, Murphy G, Aggeler J (1986) Commitment to expression of the metalloendopeptidases, collagenase and stromelysin: relationship of inducing events to changes in cytoskeletal architecture. J Cell Biol 102: 697–702

Potential Role of Human Cytomegalovirus and Its Interaction with p53 in Coronary Restenosis

E. Speir[1], R. Modali[2], E.S. Huang[3], and S.E. Epstein[1]

Introduction

A subset of patients undergoing coronary angioplasty subsequently develop recurrent narrowing (restenosis), characterized by excessive proliferation of smooth muscle cells (SMCs). Of 60 restenosis lesions examined, 23 (38 percent) had accumulated high amounts of the wild-type form of the tumor suppressor protein p53. Accumulation of p53 correlated with the presence of human cytomegalovirus (HCMV) in the lesions. SMCs grown from lesions expressed the HCMV protein IE84 and exhibited elevated p53 levels. HCMV infection of cultured SMCs increased p53 accumulation, which correlated temporally with IE84 expression. IE84 also directly binds with p53 and abolishes p53's ability to transcriptionally activate a reporter gene. Thus HCMV, and IE84 mediated inhibition of p53 function, may contribute to the development of restenosis.

Coronary angioplasty causes vessel wall injury and induces a SMC proliferative response similar to the healing response of other tissues to injury. This response is so excessive in 25%–50% of patients that it leads to coronary restenosis. On the basis of an earlier proposal that atherosclerosis (also characterized by SMC proliferation) might be a form of benign neoplasia, [1], we hypothesized that formation of the neointimal lesion during restenosis may be driven by alterations that confer to cells a selective growth advantage; upon activation, as by injury, such cells would undergo excessive proliferation.

We investigated two molecular mechanisms that might contribute to the abnormal SMC proliferation: (i) aberrant expression of p53, a tumor suppressor protein that inhibits cell cycle progression and that is functionally inactivated in many human cancers [2] and (ii) activation of latent HCMV, a herpesvirus that has been associated with the development of atherosclerosis [3]. Conceivably, an interaction between an HCMV protein(s) and p53 could impair the latter's growth suppressor function, as is the case for proteins encoded by several DNA tumor viruses, including adenovirus, human papillomavirus, simian virus 40 (SV40), and Epstein-Barr virus [4–9].

[1]Cardiology Branch, Bldg. 10, Room 7B04, National Institutes of Health, Bethesda, MD 20892, USA
[2]Bioserve Biotechnologies Ltd., Laurel, MD 20707, USA
[3]Lineberger Comprehensive Cancer Center, University of North Carolina, Chapel Hill, NC 27599, USA

Methods

We studied 60 patients (age 36–89 years; mean 59) who had undergone primary balloon angioplasty for severe symptoms secondary to coronary artery disease. Each had a satisfactory angiographic result at the time of angioplasty, but later developed recurrent angina and were subsequently found to have stenosis at the site of angioplasty. Coronary atherectomy was performed 1–6 months after angioplasty and the specimens obtained from such patients are referred to here as "restenosis lesions". Atherectomy tissue was also obtained from an additional 20 patients who were undergoing atherectomy for angina, but who had no prior angioplasty. These specimens are referred to as "primary lesions".

The lesions were firm, cylindrical fragments, 1–5 mm long and 0.2–0.4 mm in diameter. The restenosis lesions were typically much more cellular than the primary lesions, and nearly all cells were identifiable as SMCs by immunostaining with a monoclonal antibody to muscle actin [10].

Immunohistochemistry

Wild-type p53 has a very short half-life (5–20 min) in normal cells [11–13] contributing to steady-state protein levels below the detection limits of immunohistochemical methods [14]. In cancers in which p53 is believed to play a contributory role, the protein loses its inhibitory function; it also displays enhanced stability and increased steady-state levels, detectable by immunostaining with antibodies to p53 [14]. We therefore determined whether the restenosis lesions were p53 immunopositive (defined as such when $\geq$ 10% of the SMCs in the lesions stained with p53-specific antibodies).

DNA Extraction and PCR

DNA was extracted from one 50 μm frozen section and extracts (5 μl) were tested for HCMV sequences by PCR. A 511 bp product of the transforming region or a 240 bp product of the IE2 region of HCMV was amplified (95 ° C for 25 s, 42 °C for 15 s, 72 °C for 60 s; 40 cycles) with following primers: AAGCTTGTGTTTTCGAACAT and TTTATTGTTCTGTCTCCTCTC [15] or for the IE2 region: TCCTCCTGCAGTTCGGCTTC and TTTCATGATATTGCGCACCT and [16]. The conditions for each 100 μl reaction mixture were: 50 mM tris-HCL (pH 9.0), 3 mM $MgCl_2$, 40 pmol of each primer, 200 μM of each deoxynucleotide triphosphate, 5 U Amplitaq (Cetus) and 50 ng genomic DNA. The following controls were amplified with each PCR run: DNA previously demonstrated to be CMV-positive, DNA previously demonstrated to be CMV-negative, and samples without added DNA.

The sensitivity of PCR direct sequencing to detect a mutant allele in the presence of wild-type sequences was established in a mixing experiment (Curt Harris, personal communication) using serial dilutions of a mutant p53 gene in the presence of the wild-type gene. The mutant sequence could be detected in a background of 90% wild-type sequences. This result was confirmed by a prior experiment conducted by one of the present authors (R. Modali). Since most lesions analyzed had 50%–75% of cells immunopositive for p53, if a mutated allele were present It could comprise 25%–35% of the total p53 DNA population. Based on the mixing experiments, it can be concluded that a mutant p53 allele could have been detected in lesions, if such existed.

Vectors and Immunoprecipitation

Expression vectors were constructed as follows. The coding region of p53 was cloned into pAcUW51 (Pharmigen) baculovirus transfer vector under control of the p10 promoter. The coding region of CMV was cloned into pVL 1392 (Pharmigen) vector under control of the polyhedrin promoter. *Spodoptera frugiperda* insect cells (Sf9 cells) were grown at 27 °C in Graces media (GIBCO) containing 10% heat inactivated fetal bovine serum. The Invitrogen XPRESS SYSTEM was used, as recommended by the manufacturer, for transfection and generation of high titer virus stock. Sf9 cells (2×10^7 per 100 mm dish) were infected with recombinant viruses and harvested 72 h post infection. Cultures were washed in cold PBS and lysed in 0.4 ml of lysis buffer (50 mM Tris-HCl pH 8.0, 150 mM NaCl, 0.5% NP-40, 25 mg/ml Leupeptin and 0.35 mM PMSF). Lysates were clarified by centrifugation and used for immunoprecipitations.

Approximately 400 µg of insect lysate was used for each immunoprecipitation. Lysates were first incubated at 4 °C overnight with 1 µg of the p53 specific antibody 1801. The antigen–antibody complexes were collected by adding and then pelleting protein A sepharose CL-4B (Pharmacia). Pellets were washed four times in lysis buffer. The final pellets were resuspended in 40 µl of loading buffer and run on an SDS-PAGE. Proteins were electroblotted onto a nitrocellulose membrane in cold transfer buffer (200 mM glycine, 25 mM Tris-base and 20% methanol) and run on ice at 65 volts for 3 h. Blots were blocked at 4 °C overnight in TBST (10 mM Tris pH 8.0, 150 mM NaCl, 0.05% Tween 20) plus 5% nonfat dry milk. Filters were then incubated for 2 h in TBST buffer with an IE84 antibody (12E2; 1µg/ml). Filters were subsequently washed three times in TBST and then incubated with an anti-mouse IgG coupled to HRP (1:25 000 dilution). The blot was washed subsequently three times in TBST and then developed using EcL detection kit (Amersham).

Tissue Specimens

Fresh atherectomy specimens were obtained in the catheterization laboratory from 60 patients with restenosis. Tissue fragments (1–5 mg) were embedded in freezing compound, frozen in isopentane/dry ice and cut into 10–20 sections of 6 µm; two sections of 50 µm thickness were cut for DNA isolation and PCR [17]. Sections were placed on polylysine-coated slides and stored at –80 °C until processed for staining. The sections were thawed at 22 °C, fixed in methanol at 20 °C, air dried for 30 min, rehydrated in phosphate-buffered saline and processed as described before [18]. The first and second section was stained with hematoxylin/eosin and Movat pentachrome respectively. Subsequent sections were stained with two to four of the following anti-p53 antibodies: monoclonal PAb 1801, 421, 240 at 2 µg/ml (Oncogene Science, Uniondale, N.Y.) and polyclonal CM1 at 1:1000 (C. A. Midgley, University of Dundee, Dundee, Scotland). Nonimmune controls used were mouse myeloma protein, Mopc21 (Cappel, Durham, N.C.) and normal rabbit serum (Sigma); we used smooth muscle cell-specific HHF35 at 1:12 000 [10].

Cell Culture Experiments

SMC (at passage 5, grown from explants of a 1-cm segment of human coronary artery obtained at autopsy of an 18-year-old trauma victim, from National Disease Research Interchange, Philadelphia, PA) were seeded at 20 000 cells per well in eight-chamber glass slides (Nunc) and grown in Medium 199, 20% FBS, 1% antibotic-antimycotic for 72 h. After removal of the medium, the cells were infected with 50 µl of viral supernatant for 2 h. The virus suspension was then removed and replaced with 0.4 ml growth medium. Four wells each of infected or uninfected controls for each time point were analyzed by immunocytochemistry. Cells were fixed as described above, at 24 or 48 h and at 7 or 14 days post-infection. They were then incubated with monoclonal anti-CMV 6E1 (IE72) or 12E2 (IE84) 6El (IE72) or 12E2 (IE84) (Vancouver Biotech, Vancouver, Canada or with anti-p53 1801 or 421 overnight at 4 °C and subsequently reacted with biotinylated antimouse IgG and ABC complex (Vector Labs) and with diaminobenzidine as described before [18]. Whereas IE1 (72) expression was maximal at 48 h post infection and then declined, IE2 (84) expression was low at 48 h, but was apparent in 70% of the infected cells at 7 days and in 100% of the cells at 14 days post-infection. Expression of p53 protein paralleled the time course of IE2 (84) expression.

Immunofluorescence

For the indirect immunofluorescence method, human coronary SMCs at passage 5 were seeded at 30 000 per cm^2 in eight-well glass chamber slides in Medium 199, 10% FBS and grown for 48 h. After removal of the medium and three washes with warm PBS, cells were fixed first in 1% paraformaldehyde for 2 min and then in 50% acetone/methanol at –10 °C for 7 min. The cells were then air dried, washed three times in PBS for 3 min, and blocked with 1% goat serum (Vector Labs) for 20 min. After suctioning the blocking sera, 50 µl of monoclonal anti-IE2 antibody 12E2, diluted 1:200 in 0.1% crystalline bovine serum albumin, was added to the wells for 1h at 22 °C. This was followed by three 3- min washes in warm PBS. The lissamine-rhodamine conjugated goat-antimouse secondary antibody (Jackson ImmunoResearch, West Grove, PA) was diluted in 1% rabbit serum/PBS at 1:50 and layered over the cells for 30 min at 37 °C. After three washes with warm PBS, polyclonal anti-p53 antibody (CM1, Signet, Dedham, MA) diluted 1:200 in 0.1% BSA was added to the wells for 1 h at 22 °C. Cells were washed in PBS 3 times and the FITC-conjugated secondary goat-antirabbit antibody diluted in 1% rabbit IgG/PBS (Vector Labs) at 1·50 was added for 30 min. After 3 washes with warm PBS, the cells were mounted in 0.1% p-phenylenediamine dissolved in PBS pH 8, and adjusted with carbonate buffer pH 9. This retards fading of the fluorescence for 48–72 h [19].

CAT-Assays

The complete coding region and domains of IE2 were PCR amplified from an IE2 cDNA and cloned into a eukaryotic expression vector pRc/RSV with Hind III and XbaI linkers (from E.S. Huang). Human coronary SMCs were grown in Medium 199 and 10% fetal bovine serum for 48 h, then synchronized with 5 mM thymidine for 24 h [20] and transiently transfected by lipofection (Dotap, Boehringer) with 2 µg of each plasmid and 1 µg of the reporter plasmid p50-2. The results are the average CAT activity of duplicate samples of equal protein content from 10 cm plates from a single experiment. Three separate transfections were performed. Duplicate plates within any experiment varied less than 10% from the average although variation between experiments was considerably larger. Five separate transfections were initially performed in Chinese hamster ovary cells (DUKXB1) with similar results. Cell extracts were prepared using three freeze-thaw cycles and then measured for CAT activity using [^{14}C] Chloramphenicol and butyryl coenzyme A. Quantitation was achieved by the phase extraction assay [21].

Results and Discussion

Of the 60 restenosis patients, 23 (38%) had p53 immunopositive lesions (Fig. 1), with 83% containing $\geq$ 25% immunopositive cells and 60% containing $\geq$ 50% immunopositive cells. In contrast, none of the 20 primary lesions were p53 immunopositive.

The possibilities that p53 immunopositivity is a consequence of either rapid proliferation of SMCs or is normally present in the vessel wall are unlikely, in that no p53 immunopositivity was found in: (i) primary rat and human aortic SMCs grown in culture when growth was stimulated by addition of serum (E. Speir, unpublished results); (ii) tissue derived from a rat internal carotid artery obtained 2, 4, 7, 14, 21, 28, and 75 days after balloon-induced injury, and treated identically to the patient atherectomy specimens (E. Speir, unpublished results); (iii) frozen sections of "normal" human coronary arteries from two 18-year-old trauma victims, each demonstrating concentric accumulation of SMCs in the neointima (Fig. 1g); and (iv) frozen sections from normal internal mammary arteries obtained from 11 patients undergoing coronary bypass surgery (not shown).

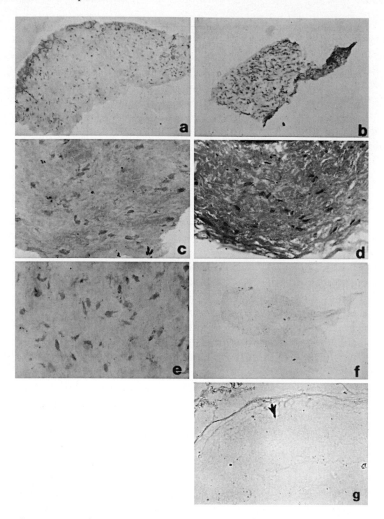

Fig. 1a–g. p53 immunopositivity in a restenosis lesion from a patient who had undergone coronary angioplasty 4 months earlier. Tissue was stained with antibody 1801 to p53 (**a, e and g**), antibody HHF35 to muscle actin (**b**), antibody CM-1 to p53 (**c**), Movat pentachrome (extracellular matrix is stained blue, collagen yellow, muscle red) (**d**), and MOPC 21 (nonimmune mouse myeloma protein) (**f**). Normal human coronary artery (**g**). Magnification: **a, b, f,** ×40; **c, d, e,** ×250; **g,** 10×

To determine whether the accumulation of p53 in the restenosis lesions was due to mutations in the p53 gene, which typically result in the expression of a protein with impaired function and increased stability, we amplified by polymerase chanin reaction (PCR) the genomic DNA of ten p53-immunopositive lesions (selected if > 35% of the SMCs in the lesion were p53 immunopositive) using primers complementary to the introns surrounding each of the translated exons (exons 2–11) of the p53 gene [22]. Sequencing of the PCR products demonstrated that the lesions contained only wild-type p53.

In certain tumors that are immunopositive for wild-type p53, the protein has been shown to be inactivated and stabilized by interaction with cellular or virally-encoded transforming proteins [5–9, 23]. We investigated whether the herpesvirus HCMV was present in the atherectomy specimens because several previous studies have demonstrated an association between CMV infection and atherosclerosis or SMC proliferation. Thus, HCMV nucleic acid sequences have been detected in atherosclerotic arteries, and HCMV antigens have been detected in SMCs derived from atherosclerotic arteries [3]. Moreover, other herpesviruses have been shown to induce SMC proliferation and atherosclerotic-like lesions in the coronary arteries and the aorta of chickens (Marek's disease virus) [24] and in aortic allografts placed into rats (rat CMV) [25].

We used PCR analysis to search for HCMV sequences in 24 human restenosis lesions, 13 of which were immunopositive for wild-type p53 (selected because > 35% of the SMCs in the lesion were immunopositive for p53) and 11 of which were p53-immunonegative. There was a significant concordance between p53 immunoreactivity and the presence of the HCMV genome; amplified viral-specific PCR products were found in 11 of 13 (85%) of the p53-immunopositive lesions, but in only three of 11 (27%) of the p53 immunonegative lesions ($p < 0.01$). Conversely, almost 80% of the HCMV-positive lesions (11 of 14) were p53-immunopositive. The PCR products were confirmed to be derived from HCMV by size analysis, by cross-hybridization with an HCMV-specific probe, and by direct sequencing of the PCR products from two of the lesions. In contrast, none of the 11 primary lesions analyzed by PCR contained HCMV sequences [15, 16].

To determine whether HCMV sequences present in the restenosis lesions could express viral gene products, we attempted to culture SMCs from 12 atherectomy specimens. We were particularly interested in the gene products of the two major immediate-early genes of HCMV, IE1 and IE2 (IE72 and IE84, the 72 and 84kD products of IE1 and IE2, respectively). We focused on these, as in other DNA tumor viruses that encode proteins binding to and inactivating p53, it is the immediate early or early gene products that possess such activity [4–9, 24]. Furthermore, IE72 and IE84 are expressed in many cell types whether or not viral replication ensues, and they are believed to be involved in activating cellular DNA replication machinery [26]. Finally, we chose to focus mainly on IE84 because it transactivates a wide variety of heterologous promoters [27].

We succeeded in culturing SMCs from nine of the 12 specimens; SMCs from four of the cultures were immunopositve for IE84 and for p53 at passages 1 and 2. The remaining five cultures were negative for IE84 and p53.

The concordance between p53 accumulation and IE84 expression raised the possiblity that IE84 might functionally interact with p53. To test this idea, we determined whether HCMV infection of SMCs causes p53 accumulation, and if so, whether the time course of IE84 expression and p53 accumulation correlate, and whether there is cellular co-localization of these two proteins. Normal human coronary SMCs were infected with HCMV and assayed for immunohistochemically detectable p53 and IE84. The SMCs, initially immunonegative for p53 and IE84, became immunopositve for both proteins

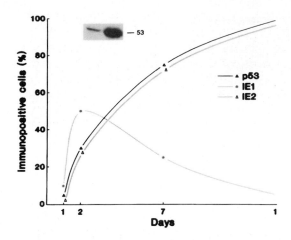

Fig. 2. Time dependent expression of IE1 (IE72), IE2 (IE84), and p53 accumulation in human coronary SMCs infected with HCMV at a multiplicity of infection of ten plaque forming units. After fixation and staining with immunoperoxidase, the cells were dehydrated in graded alcohols, and then in xylenes, and mounted on coverslips. The ratio of infected cells (brown nuclei) to uninfected cells was determined by counting 100 cells per well, in duplicate wells

within two days after infection. Notably, there was a striking similarity in the kinetics of accumulation of the two proteins (Fig. 2). Western blotting for p53 confirmed that HCMV infection leads to p53 accumulation. IE72, as expected, was expressed earlier than IE84 and more transiently [28]. Double immuno-fluorescence staining revealed that IE84 and p53 accumulated in the same cells (Fig. 3).

We next determined whether IE84 alters p53 function. We investigated the effect of IE84 on the ability of wild-type p53 to stimulate transcription of a chloramphenicol acetyl transferase (CAT) reporter construct containing a minimal promoter and two 50-bp repeats derived from the muscle creatine kinase (MCK) promoter [29]. Human coronary SMCs were co-transfected with plasmids encoding p53, the HCMV IE84 gene, and the CAT reporter gene construct. As previously demonstrated [29], wild-type p53 alone efficiently transactivated the reporter gene. In contrast, when p53 was co-expressed with IE84, its transactivational activity was abolished (Fig. 4).

To determine whether IE84's ability to inhibit p53 transcriptional activity resulted from a direct interaction between the two proteins, both proteins were expressed individually or together in insect cells using a baculovirus expression system.

Insect cell lysates were first immunoprecipitated with an antibody to p53 (Fig. 4, insert; lanes 1–4) and then probed with an IE2 antibody by Western blot analysis. Evidence that IE84 and p53 interact is demonstrated by co-immunoprecipitation of IE84 using a p53 specific antibody (Fig. 4, lane 2). A detectable, but consistently smaller amount of IE84 was evident on Western blot analysis even without p53 being present in the extract (Fig. 4, insert; compare lanes 2 and 3) suggesting that some IE84 bound nonspecifically to the

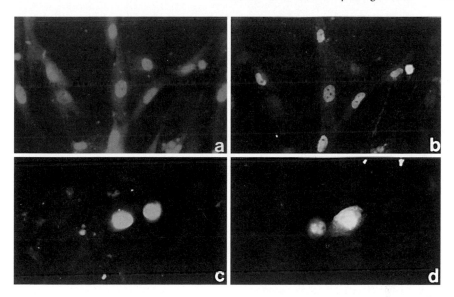

Fig. 3a–d. Double immunofluorescence staining of HCMV-infected human coronary SMCs for IE84 (red) and p53 (green). **a, b** A colony of SMCs with normal morphology 24 h after infection. Most of the cells that were immunopositive for IE84 were also immunopositive for p53. **c, d** SMCs 72 h after infection. Two cells with virus-mediated cytomegaly are intensely stained for both IE84 and p53. As controls, infected cells were treated with nonimmune primary antibodies and uninfected cells were treated with immune primary antibodies (not shown). ×40

protein A sepharose beads. Similar nonspecific binding was seen when an irrelevant first antibody was used (data not shown). Analysis of the levels of p53 and IE84 in the insect cells suggest that less than 10% of the proteins are in a stable complex under the conditions used. Thus, these results are consistent with the concept that IE84 mediates its effects on p53, at least in part, through a protein–protein interaction.

Conclusion

Given that CMV infection can cause proliferation of a wide variety of cells [26] including SMCs [30], that herpesviruses can cause atherosclerotic-like lesions in animal models [25], and that various stimuli have been associated with reactivation of latent herpesviruses [31], we propose the following model. Angioplasty-induced injury to the vessel wall reactivates latent HCMV, which in turn causes multiple cellular changes and predisposes SMCs to proliferate. As HCMV encodes numerous proteins, there are undoubtedly many mechanisms by which HCMV may potentiate the development of the restenotic lesion. However, expression of IE84 may importantly potentiate the development of restenosis by blocking p53's inhibitory effect on cell cycle progression. It is of interest that restenosis shares many pathophysiologic features with

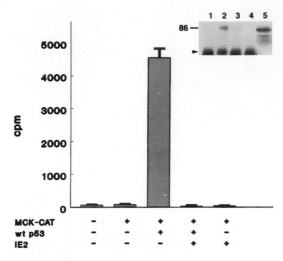

Fig. 4. Detection of a functional interaction between p53 and HCMV in primary human coronary SMCs. The p50-2 plasmid contains two copies of the 50-bp p53-responsive element of the murine MCK promoter positioned upstream of the CAT reporter gene; the p11-4 plasmid encodes a murine wild-type p53 cDNA under the control of the SV40 promoter [24]; Plasmid pRc/RSVIE84 encodes the HCMV-IE84 cDNA under the control of the RSV promoter. Separate transfection studies demonstrated that IE84 does not inhibit the transcriptional activity of the SV40 promoter (not shown). The insert shows a Western blot for the detection of co-immunoprecipitated IE84. Equal amounts of cell lysates were prepared from insect cells (lanes *1–4*) that were uninfected (lane *1*), doubly infected with a baculovirus encoding p53 and IE84 (lane *2*), infected with IE84 only (lane *3*) or infected with p53 only (lane *4*). Lysates were precipitated with anti-p53 antibody (1801), analyzed by SDS-PAGE, transferred to nitrocellulose, and then probed with anti IE84 (12E2). The presence of the IgG heavy chain at 50–55 kD (*arrowhead*) restricted the ability to perform the reciprocal co-immunoprecipitation. Total cell lysate (100 µg) from CMV-infected HEL cells was loaded in lane 5 as a positive control for IE84. *Insert*, Western blotting of SMC lysates with anti-p53: uninfected, lane *1*; 72 h after HCMV infection, lane *2*

atherogenesis, and that atheroscleortic vessels often contain HCMV. Conceivably, HCMV-mediated inhibition of p53's growth suppressor function may also be important in the development of atherosclerosis, and may in part explain the monoclonality observed in some atheroscleortic lesions. [1].

References

1. Benditt EP, Benditt JM (1973) Evidence for a monoclonal origin of human atherosclerotic plaques. Proc Natl Acad Sci USA 70: 1753–1756
2. Vogelstein B (1990) Cancer. A deadly inheritance. Nature 348: 681–682
3. Melnick RJ, Adams E, DeBakey M (1993) In: Becker Y, Darai G, Huang ES (eds) Frontiers of Virology, 2 vol, chapter 4. Springer, Berlin Heidelberg New York
4. Werness BA, Levine AJ, Howley PM (1990) Association of human papillomavirus types 16 and 18 E6 proteins with p53. Science 248: 76–79
5. Linzer DI, Levine AJ (1979) Characterization of a 54K dalton cellular SV40 tumor antigen present in SV40-transformed cells and uninfected embryonal carcinoma cells. Cell 17: 43–52

6. Lane DP, Crawford LV (1979) T-antigen is bound to a host protein in SV40-transformed cells. Nature 278: 261–263
7. Sarnow P, Ho YS, Williams J, Levine AJ (1982) Adenovirus E1b-58kd tumor antigen and SV40 large tumor antigen are physically associated with the same 54kd cellular protein in transformed cells. Cell 28: 387–394
8. Szekely L, Selivanova G, Magnusson KP, Klein G, Wiman KG (1993) EBNA-5 an Epstein-Barr virus-encoded nuclear antigen binds to the retinoblastoma and p53 proteins. Proc Natl Acad Sci USA 90: 5455–5459
9. Zhang QD, Gutsch D, Kenney S (1994) Functional and physical interaction between p53 and BZLF1: implication for Epstein-Barr virus latency. Mol Cell Biol 14: 1929–1938
10. Tsukada T, Tippens D, Gordon D, Ross R, Gown AM (1987) HHF35 a muscle-actin-specific monoclonal antibody. I. Immunocytochemical and biochemical characterization. Am J Pathol 126: 51–60
11. Oren M, Maltzman W, Levine AJ (1981) Post-translational regulation of the 54K cellular tumor antigen in normal and transformed cells. Mol Cell Biol 1: 101–110
12. Reich NC, Oren M, Levine AJ (1983) Two distinct mechanisms regulate the levels of a cellular tumor antigen. Mol Cell Biol 3: 2143–2150
13. Rogel A, Popliker M, Webb CG, Oren M (1985) p53 cellular tumor antigen: analysis of mRNA levels in normal adult tissues, embryos, and tumors. Mol Cell Biol 5: 2851–2855
14. Bennett WP, Hollstein MC, He A, Zhu SM, Resau JH, Trump BF, Metcalf RA, Welsh JA, Midgley C, Lane DP (1991) Archival analysis of p53 genetic and protein alterations in Chinese esophageal cancer. Oncogene 6: 1779–1784
15. Nelson JA, Fleckenstein B, Jahn G, Galloway DA, McDougall JK (1984) Structure of the transforming region of human cytomegalovirus. J Virol 49: 109–115
16. Huang ES, Kowalik TF (1993) In: Becker Y, Darai G, Huang ES (eds) Frontiers of Virology, 2 vol Springer, Berlin Heidelberg New York, pp 247
17. Gumerlock PH, Poonawallee UR, Meyers FJ, White RWD (1991) Activated ras alleles in human carcinoma of the prostate are rare. Cancer Res 51: 1632–1637
18. Speir E, Tanner V, Gonzalez AM, Farris J et al (1992) Acidic and basic fibroblast growth factors in adult rat heart myocytes. Circ Res 71: 251–259
19. Johnson GD, de Nogueira Araujo GM (1981) A simple method of reducing the fading of immunofluorescence during microscopy. J Immunol Methods 43: 349–350
20. Speir E, Epstein SE (1992) Inhibition of smooth muscle cell proliferation by an antisense oligodeoxynucleotide targeting the messenger RNA encoding proliferating cell nuclear antigen. Circulation 86: 538–547
21. Seed B, Sheen JY (1988) A simple phase-extraction assay for chloramphenicol acetyl transferase activity. Gene 67: 271–277
22. Lehman TA, Bennett WP, Metcalf RA, Welsh JA, Ecker J Modali RV, Ullrich S, Romano JW, Appella E, Testa JR, Gerwin BI, Harris CC (1991) p53 mutations, ras mutations, and p53-heat shock 70 protein complexes in human lung carcinoma cell lines. Cancer Res 51: 4090–4096
23. Oliner JD, Kinzler KW, Meltzer PS, George DL, Vogelstein B (1992) Amplification of a gene encoding a p53-associated protein in human sarcomas. Nature 358: 80–83
24. Fabricant CG, Fabricant J, Litrenta MM, Minick CR (1978) Virus-induced atherosclerosis. J Exp Med 148: 335–340
25. Lemstrom KB, Bruning JH, Bruggeman CA, Lautenschlager IT, Häyry PJ (1993) Cytomegalovirus infection enhances smooth muscle cell proliferation and intimal thickening of rat aortic allografts. J Clin Invest 92: 549–558
26. Albrecht T, Boldogh I, Fons MP, Valyin-Nagy T (1993) In: Becker Y, Darai G, Huang ES (eds) Frontiers of Virology, 2 vol, chapter 9. Springer, Berlin Heidelberg New York
27. Hagemeier C, Walker S, Caswell R, Kouzarides T, Sinclair J (1992) The human cytomegalovirus 80-kilodalton but not the 72-kilodalton immediate-early protein transactivates heterologous promoters in a TATA box-dependent mechanism and interacts directly with TFIID. J Virol 66: 4452–4456
28. Stenberg RM, Depto AS, Fortney J, Nelson JA (1989) Regulated expression of early and late RNAs and proteins from the human cytomegalovirus immediate-early gene region. J Virol 63: 2699–2708

29. Zambetti GP, Bargonetti J, Walker K, Prives C, Levine AJ (1992) Wild-type p53 mediates positive regulation of gene expression through a specific DNA sequence element. Genes Dev 6: 1143–1152
30. Tumilowicz JJ, Gawlik ME, Powell BB, Trentin JJ (1985) Replication of cytomegalovirus in human arterial smooth muscle cells. J Virol 56: 839–845
31. Gurevich I (1992) Varicella zoster and herpes simplex virus infections. Heart Lung 21: 85–91

Therapeutic Approaches for Immune - Mediated Cardiovascular Diseases

Protective Effects of Monoclonal Antibodies to Cell Adhesion Glycoproteins in Models of Cardiac Reperfusion Injury and Leukocyte/Vascular Responses

R.J. Winquist, J.B. Madwed, P.P. Frei, P.C. Harrison, S.W. Kerr, and R. Rothlein

Introduction

Prompt reperfusion of an ischemic tissue is necessary for restoration of function but can be associated, paradoxically, with the progressive deterioration of reversibly damaged cells resulting in dysfunction and necrosis (Braunwald 1985; Heras et al. 1988). This reperfusion injury has been studied extensively in models of myocardial ischemia (Lehr et al. 1993; Lefer et al. 1994) but has also been implicated in delayed graft function and rejection following cardiac allograft transplantation (Land 1994). The cause of reperfusion injury is no doubt multifactorial and is believed to involve an inappropriate infiltration of leukocytes and the subsequent release of their cytotoxic mediators into the previously ischemic tissue (Pinckard et al. 1983; Mullane et al. 1984). The leukocytic infiltrate has been implicated in the alteration of tissue function which can lead to cell death and organ failure. Leukocyte adhesion to the vascular endothelium, and subsequent migration into the ischemic myocardium or into a transplanted heart is orchestrated by a series of ligand–receptor events between leukocyte and endothelial cell surface glycoproteins (Lipsky et al. 1993). The importance of the various cell adhesion glycoproteins in mediating tissue damage in preclinical models of these disease states has been addressed with the administration of monoclonal antibodies (MAbs) which recognize and neutralize the function of the particular glycoproteins.

Leukocyte–endothelium adhesion events are mediated by several classes of glycoproteins including the leukocyte integrins (CD11/CD18), the immunoglobulin supergene family (intercellular adhesion molecule-1, ICAM-1; vascular cell adhesion molecule-1, VCAM-1) and the selectins (L-, P- and E-selectin) (reviewed in Lipsky et al. 1993). The leukocyte integrins are heterodimers composed of distinct α chains (CD11a, CD11b and CD11c) and a common β chain (CD18), and are distributed on all leukocytes (CD11a/CD18, lymphocyte function associated antigen-1 LFA-1); CD11c/CD18, gp 150/95) and on neutrophils and monocytes (CD11b/CD18, Mac-1). The leukocyte integrins are involved in the firm adhesive attachment to the vascular endothelium typically via ICAM-1. ICAM-1 is constitutively expressed on the endothelium and is up-

Department of Immunological Diseases, Boehringer Ingelheim Pharmaceuticals Inc., P. O. Box 368, 900 Ridgebury Road, Ridgefield, CT 06877, USA

regulated in inflammed tissue. L-selectin is also found on most leukocytes and is involved in the "rolling"of these cells along the microvasculature. Shedding of L-selectin occurs concommitantly with the firm adhesion mediated by CD11/CD18. P- and E- selectin and VCAM-1 are endothelial adhesive glycoproteins which can be up-regulated during inflammatory conditions with different kinetics, and mediate some of the leukocyte–endothelium adhesive events. The efficacy of the various MAbs tested to date suggest that several of these ligand–receptor interactions are involved in the trafficking of leukocytes into the previously ischemic myocardium, and that blockade of these interactions may be of benefit in alleviating the injury associated with cardiac reperfusion injury and chronic rejection.

In addition, we have also studied the efficacy of these monoclonal antibodies in preventing the ability of leukocytes to influence the contractile force in isolated, intact human vascular segments. These in vitro findings demonstrate that adherence of leukocytes to the vessel wall can modulate vascular dynamics which, by itself, would be predicted to affect organ function.

Myocardial Ischemia–Reperfusion Injury

Several studies have implicated the adhesion of granulocytes as an important early event for the injury observed following reperfusion of ischemic myocardium in animal models. Neutrophil adhesion and accumulation in the microcirculatory vascular bed may cause the stasis ("no-reflow") observed in some models upon reperfusion after brief periods of ischemia (Engler et al. 1986a). The sequestration of neutrophils in previously ischemic myocardial tissue, ostensibly a prodromal event for tissue destruction by the release of cytotoxic substances, has been documented during the early time points of reperfusion (Dreyer et al. 1991). In addition, treatments directed at either depleting circulating neutrophils or preventing neutrophil accumulation in the ischemic myocardium were shown to be effective in limiting myocardial necrosis which is used as an index of reperfusion injury (Romson et al. 1983; Engler et al. 1986b; Litt et al. 1989).

Several laboratories have contributed to the evaluation of MAbs, selective for particular cell adhesion glycoproteins, in animal models of myocardial ischemia–reperfusion injury. A key issue in determining the efficacy of these MAbs is the time point of administration of the MAbs, i.e., whether the MAbs are administered prophylactically (prior to or during the ischemic period) or "therapeutically"(upon reperfusion). The latter is of obvious interest when considering advancing a particular entity into clinical trials.

The initial studies examining the efficacy of MAbs directed against leukocyte integrins were performed by Simpson et al. (1988) in dogs and Seewaldt-Becker et al. (1990) in rabbits. Simpson et al. found that a MAb to Mac-1 (904; 1 mg/kg i.v.), administered at the 45-min time point during a 90-min occlusion of the left circumflex artery, caused a significant (46%) reduction, compared to vehicle, in the myocardial necrosis observed with a 6-h reperfusion protocol. The anti-Mac-1 also effectively prevented tissue infiltration by neutrophils. Seewaldt-Becker et al. found that MAb to either LFA-1 (R3.1, 0.5 mg/kg i.v.) or CD18 (R3.3, 0.5 mg/kg i.v.), when administered just prior to the ischemic event (60 min occlusion of the left anterior descending artery, LAD), effectively reduced (50% or 68%, respectively) the myocardial necrosis following a 5-h reperfusion. The anti-LFA-1 was not effective, however, when administered 3 min prior to reperfusion. Ma et al. (1991a) evaluated an anti-CD18 (R15.7, 1 mg/kg i.v.) administered 10 min prior to reperfusion in a feline model of ischemia (1.5 h) followed by reperfusion (4.5 h). These authors found that the anti-CD18 (94%) nearly abolished the necrosis which developed in the previously ischemic myocardium during vehicle treatment. Endothelial injury, as indicated by the extent of endothelial-dependent vasorelaxant response in isolated LAD ring segments, and neutrophil infiltration (myeloperoxidase, MPO) assay were also reduced by treatment with the anti-CD18 in the feline model. Yamazaki et al. (1993) found that an anti-LFA-1 (WT.1; 5 mg/kg i.v.), an anti-Mac-1 and gp 150/95 (OX42; 5 mg/kg i.v.) and an anti-CD18 (WT.3; 5 mg/kg i.v.) all had a similar efficacy (43%–76%) in reducing myocardial infarct size in a rat model of 30 minutes ischemia of the left coronary artery followed by 48 hours of reperfusion. The MAbs were administered five minutes prior to the ischemic insult.

Tanaka et al. (1993) examined the efficacy of an anti-CD18 (F[ab]'2 fragments of IB$_4$, 0.33 mg/kg i.v.) in dogs administered both before a 90-min occlusion of the left circumflex artery and 30 min after the beginning of a 3-h reperfusion period. This dosing regimen was found to prevent neutrophil infiltration but failed to significantly prevent the degree of necrosis observed with vehicle administration. Tanaka et al. also found that the anti-CD18-MAb-treated animals exhibited an improved perfusion of mid- and subepicardium during the reperfusion period which the authors ascribed to the prevention of neutrophil accumulation or plugging. However, the report by Tanaka et al. shows a dissociation between prevention of neutrophil accumulation into ischemic myocardium and beneficial effects of treatment on myocardial necrosis following ischemia-reperfusion. The reasons why the findings of Tanaka et al. differ from those of Simpson et al. are not clear.

Several laboratories have assessed the efficacy of MAbs directed at endothelial adhesion glycoproteins in preventing myocardial ischemia–reperfusion injury. Using the rabbit model described above, Seewaldt-Becker et al. (1990) showed that treatment with a MAb to ICAM-1 (R6.5, 1 mg/kg i.v.), administered 15 min prior to occlusion, resulted in a significant attenuation (51%) of the infarct size found with reperfusion. Ma et al. (1992) reported that an anti-ICAM 1 (RR1/1; 2 mg/kg i.v.) decreased (64%) the extent of necrosis found with control MAb treatment during reperfusion in cats. The anti-ICAM-1 was administered during the ischemic period, 10 min prior to a 4.5-h reperfusion. Ioculano et al. (1994) examined a MAb to ICAM-1 (1A29, 1mg/kg i.v.) in a rat model of myocardial ischemia–reperfusion, administering the antibody 3 h prior to a 1-h occlusion of the main coronary artery followed by a 1-h reperfusion period. These authors found that the anti-ICAM-1 treatment improved survival and myocardial function (mean blood pressure-heart rate index) and decreased myocardial necrosis (48%), injury (serum creatine phosphokinase) and neutrophil sequestration (MPO activity). Interestingly, this same laboratory group (Altavilla et al. 1994) found that a similar treatment regimen (3 h prior to occlusion) with a murine anti-human MAb to E-selectin (BBIG-E5; 2 mg/kg i.v.) produced near-identical efficacy as with IA29 in the rat model of myocardial ischemia–reperfusion injury. Yamazaki et al. (1993) also found that the same anti-ICAM-1 (1A290; 5 mg/kg i.v. administered 5 min prior to a 30-min ischemia period) effectively reduced (60%) the myocardial infarct size recorded with the control antibody in the rat following 48 h of reperfusion.

MAbs to either L-(DREG 200; 1 mg/kg i.v.; Ma et al., 1993) or P-(PB1.3; 1 mg/kg i.v.; Weyrich et al. 1993) selectin have been demonstrated to reduce myocardial infarct size (approximately 60%) in the feline model of ischemia–reperfusion injury. The MAbs were administered at the 80-min time point of a 90-min ischemia period prior to 4.5 h of reperfusion. Treatment with either MAb also reduced neutrophil accumulation and/or adhesion in addition to preventing the loss of endothelial-dependent relaxation in isolated coronary ring segments removed after the reperfusion period.

We have compared the efficacy of an anti-ICAM-1 (R6.5, 1 mg/kg i.v.), an antiCD18 (R15.7; 1 mg/kg i.v.) and an anti-E-Selectin (CL2; 2 mg/kg i.v.) in a primate model of ischemia–reperfusion injury. Cynomolgus monkeys were dosed with the antibody 30 min prior to a 90-min occlusion of the left anterior descending coronary artery. The ischemic period was followed by a 4-h period of reperfusion. Treatment of animals with the anti-CD18 or anti-ICAM-1 resulted in a 74% and a 44% reduction, respectively in the myocardial necrosis found with saline treatment using this protocol. In contrast animals dosed with the anti-E-selectin had similar necrotic areas of the left ventricle as found in the control animals. Myocardial contractile function, as assessed by segment shortening, was better maintained during the reperfusion period in animals dosed with either the anti-CD18 or anti-ICAM-1.

Most studies to date find that prophylactic treatment with MAbs to cell adhesion glycoproteins affords protection against the myocardial necrosis typically observed following ischemia–reperfusion protocols. Several studies have found that the MAbs are protective when administered in a more "therapeutic"protocol, i.e. just prior to the reperfusion period.

Cardiac Heterotopic Transplantation

MAbs to cell adhesion glycoproteins may prolong allograft survival by preventing the occurrence of a reperfusion injury and/or by blocking the ability of adhesion molecules to function as costimulatory agents in T-cell signaling. A retrospective analysis of human post-transplantation myocardium showed that ICAM-1, but neither VCAM-1 nor E-selectin expression was strongly correlated with indices of rejection (Tanio et al. 1994). However, in mouse heterotopic models, MAb to ICAM-1 alone does not appear to be an effective therapeutic for prolonging allograft survival. Isobe et al. (1992) found that co-administration of an anti-LFA-1 (KBA) and an anti-ICAM-1 (YNI/1.7; 50 µg/kg per day of each MAb for 7 days) resulted in an indefinite survival of cardiac allografts (BALB/c [H-2^d] hearts into C3H/He recipients) in mice. Treatment of mice with either MAb alone (at 100 µg/kg per day) had no significant effect on graft survival. Russell et al. (1995) found that this co-administration regimen significantly suppressed the development of accelerated graft atherosclerosis in mice, whereas treatment with either MAb alone did not. Consistent with these findings are the results of Schowengerdt et al. (1995) who found that cardiac allografts were rejected with a similar time course in ICAM-1 knockout mice as in wild-type mice. However, Stepkowski et al. (1994) found that administration of an ICAM-1 antisense oligodeoxynucleotide, IP-3082 (i.v. via an osmotic minipump over 7 or 14 days), resulted in a dose-dependent increase in the survival time of hearts from C57BL/10 (H-2^b) transplanted into C3H (H-2^k) mice. Co-administration of the ICAM-1 antisense probe (5 mg/kg per day for 7 days) with an anti-LFA-1 (KBA, 50 µg/day i.p. for 7 days) resulted in prolonged allograft tolerance (> 150 days).

Isobe et al. (1994) also examined a combination of MAbs to VCAM-1 (M/K-2) and VLA-4 (PS/2) in the mouse cardiac heterotopic model. With monotherapy, the MAbs to either VCAM-1 (100 µg/day i.p. for 6 days) or VLA-4 (same dosage regimen) were found to prolong the survival of hearts (from 7–20 or 30 days). Combined therapy (50 µg/day of each MAb) resulted in survival for at least 65 days. Therefore, the monotherapy regimen provided an improved protection compared with the anti-LFA-1 or anti-ICAM-1 dosage regimen discussed above. The combined therapy was effective but less so than the anti-LFA-1/anti-ICAM-1 regimen.

In rat heterotopic models of cardiac transplantation, treatment with an anti-LFA-1 (WT.1, 1.0 mg/kg i.v. for 7 days) prolonged the survival of Fischer rat hearts transplanted into WKAH rat recipients (Morikawa et al. 1994). Treatment with an anti-ICAM-1 (1A29, 1mg/kg i.v. for 7 days) prolonged graft survival (> 100 days) in only one of eight animals. Interestingly, co-administration of the anti-ICAM-1 and anti-LFA-1 resulted in an accelerated graft loss. Paul et al. (1993) also found that an anti-LFA-1 (TA-3; 750 µg/day i.p. for 13 days) prolonged the survival of (LEW × BN) F1 hearts transplanted into Lewis recipient rats (from 7 to 24.5 days). Monotherapy with an anti-VLA-4 (TA-2; same dosage regimen) was not as efficacious (14.5 days) but also prolonged survival of allografts. Combined treatment was similar to the efficacy achieved with the anti-LFA-1 alone.

Monotherapy with an anti-ICAM-1 (R6.5) has been shown to delay cardiac allograft rejection in a heterotopic protocol using cynomolgus monkeys (Flavin et al. 1991). R6.5 at either 1 or 2 mg/kg per day, i.v., starting 2 days prior to transplantation and continuing for ten days post-transplantation resulted in a significant prolongation of allograft survival (from 8.8 to either 23.4 or 26.8 days).

We further assessed the efficacy of a MAb to ICAM-1 (1A29), alone and in combination with cyclosporin A, in a rat model of heterotopic cardiac transplantation (Table 1). Donor hearts from ACI rats were transplanted into the abdomens of Lewis recipient rats. Administration of the anti-ICAM-1 (2 mg/kg i.v. loading dose followed by 2 mg/kg i.p. for 10 days) failed to significantly

Table 1. Effects of cyclosporin A and anti-ICAM-1 monoclonal antibody on cardiac allografts in rats

Group	Treatment (mg/kg, days)	Patients (n)	Individual rejection time (days)	MRT[a]	p
1	Olive oil (days 0–10)	6	7, 7, 8, 10, 13, 13	9.7 ± 1.1	–
2	CsA (1.5, days 0–10)	6	8, 8, 8, 8, 9, 10	8.5 ± 0.3	NS
3	1A29 (2.0, days 0–10)	6	7, 8, 9, 10, 11, 11	9.3 ± 0.7	NS
4	1A29 (2.0, days 0–10)+ CsA (1.5, days 0–10)	6	8, 11, 13, 22, 23, 29	17.7 ± 3.3	< 0.05[b]

CsA, cyclosporin A; 1A29, rat anti-ICAM-1 monoclonal antibody; NS, not significant $p > 0.05$ using Kaplan-Meier survival analysis
[a]Mean rejection time ± SEM in days.
[b]Significant with respect to group 1.

alter the time to rejection observed in untreated rats (8.8 versus 9.3 days, untreated versus 1A29 treated, respectively; $n=6$ in each group). However, co-administration of 1A29 with a sub-therapeutic dose of cyclosporin A (1.5 mg/ kg per day, po, for 10 days) resulted in an approximate twofold increase in the time to rejection (17.7 days).

Therefore, although MAbs to ICAM-1 are not usually effective as a mono-therapy in animal models of cardiac transplantation, co-administration with cyclosporin A can result in a prolongation of graft survival, with lower, pos-sibly less toxic doses of cyclosporin A. This efficacy may reflect the delay or prevention of a reperfusion injury following the ischemic period during graft transplantation. Co-administration of an anti-ICAM-1 with an anti-LFA-1, or of an anti-VCAM-1 and an anti-VLA-4, typically results in an impressive prolongation of allograft survival with a diminished leukocytic infiltrate. This co-administration regimen may, however, be strain-dependent. Finally, the genesis of anti-sense probes provides a provocative technique for assessing whether the upregulation of selective cell adhesion glycoproteins is an im-portant contributor to acute graft rejection.

Leukocyte-Induced Contractile Response in Human Vascular Tissue

As discussed above, the accumulation of leukocytes at sites of inflammation may cause microvascular flow abnormalities as a result of plugging or ad-versely affecting endothelial-dependent relaxation responses. There have been reports in the literature that neutrophils affect endothelium-dependent re-sponses in isolated animal vessels (Ma et al. 1991b; Ohlstein and Nichols 1989). We further assessed the direct effects of freshly isolated human leukocytes on human umbilical venous segments. Human umbilical cords were obtained from the local hospital, and umbilical vein was carefully removed and mounted in tissue bath for monitoring contractile force. Although these vessel segments were intact (as confirmed by immunohistochemistry), we and others (Mon-uszko et al. 1990) have not been able to demonstrate endothelium-dependent

A.)

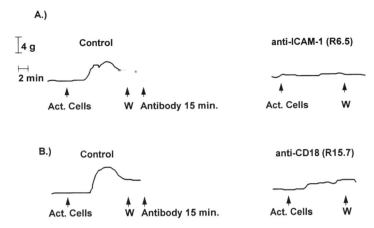

Fig. 1. Representative recorder tracing illustrating the effect of activated human polymorpho-nuclear cells (6×10^5 cells/ml) on isolated human umbilical vein rings previously stimulated with cytokines (tumor necrosis factor-α, 100 U/ml; interleukin-1β, 100 ng/ml; γ-Interferon, 100 U/ml). Panel A demonstrates the effect of anti-ICAM-1 antibody (R6.5, 50 µg/ml) added 15 min before the addition of cells. Panel B demonstrates the effect of anti-CD18 antibody (R15.7, 50 µg/ml) added to both the cell supernatant during activation (fMLP, $10^{-8}M$, 15 min, 37 °C) and to the tissue bath 15 min before the addition of cells. *Act. cells,* activated cells; *W,* wash

relaxant responses to acetylcholine, calcium ionophore or various peptides. Neutrophils were isolated from peripheral blood using dextran sedimentation followed by a Ficoll-Paque gradient and washed before being kept on ice prior to activation and addition to the tissue baths. Neutrophils activated with for-myl-methionyl-leucyl-phenylalanine generated a robust, cell-dependent con-tractile response which was abrogated by prior treatment of cells with an anti-CD18 (R15.7, 50 µg/ml) or by treating the tissues with an anti-ICAM-1 MAb (R6.5, 50 µg/ml) (Fig. 1). Neutrophils which were not activated still elicited a contractile response when added to the tissue bath, but this response was not blocked by the cell adhesion MAbs. IgG isotype controls had no effect on the contractile response of neutrophils.

Therefore, activated human neutrophils have the ability to elicit marked contractile responses in isolated human vascular segments. These contractile responses may be due to direct effects on the vascular smooth muscle, and, if they occur in the microcirculation, would be expected to exacerbate stasis during an inflammatory event.

References

Altavilla D, Squadrito F, Ioculano M, Canale P, Campo GM, Zingarelli B, Caputi AP (1994) E-selectin in the pathogenesis of experimental myocardial ischemia-reperfusion injury. Eur J Pharmacol 270: 45–51
Braunwald E (1985) The aggressive treatment of acute myocardial infarction. Circulation 71: 1087–1092

Dreyer WJ, Michael LH, West MS, Smith CW, Rothlein R, Rossen RD, Anderson DC, Entman ML (1991) Neutrophil accumulation in ischemic canine myocardium: insights into the time course, distribution, and mechanism of localization during early reperfusion. Circulation 84: 400–411

Engler RL, Schmid-Schonbein GW, Pavelec RS (1986a) Leukocyte capillary plugging in myocardial ischemia and reperfusion in the dog. Am J Pathol 111: 98–111

Engler RL, Dahlgren MD, Morris DD, Peterson MA, Schmid-Schonbein GW (1986b) Role of leukocytes in response to acute myocardial ischemia and reflow in dogs. Am J Physiol 251: H314–H322

Flavin T, Ivens K, Rothlein R, Faanes R, Clayberger C, Billingham M, Starnes VA (1991) Monoclonal antibodies against intercellular adhesion molecule-1 prolong cardiac allograft survival in cynomolgus monkeys. Transplant Proc 23: 533–534

Heras M, Chesebro JH, Gersh BG, Holmes DR, Mock MB, Fuster V (1988) Emergency thrombolysis in acute myocardial infarction. Ann Emerg Med 17: 1168–1175

Ioculano M, Squadrito F, Altavilla D, Canale P, Squadrito G, Campo GM, Saitta A, Caputi AP (1994) Antibodies against intercellular adhesion molecule-1 protect against myocardial ischemia–reperfusion injury in rat. Eur J Pharmacol 264: 143–149

Isobe M, Yagita H, Okumura K, Ihara A (1992) Specific acceptance of cardiac allograft after treatment with antibodies to ICAM-1 and LFA-1. Science 255: 1125–1127

Isobe M, Suzuki J-I, Yagita H, Okumura K, Yamazaki S, Nagai R, Yazaki Y, Sekiguchi M (1994) Immunosuppression to cardiac allografts and soluble antigens by anti-vascular cellular adhesion molecule-1 and anti-very late antigen-4 monoclonal antibodies. J Immunol 153: 5810–5818

Land W (1994) The potential impact of the reperfusion injury on acute and chronic rejection events following organ transplantation. Transplant Proc 26: 3169–3171

Lefer AM, Weyrich AS, Buerke M (1994) Role of selectins, a new family of adhesion molecules, in ischemia-reperfusion injury. Cardiovasc Res 28: 289–294

Lehr H-A, Menger MD, Messmer K (1993) Impact of leukocyte adhesion on myocardial ischemia/reperfusion injury: conceivable mechanisms and proven facts. J Lab Clin Med 121: 539–545

Lipsky PE, Rothlein R, Kishimoto TK, Faanes RB, Smith CW (1993) Structure, function, and regulation of molecules involved in leukocyte adhesion. Springer Berlin Heidelberg New York

Litt MR, Jeremy RW, Weisman HF, Winkelstein JA, Becker LC (1989) Neutrophil depletion limited to reperfusion reduces myocardial infarct size after 90 minutes of ischemia: evidence for neutrophil-mediated reperfusion injury. Circulation 80: 1816–1827

Ma XL, Johnson G III, Tsao PS, Lefer AM (1991a) Antibody to CD-18 exerts endothelial and cardiac protective effects in myocardial ischemia and reperfusion. J Clin Invest 88: 1237–1243

Ma XL, Lefer DJ, Lefer AM, Rothlein R (1992) Coronary endothelial and cardiac protective effects of a monoclonal antibody to intercellular adhesion molecule-1 in myocardial ischemia and reperfusion. Circulation 86: 937–946

Ma XL, Weyrich AS, Lefer DJ, Buerke M, Albertine KH, Kishimoto TK, Lefer AM (1993) Monoclonal antibody to L-selectin attenuates neutrophil accumulation and protects ischemic reperfused cat myocardium. Circulation 88: 649–658

Monuszko E, Halevy S, Freese KJ, Shih HJ, Parikh NS, Jelveh Z, Liu-Barnett M, Cybulska J (1990) Umbilical vessels, endothelium and vascular reactivity. Microcirc Endothelium Lymphatics 6: 183–208

Morikawa M, Tamatani T, Miyasaka M, Uede T (1994) Cardiac allografts in rat recipients with simultaneous use of anti-ICAM-1 and anti-LFA-1 monoclonal antibodies leads to accelerated graft loss. Immunopharmacology 28: 171–182

Mullane KM, Read N, Salmon JA, Moncada S (1984) Role of leukocytes in acute myocardial infarction in anesthetized dogs: relationship to myocardial salvage by antiinflammatory drugs. J Pharmacol Exp Ther 228: 510–522

Paul LC, Davidoff A, Benediktsson H, Issekutz TB (1993) The efficacy of LFA-1 and VLA-4 antibody treatment in rat vascularized cardiac allograft rejection. Transplantation 55: 1196–1199

Pinckard RN, McManus LM, Crawford MH, Kolb WP, Grover FL, Webster SA, O'Rourke RA (1983) The role of the acute inflammatory process in the pathogenesis of ischemic myocardial tissue injury. In: DeBakey ME, Gotto A (eds) Factors influencing the course of myocardial ischemia. Elsevier, Amsterdam, pp 173–187

Romson JL, Hook BG, Kunkel Sl, Abrams GD, Schork A, Lucchesi BR (1983) Reduction of the extent of ischemic myocardial injury by neutrophil depletion in the dog. Circulation 67: 1016–1023

Russell PS, Chase CM, Colvin RB (1995) Coronary atherosclerosis in transplanted mouse hearts. IV Effects of treatment with monoclonal antibodies to intercellular adhesion molecule-1 and leukocyte function-associated antigen-1. Transplantation 60: 724–729

Schowengerdt KO, Zhu JY, Stepkowski SM, Tu Y, Entman ML, Ballantyne CM (1995) Cardiac allograft survival in mice deficient in intercellular adhesion molecule-1. Circulation 92: 82–87

Seewaldt–Becker E, Rothlein R, Dammgen J (1990) CDw18 dependent adhesion of leukocytes to endothelium and its relevance for cardiac reperfusion. In, Springer TA, Anderson DC, Rosenthal AS, Rothlein R (eds) Leukocyte adhesion molecules. Springer, Berlin Heidelberg New York, pp 138–148

Simpson PJ, Todd RF, Fantone JC, Michelson JK, Griffin JD, Lucchesi BR (1988) Reduction of experimental canine myocardial reperfusion injury by a monoclonal antibody (anti-Mol, anti-CD11b) that inhibits leukocyte adhesion. J Clin Invest 81: 624–629

Stepkowski SM, Tu Y, Condon TP, Bennett CF (1994) Blocking of heart allograft rejection by intercellular adhesion molecule-1 antisense oligonucleotides alone or in combination with other immunosuppressive modalities. J Immunol 153: 5336–5346

Tanaka M, Brooks SE, Richard VJ, FitzHarris GP, Stoler RC, Jennings RB, Arfors K-E, Reimer KA (1993) Effect of anti-CD18 antibody on myocardial neutrophil accumulation and infarct size after ischemia and reperfusion in dogs. Circulation 87: 526–535

Tanio YW, Chandrasekar BB, Albelda SM, Eisen HJ (1994) Differential expression of the cell adhesion molecules ICAM-1, VCAM-1, and E-selectin in normal and posttransplantation myocardium. Circulation 89: 1760–1768

Weyrich AS, Ma XY, Lefer DJ, Albertine KH, Lefer AM (1993) In vivo neutralization of P-selectin protects feline heart and endothelium in myocardial ischemia and reperfusion injury. J Clin Invest 91: 2620–2629

Yamazaki T, Seko Y, Tamatani T, Miyasaka M, Yagita H, Okumura K, Nagai R, Yazaki Y (1993) Expression of intercellular adhesion molecule-1 in rat heart with ischemia/reperfusion and limitation of infarct size by treatment with antibodies against cell adhesion molecules. Am J Pathol 143: 410–418

Prevention of Arterial Restenosis by Rapamycin and Mycophenolate Mofetil: A New Role for Novel Immunosuppressants in the Prevention of Post-Balloon Angioplasty Restenosis?

R.V. Nair[1,2], C.R. Gregory[1,3], X. Huang[1,4], W. Cao[1,5], and R.E. Morris[1]

Introduction

Angioplasty is a minimally invasive method for widening both stenotic coronary and peripheral atherosclerotic vessels. Restenosis is a late complication that affects almost 50% of vessels undergoing angioplasty within six months after the procedure (Nobuyoshi et al. 1988) and is characterized by vascular smooth muscle cell proliferation in the area of balloon catheter-induced injury. There has been a concerted effort to identify effective therapy for preventing or limiting this complication (Handley 1995), but despite a number of successful pharmacologic interventions in a variety of animal models of vascular injury, none of the agents (with perhaps the exception of angiopeptin (Eriksen et al. 1995)) has proven to be effective in clinical trials.

A conceptual framework which has guided work with novel immunosuppressants in our laboratory is the *Response-to-Injury Paradigm* proposed by R. Ross (1995). In its simplified form, it hypothesizes that in response to a variety of injuries (ischemia, mechanical injury, immune-mediated damage, etc.), there is production and release of growth factors which results in cellular activation and proliferation, secondarily triggering a cytokine cascade, causing fibroproliferative remodeling which can result in luminal narrowing. In this paper, we will review how this paradigm has been used to discover applications for novel immunosuppressants that extend beyond their conventional use to suppress graft rejection.

[1]Laboratory for Transplantation Immunology, Department of Cardiothoracic Surgery, Stanford University School of Medicine, Stanford, CA 94305–5247, USA
[2]Department of General Surgery, University of Arizona, College of Medicine, Tucson, AZ 85724–5058, USA
[3]Department of Surgery and Radiological Sciences, School of Veterinary Medicine, University of California, Davis, CA 95616–8745, USA
[4]Current address: Fibrogen, Inc., 772 Lucerne Drive, Sunnyvale, CA 94086, USA
[5]Current address: Chiron Corp., D-233, Department of Nucleic Acid Systems, Division of Probe Identification, 4560 Horton Street, Emeryville, CA 94608–2916, USA

The Immunosuppressants

A variety of new small molecular immunosuppressants have been discovered
and developed since the mid-1980s, and all have been shown to prolong allograft survival in different animal models of organ transplantation (Fig. 1;
Morris 1996). These agents are enzyme inhibitors and can be very broadly
classified by their sites of action.

Cyclosporine A (CsA) and tacrolimus (FK506) are known to bind intracellular binding proteins known as immunophilins in lymphocytes ("cy-
clophilins" for CsA and "FK binding proteins (FKBPs)" for FK506). In each
case, the drug-immunophilin complex inhibits the activity of a serine-threonine phosphatase called calcineurin that is linked to the dephosphorylation
and subsequent nuclear translocation of the cytoplasmic component of the
transcription factor NF-AT; this and other transcription factors are prerequisites for early lymphokine (interleukin (IL)-1,-2, tumor necrosis factor-α)
gene transcription. Another new immunosuppressant, sirolimus (rapamycin;
RPM), is known to bind competitively with tacrolimus for FKBP, but its mechanism of action following immunophilin binding is distinctly different from

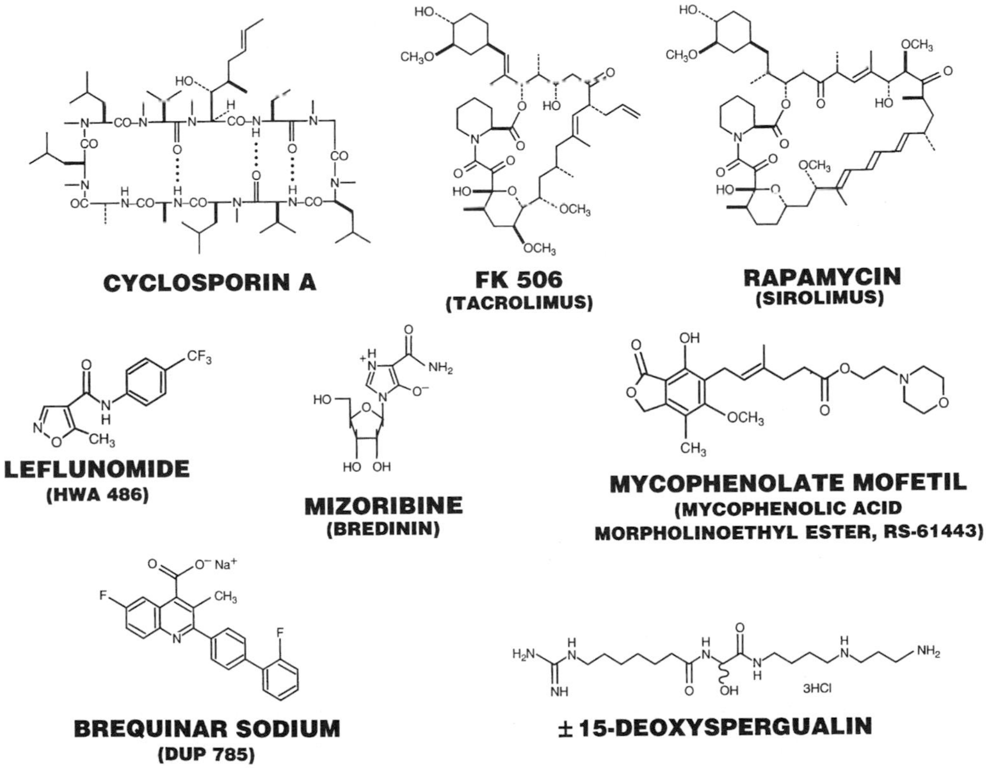

Fig. 1. The molecular structures of novel small immunosuppressants

that of tacrolimus (see below). Other new agents appear to affect the de novo pathways for nucleotide biosynthesis. The purine analogue prodrug, mizoribine (MZR), as well as mycophenolate mofetil (MMF) inhibit the same target enzyme in de novo purine biosynthesis (inosine monophosphate dehydrogenase; IMPDH). On the other hand, the therapeutic target of brequinar sodium (BQR) is the enzyme dihydroorotate dehydrogenase (DHODH) in the de novo pyrimidine biosynthetic pathway; leflunomide (LFM), another novel immunosuppressant, also appears to inhibit this enzyme in vitro. Based on currently available data, LFM also appears to have a second site of action as an inhibitor of protein tyrosine kinases (e.g., src) involved in signal transduction from cytokine receptors. The mechanism of action of the agent deoxyspergualin (DSG) remains incompletely understood; it appears to interfere with antigen processing and presentation by macrophages and other antigen presenting cells (APCs) by binding to a member of the cytosolic heat shock protein family (Hsp 70) which is linked to antigen processing.

The remainder of this paper will focus on work we have done in animal models of both chronic vascular rejection and vascular injury using RPM and MMF; therefore, a more detailed introduction to these two compounds will be given. RPM is a macrocyclic lactone initially isolated from a *Streptomyces* species broth by S. Sehgal at Ayerst Pharmaceuticals in the early-1970s during a screen for anti-fungal activity (Morris 1991; Sehgal et al. 1995). Despite its efficacy for this application, in vivo studies showed that it caused involution of lymphoid tissue in treated animals, and its further development was discontinued due to concern that its effects on the immune system might undermine its use as an antibiotic. Later, when the efficacy of tacrolimus as an immunosuppressant was shown, the structural similarity between RPM and tacrolimus prompted a reinvestigation of RPM as an immunosuppressive agent (Morris and Meiser 1989; Calne et al. 1989).

As mentioned above, in vitro work showed that in lymphocytes, RPM shares the binding site on FKBP with tacrolimus due to the structural identity of the two agents in the FKBP-binding domains (Sehgal et al. 1995). In contrast to tacrolimus, however, the RPM–FKBP complex, rather than inhibiting early gene transcription through inhibition of calcineurin, instead inhibits signal transduction from the IL-2 receptor and other growth factor receptors to the nucleus. This novel action, presumably due to differences in the effector domains of the RPM molecule, leads to inhibition of cellular processes which are responsible for cell cycle transition from G_1 to S phase. Although the target of RPM–FKBP complex in mammalian cells has still not been clearly identified, recent work suggests that the complex may bind and prevent release of a cyclin-dependent kinase (cdk) inhibitor p27^{Kip1} from its cdk substrate, thereby inducing cell cycle arrest (Molinar-Kimber and Sehgal, in press, Cardenas et al. 1995).

Work with RPM in preclinical models of organ transplantation showed that RPM is a potent immunosuppressant capable of prolonging graft survival in a variety of small and large animals and of inducing long-term donor specific tolerance (Morris et al. 1991a; Morris 1993). Moreover, RPM has the added advantage that it is able to reverse ongoing acute rejection (Morris 1993). These and other promising preclinical results led to phase I and II clinical trials in renal and heart transplantation. Phase III trials in renal transplant patients will begin in 1996.

Another novel immunosuppressive agent is the morpholinoethyl ester of mycophenolic acid (MPA) known as mycophenolate mofetil (MMF). MMF, a prodrug of MPA, was approved by the FDA for use as an immunosuppressant for transplantation in May 1995. MPA was initially developed as an antitumor agent, but it has long been known to have immunosuppressive properties (Franklin and Cook 1969; Allison and Eugui 1993). In vitro experiments have demonstrated that MPA is an effective and specific inhibitor of activated lymphocyte proliferation. It is believed that activated lymphocytes rely on up-regulation of both the de novo as well as the salvage purine biosynthetic pathways for clonal proliferation. The efficacy of MPA was found to reside in its ability to selectively inhibit inosine monophosphate dehydrogenase (IMPDH), a key enzyme in the de novo pathway, thereby resulting primarily in a selective depletion in guanosine nucleotides and secondarily in a down-regulation in the catalytic activities of other enzymes in the biosynthetic pathway.

The relatively specific immunosuppressive properties of MPA (Allison et al. 1993) and its previously known clinical safety and selectivity in the treatment of psoriasis patients prompted our group to explore the efficacy of MPA and its analogues as immunosuppressants in animal models of transplantation. MMF, which is hydrolyzed in vivo to its active metabolite MPA, and subsequently inactivated through hepatic beta-glucuronidation, prolongs rat heart allograft survival and induces donor specific tolerance (Morris et al. 1989; Morris et al. 1990). As with RPM, MPA reverses ongoing acute rejection in rodent models of heart transplantation as well as preventing acute rejection in non-human primate cardiac allografts (Morris et al. 1991b). Unlike other purine biosynthetic inhibitors currently in clinical use (e.g., azathioprine), trials with MMF in patients showed minimal toxicity and showed that the drug prevents recurrent cardiac rejection (Kirklin et al. 1994). Based on its efficacy for reducing the incidence and severity of cadaveric renal allograft rejection, MMF was approved for use in clinical transplantation by the FDA in May 1995, and is currently marketed under the trade name of Cellcept by Syntex-Roche.

Efficacy of Rapamycin and Mycophenolic Acid in Graft Vascular Disease

The advent of CsA in the early 1980s revolutionized clinical organ transplantation by offering a highly effective agent for prolonging graft survival by decreasing the incidence and severity of acute rejection episodes, while concomitantly decreasing infectious complications related to immunosuppression. Many of the newer agents mentioned above show even more promise, by *reversing* ongoing acute rejection in both preclinical and clinical settings. Unfortunately, although these interventions have a favorable impact on short-term allograft survival, transplanted organs continue to suffer from chronic rejection. In vascularized allografts such as heart and kidney, this process is characterized by initial perivascular inflammatory and immune infiltrates and subsequent endothelial injury. The end result is mural vascular smooth muscle cell (VSMC) proliferation and migration to form a concentric, fibroproliferative neointima causing luminal stenosis and obliterative arteriopathy (Häyry et al. 1993; Billingham 1995). This form of chronic rejection (which has been variously termed "accelerated graft atherosclerosis", "chronic vascular rejection", or "graft vascular disease") is clinically relevant; based on angiographic criteria, it affects approximately 50% of cardiac transplants by 5 y posttransplantation (Ardehali 1995). Unfortunately, apart from retransplantation, no currently available therapy has been safe and effective for preventing or halting progression of chronic rejection.

In our laboratory, we have used two animal models of graft vascular disease (GVD) to assess the efficacy of novel immunosuppressants in preventing the onset or progression of chronic rejection. The classical model involves examination of the coronary vessels of intra-abdominal heterotopic cardiac allografts transplanted between histo-incompatible rat strains (in our laboratory, Brown Norway, BN, donors to Lewis, LEW, recipients) and removed at various times posttransplantation. A second model that we have developed more recently is the transplantation of a BN donor femoral artery segment orthotopically as an interposition allograft into a LEW recipient. After 40 days, grafts in this model undergo concentric neointimal hyperplasia which mirrors the changes seen in clinical GVD (Gregory et al. 1993b). More importantly, the femoral artery allograft has been found to be a more stringent model of chronic vascular rejection, since the lesion is more resistant to pharmacologic therapy (Meiser et al. 1991; Gregory et al. 1993b).

Our lab first began to examine the effect of novel immunosuppressants on the development of GVD using the rat heterotopic heart transplant model. We were able to show that treatment from post-operative day (POD) 1 to 50 with 1.5 mg/kg per day of RPM not only significantly decreases the acute rejection score compared with treatment with CsA or FK506, but perhaps more importantly, it is just as effective as CsA (and significantly more effective than FK506) in preventing GVD (Meiser et al. 1991).

Using the same model, we also examined the effect of MPA on the development of GVD (Morris et al. 1991b). In this experiment, the LEW recipients were treated with 30 mg/kg per day of MPA from POD 1 to 50, then with 20 mg/kg per day of MPA from POD 51 to 100, and the BN allografts were harvested between POD 101 and 109. Our results showed that while MPA decreases the incidence and severity of GVD, it is unable to completely prevent the lesion. The conclusion was drawn that the extent of GVD in any given animal correlates best with the extent of interstitial cellular infiltrate seen by histology.

We reinvestigated the effect of RPM in the more stringent isolated femoral arterial allograft model (Gregory et al. 1993b). As shown in Fig. 2, treatment with RPM at a dose of 1.5 mg/kg per day for 40 days posttransplantation significantly (but not completely) reduces neointimal area compared to untreated control grafts. A tapering-dose treatment schedule of RPM at 6 mg/kg per day for the first week posttransplantation, followed by 3 mg/kg per day

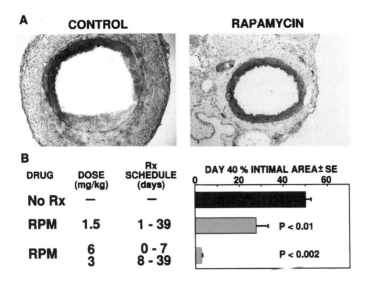

Fig. 2. A Histologic comparison of untreated (*left*) and rapamycin-treated (*right*) BN-LEW femoral artery allografts harvested on post-operative day (POD) 40, prepared as 6 μm transverse sections, and examined at 100× magnification. The section on the *right* was obtained from an animal treated with rapamycin at 6 mg/kg per day from POD 0–7, followed by 3 mg/kg per day from POD 8–39. B Graphical representation of improvement in mean percent intimal area following low-dose and tapering rapamycin treatment regimens. Intimal cross-sectional areas were estimated by micrometer grid point counting, and mean percent intimal area was calculated as follows: intimal area (mm^2)/medial area (mm^2) + intimal area $(mm^2) \times 100$; *Rx*, treatment

until POD 39 results in almost complete abrogation of the neointimal response. The pathophysiology of GVD has been attributed at least in part to expression of growth factors and cytokines mitogenic for mural VSMC (Reidy and Jackson 1990). In situ hybridization with probes for platelet-derived growth factor (PDGF), basic fibroblast growth factor (bFGF), and transforming growth factor-β showed that the expression of mRNAs for all of these mitogenic growth factors is significantly decreased in the vessels of RPM-treated allografts compared with those from untreated controls.

Similar results have been demonstrated by Steele et al. (1993) using MMF to prevent neointimal formation in aortic segment allografts between ACI donors and LEW recipients. Unlike syngeneic grafts which develop minimal stenotic lesions, allografts develop lesions which progress over the first three months following transplantation and become stable thereafter. When they evaluated the allografts at 3 months post-transplantation, treatment with MMF was found to cause a significant decrease in intimal proliferation compared either with untreated controls or those treated with a variety of other immunosuppressants including CsA.

Effect of Rapamycin and Mycophenolic Acid on Vascular Smooth Muscle Cell Proliferation In Vitro

Based on the results of transplantation in animal models, we concluded that RPM and MPA are effective in preventing GVD in vivo in response to immune-mediated injury. This led us to hypothesize that these agents may be effective in preventing GVD based not solely on their suppressive effects on the recipient immune system, but also due to direct antiproliferative effects on growth factor-stimulated proliferation of mesenchymal cells in the donor organ. In other words, if these agents are so effective in inhibiting proliferation of lymphocytes activated by lymphokines, could they also be effective in inhibiting the proliferation of VSMCs stimulated by mitogenic cytokines such as PDGF and bFGF (Fig. 3)?

Using cultures of rat vascular smooth muscle cells stimulated with bFGF or PDGF, Cao and colleagues were able to show that RPM potently (IC_{50} of 0.8–5 nM) and dose-dependently inhibits the proliferation of these growth factor-stimulated cells (Cao et al. 1995). The authors demonstrated that the effect of the drug was *cytostatic* (not cytotoxic), and that even relatively late addition of the drug (as late as 46 h following stimulus) still inhibits growth factor-stimulated proliferation. Perhaps most importantly, the antiproliferative effect of RPM is reversed by increasing concentrations of FK506 in the culture medium, suggesting that in mesenchymal cells as in lymphocytes, these two immunosuppressants share the same intracellular binding protein (FKBP) that is responsible for the effects of RPM.

Members of our laboratory at Stanford (Gregory et al. 1993a) and Allison et al. (1993) at Syntex have examined the effects of MPA on vascular smooth muscle cell proliferation. Using either ^{3}H-thymidine or ^{3}H-leucine as markers for proliferation, it has been shown that MPA (the active metabolite of the

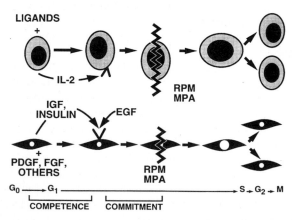

Fig. 3. Schematic representation of the hypothesis that novel immunosuppressants may inhibit both lymphokine-stimulated lymphocyte proliferation (*top*) and growth factor-stimulated mesenchymal cell (VSMC) proliferation (*bottom*). *IGF*, insulin-like growth factor; *EGF*, epidermal growth factor. (see text for other abbreviations)

prodrug MMF) is able to inhibit proliferation of these cells within a clinically achievable range of 1–10 μM. Again, as in the case of RPM, cytotoxicity was *not* responsible for the antiproliferative effect of the drug.

Efficacy of Rapamycin and Mycophenolate Mofetil
in Balloon-Injured Rat Carotid Model of Post-angioplasty Restenosis

From the data presented, we could conclude that at least in vitro, these novel immunosuppressive agents inhibit cytokine-stimulated proliferation of mesenchymal cells as well as lymphocytes. It is not entirely clear, however, that this is what really takes place in vivo. By invoking the *Response-to-Injury Paradigm* of Ross, we would surmise that the similar concentric, hyperplastic neointimal lesions seen in GVD and post-angioplasty restenosis are a result of initial immune injury in the case of GVD or initial mechanical injury in the case of restenosis (Clowes et al. 1989). Although somewhat controversial (Hansson et al. 1991), the consensus of opinion seems to suggest that the smooth-muscle-cell-rich, proliferative restenotic lesion seen in the balloon-injured rat carotid model is one that is divorced from immune mechanisms (Ferns et al. 1991; Hancock et al. 1994). Based on these premises, one could ask the following question: Do RPM and/or MPA inhibit lesion formation in a rodent model of restenosis where the effects of the drug cannot be attributed to suppressive effects on the immune system?

Gregory et al. examined this hypothesis by injuring the left common carotids of Sprague-Dawley rats using a 2-Fr embolectomy catheter, treating the animals with vehicle or drug (RPM, MPA, or both) at various dosages and schedules, and assessing the intimal proliferation by morphometric analysis (Fig. 4; Gregory et al. 1995). In untreated animals, the intimal area occupies approximately 45% of the total intimal and medial area by 2 weeks following injury, and progresses to 63% by POD 44. Immunohistochemistry at both of these time points in untreated control animals demonstrated that staining for endothelial cells using von Willebrand's Factor (vWF) was absent. Moreover, similar to other previously published data (Ferns et al. 1990), treatment with either CsA or FK506 from the day of injury to POD 14 does not decrease neointimal formation at 2 weeks relative to untreated controls. In contrast, at the same time point, treatment with either RPM or MPA alone significantly decreases the formation of hyperplastic neointima. Moreover, combination treatment with both agents even more effectively prevents the increase in intimal area (only 6% neointimal area); nevertheless, neither monotherapy nor combination therapy is able to promote restoration of endothelium 14 days following injury.

The initial success in preventing the restenotic lesion 2 weeks after combination therapy with RPM and MPA is no longer seen when the injured carotid arteries are examined on POD 44. By that time, the intimal area progresses to almost 50% following cessation of drug therapy on POD 13. Even more disappointing was the finding that prolongation of combination therapy from POD 13 to POD 30 does not significantly decrease the magnitude of the

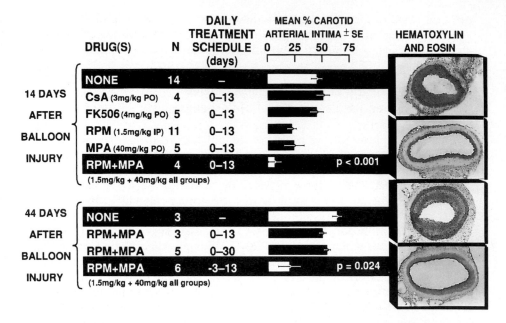

Fig. 4. Rapamycin (*RPM*) and mycophenolic acid (*MPA*) mono- and combination-therapy for prevention of balloon-injured rat carotid artery restenosis. Injured and uninjured carotid artery segments harvested at either 14 days or 44 days after injury were prepared and examined as described in the legend of Fig. 2. The mean percent intimal area [intimal area (mm^2)/medial area (mm^2) + intimal area (mm^2) × 100] was derived from morphometric analyses, and values for experimental and control tissues were compared using a one-tailed Mann Whitney U test corrected for small sample sizes

lesion. After systematic manipulation of the treatment schedules, Gregory and his colleagues concluded that pretreatment of the animals with both RPM and MPA from three days prior to injury until two weeks postinjury is sufficient not only to promote reendothelialization, but also inhibit intimal formation at POD 44 to 19% intimal area. This suggested that therapeutic blood levels of these agents may be necessary *at the time of injury (and release of growth factors)* in order to achieve a beneficial effect. Based on these results, we would conclude that RPM and MPA inhibit restenosis after mechanical injury in the rat carotid balloon injury model, presumably through direct antiproliferative effects on the growth factor-stimulated proliferation of VSMC in vivo.

Limitations

One might question how relevant these findings are to clinical restenosis seen in patients undergoing PTCA (percutaneous transluminal coronary angioplasty) or even angioplasty of peripheral artery lesions. Especially in light of the dismal failures of various treatment modalities in clinical trials (Faxon and Currier 1995), one of the greatest criticisms of preclinical studies of drug therapy in animal studies of restenosis has been wide variabilities in the models themselves. A variety of factors are thought to influence the formation of neointima in the different animal models of restenosis (Schwartz 1994), including the species of animal used, the type of vessel injured, the type, depth, and duration of injury, as well as the species-specific type of response (i.e., proliferative vs. thrombotic). It has been suggested that larger animal models may better represent the clinical condition in humans.

Another limitation of studies using the rat carotid model is a qualitative distinction between the vessels of interest. Clearly, balloon angioplasty in a clinical setting is performed on diseased and atherosclerotic vessels, rather than healthy, normal ones. As P. Libby has suggested, the mechanism of intimal thickening after balloon injury to a macrophage-rich atheroma may differ significantly from that in previously normal vessels (Libby et al. 1992). By keeping this warning in mind, we may more carefully assess the efficacy of various pharmacologic agents in different facile albeit suboptimal animal models of restenosis.

An evolving concept in the restenosis literature is the idea of "vascular remodeling" (Gibbons and Dzau 1994). This theory suggests that in responding to injury, vessels may not merely be limited to neointimal hyperplasia as the sole response, but that there may be compensatory enlargement or contraction by the entire vessel, such that, in the final analysis, luminal area may be decreased, increased, or even remain unchanged. Others have suggested that, because of this multifaceted response, the search for pharmacologic therapies for postangioplasty restenosis that solely inhibit VSMC proliferation may in fact be directed towards the wrong pathologic target (Currier and Faxon 1995). Nevertheless, due to the nature of the proliferative reparative response following stent placement, these agents may have a clearer role in preventing restenosis in this setting (Popma and Ellis 1990).

Conclusions: Thoughts About the Future
for Pharmacologic Treatments for Restenosis

Despite the limitations of animal studies, large animal work at Mount Sinai Medical School using RPM therapy in the balloon-injured pig coronary artery model is currently underway. Preliminary results suggest that this therapy is very effective in preventing luminal narrowing in this model, primarily due to a reduction in the fibrocellular component of the neointima (R. Gallo, V. Toschi, J. H. Chesebro, J. T. Fallon, V. Fuster, A. R. Marks, and J. J. Badimon, personal communication). Use of these agents in clinical trials of postangioplasty restenosis is of great interest to many investigators, as is the question of the optimal route of drug delivery (local versus systemic). In view of these exciting developments, it seems clear that if they are shown to be clinically effective after administration for a brief time before and after PTCA, these novel immunosuppressants may offer promise in the treatment of post-balloon angioplasty restenosis by going beyond their initially intended role as suppressors of immune system activation to act as inhibitors of growth factor-stimulated mesenchymal cell proliferation.

References

Allison AC, Eugui EM (1993) Inhibitors of de novo purine and pyrimidine synthesis as immunosuppressive drugs. Transplant Proc 25-3 (Suppl 2): 8-18

Allison AC, Eugui EM, Sollinger HW (1993) Mycophenolate mofetil (RS-61443): mechanisms of action and effects in transplantation. Transplant Rev 7 (3): 129-139

Ardehali A (1995) Heart transplantation: accelerated graft atherosclerosis. Adv Card Surg 6: 195-205

Billingham ME (1995) Pathology of graft vascular disease after heart and heart–lung transplantation and its relationship to obliterative bronchiolitis. Transplant Proc 27 (3): 2013-2016

Calne RY, Lim S, Samaan A, Colier DSJ, Pollard SG, White DJG, Thiru S (1989) Rapamycin for immunosuppression in organ allografting. Lancet 2: 227

Cao W, Mohacsi P, Shorthouse R, Pratt R, Morris RE (1995) Effects of rapamycin on growth factor-stimulated vascular smooth muscle cell DNA synthesis: inhibition of basic fibroblast growth factor and platelet-derived growth factor action and antagonism of rapamycin by FK506. Transplantation 59 (3): 390-395

Cardenas ME, Zhu D, Heitman J (1995) Molecular mechanisms of immunosuppression by cyclosporine, FK506, and rapamycin. Curr Opin in Nephrol Hypertens 4 (6): 472-477

Clowes AW, Clowes MM, Fingerle J, Reidy MA (1989) Regulation of smooth muscle cell growth in injured artery. J Cardiovasc Pharmacol 14 (Suppl 6): S12-S15

Currier JW, Faxon DP (1995) Restenosis after percutaneous transluminal coronary angioplasty: have we been aiming at the wrong target? J Am Coll Cardiol 25: 516-520

Eriksen UH, Amtorp O, Bagger JP, Emanuelsson H, Foegh M, Henningsen P, Saunamäki K, Schaeffer M, Thayssen P, Ørskov H, Kuntz RE, Popma JJ (1995) Randomized double-blind Scandinavian trial of angiopeptin versus placebo for the prevention of clinical events and restenosis after coronary balloon angioplasty. Am Heart J 130: 1-8

Faxon DP, Currier JW (1995) Prevention of post-PTCA restenosis. Ann NY Acad Sci 748: 419-428

Ferns G, Reidy M, Ross R (1990) Vascular effects of cyclosporine A in vivo and in vitro; Am J Pathol 137 (2): 403-413

Ferns GA, Reidy MA, Ross R (1991) Balloon catheter de-endothelialization of the nude rat carotid: response to injury in the absence of functional T lymphocytes. Am J Pathol 138 (4): 1045-1057

Franklin T, Cook JM (1969) The inhibition of nucleic acid synthesis by mycophenolic acid. Biochem J 113: 358-363

Gibbons GH, Dzau VJ (1994) The emerging concept of vascular remodeling. N Engl J Med 330 (20): 1431-1438

Gregory CR, Pratt RE, Huie P, Shorthouse R, Dzau VJ, Billingham ME, Morris RE (1993a) Effects of treatment with cyclosporine, FK506, rapamycin, mycophenolic acid, or deoxyspergualin on vascular smooth muscle proliferation in vitro and in vivo. Transplant Proc 25-1 (1): 770-771

Gregory CR, Huie P, Billingham ME, Morris RE (1993b) Rapamycin inhibits arterial intimal thickening caused by both alloimmune and mechanical injury: its effect on cellular, growth factor, and cytokine responses in injured vessels. Transplantation 55 (6): 1409-1418

Gregory CR, Huang X, Pratt RE, Dzau VJ, Shorthouse R, Billingham ME, Morris RE (1995) Treatment with rapamycin and mycophenolic acid reduces arterial intimal thickening produced by mechanical injury and allows endothelial replacement. Transplantation 59 (5): 655-661

Hancock WW, Adams DH, Wyner LR, Sayegh MH, Karnovsky MJ (1994) CD4+ mononuclear cells induce cytokine expression, vascular smooth muscle cell proliferation, and arterial occlusion after endothelial injury. Am J Pathol 145 (5): 1008-1014

Handley DA (1995) Experimental therapeutics and clinical studies in (re)stenosis. Micron 26 (1): 51–68

Hansson GK, Holm J, Holm S, Fotev Z, Hedrich H-J, Fingerle J (1991) T lymphocytes inhibit the vascular response to injury. Proc Natl Acad Sci USA 88: 10530–10534

Häyry P, Isoniemi H, Yilmaz S, Mennander A, Lemström K, Räisänen-Sokolowski A, Koskinen P, Ustinov J, Lautenschlager I, Taskinen E, Krogerus L, Aho P, Paavonen T (1993) Chronic allograft rejection. Immunol Rev 134: 33–81

Kirklin JK, Bourge RC, Naftel DC, Morrow WR, Deierhoi MH, Kauffman RS, White-Williams C, Nomberg RI, Holman WL, Smith DC Jr. (1994) Treatment of recurrent heart rejection with mycophenolate mofetil (RS-61443): initial clinical experience. J Heart Lung Transplant 13: 444–450

Libby P, Schwartz D, Brogi E, Tanaka H, Clinton SK (1992) A cascade model for restenosis: a special case of atherosclerosis progression. Circulation 86 (Suppl III): III-47–III-52

Meiser BM, Billingham ME, Morris RE (1991) Effects of cyclosporin, FK506, and rapamycin on graft-vessel disease. Lancet 338: 1297–1298

Morris RE (1991) Rapamycin: FK506's fraternal twin or distant cousin? Immunol Today 12 (5): 137–140

Morris RE (1993) Prevention and treatment of allograft rejection in vivo by rapamycin: molecular and cellular mechanism of action. Ann NY Acad Sci 685: 68–72

Morris RE (1996) Mechanisms of action of new immunosuppressive drugs. Kidney Int 49 (Suppl 53): S26–S38

Morris RE, Meiser BM (1989) Identification of a new pharmacologic action for an old compound. Med Sci Res 17: 609–610

Morris RE, Hoyt EG, Eugui EM, Allison AC (1989) Prolongation of rat heart allograft survival by RS-61443. Surg Forum 40: 337–338

Morris RE, Hoyt EG, Murphy MP, Eugui EM, Allison AC (1990) Mycophenolic acid morpholinoethylester (RS-61443) is a new immunosuppressant that prevents and halts heart allograft rejection by selective inhibition of T- and B-cell purine synthesis. Transplant Proc 22 (4): 1659–1662

Morris RE, Meiser BM, Wu J, Shorthouse R, Wang J (1991a) Use of rapamycin for the suppression of alloimmune reactions in vivo: Schedule dependence, tolerance induction, synergy with cyclosporine and FK506, and effect on host-versus-graft and graft-versus-host reactions. Transplant Proc 23 (1): 521–524

Morris RE, Wang J, Blum JR, Flavin T, Murphy MP, Almquist SJ, Chu N, Tam YL, Kaloostian M, Allison AC, Eugui EM (1991b) Immunosuppressive effects of the morpholinoethyl ester of mycophenolic acid (RS-61443) in rat and nonhuman primate recipients of heart allografts. Transplant Proc 23-2 (Suppl 2): 19–25

Nobuyoshi M, Kimura T, Nosaka H, Mioka S, Ueno K, Yokoi H, Hamasaki N, Horiuchi H, Ohishi H (1988) Restenosis after successful percutaneous transluminal coronary angioplasty: Serial angiographic follow-up of 229 patients. J Am Coll Cardiol 12 (3): 616–623

Popma JJ, Ellis St. G (1990) Intracoronary stents: clinical and angiographic results. Herz 15 (5): 307–318

Reidy MA, Jackson CL (1990) Factors controlling growth of arterial cells following injury. Toxicol Pathol 18-4 (1): 547–553

Ross R (1995) Cell biology of atherosclerosis. Annu Rev Physiol 57: 791–804

Schwartz RS (1994) Neointima and arterial injury: dogs, rats, pigs, and more (editorial). Lab Invest 71 (6): 789–791

Sehgal S, Camardo JS, Scarola JA, Maida BT (1995) Rapamycin (sirolimus, rapamune). Curr Opin Nephrol Hypertens 4 (6): 482–487

Steele DM, Hullett DA, Bechstein WO, Kowalski J, Smith LS, Kennedy E, Allison AC, Sollinger HW (1993) Effects of immunosuppressive therapy on the rat aortic allograft model. Transplant Proc 25 (1): 754–755

Treatment of Inflammatory Cardiomyopathy with Corticosteroids

U. Kühl and H.-P. Schultheiss

Introduction

Dilated cardiomyopathy (DCM) is defined as a heart disease of unknown cause with enlargement and impaired contraction of the left or both ventricles. It may be idiopathic, familial/genetic, viral and/or immune, alcoholic/toxic, or associated with recognized cardiovascular diseases in which the degree of myocardial dysfunction is not sufficiently explained by the causative disease [1]. Recent clinical and experimental data have suggested a coincidental relationship with viral myocarditis [2]. Viral persistence has been documented in both myocarditis and chronic heart failure [3–7]. While in the acute phase tissue destruction is caused by a direct cytotoxic effect of the virus, the extent of tissue damage and depression of cardiac function in the chronic state of the disease depends on the virally induced humoral and cellular immune processes. These may on one hand limit further expansion of the destructive process, but on the other hand they may themselves cause ongoing injury to the myocardium.

The assumption that this active immunologic process may cause DCM has led to the suggestion that the use of anti-inflammatory agents could be beneficial to prevent development and progression of dilatation and ventricular dysfunction in this subgroup of patients with a pathologically inflammatory process of the myocardium [8, 9]. The histologic diagnosis of chronic myocarditis, however, can be exceedingly difficult, as shown by the great variation in the diagnosis of myocarditis when based only on histologic analysis of endomyocardial biopsies [10]. Because, at the morphologic level, lymphocytes may mimic other cellular elements of the interstitium, quantification of infiltrating lymphocytes and their differentiation from noninflammatory interstitial cells is difficult by light microscopy. Additionally, cellular infiltrates can be easily missed by "sampling error," because inflammatory infiltrates in chronic myocarditis are often focally distributed [11, 12].

While routine histologic methods are unable to provide accurate diagnostic information about chronic inflammation of the heart, immunohistologic analyses have now been introduced to identify, characterize, and quantify cellular

Department of Internal Medicine/Cardiology, Benjamin Franklin Hospital, Free University of Berlin, Hindenburgdamm 32, 12200 Berlin, Germany

infiltrates and demonstrate chronically active immunologic process in the myocardium of patients with clinically suspected DCM [13–16]. With this diagnostic approach, it is possible to characterize and identify a subgroup of patients with "inflammatory cardiomyopathy" in whom immunosuppressive therapy might have beneficial effects.

Methods

Patients

Forty-nine patients (33 men, 16 women) were enrolled in this study. The mean age of the patients was 50.6 ± 11.2 years. Clinically, all patients presented with DCM with a clinical history of more than 6 months (range 6 months to 26 years). None of them had a history of viral infection in association with the onset of clinical symptoms. The usual laboratory tests and serological tests failed to prove an inflammatory process or a viral infection. All patients were examined using invasive and noninvasive techniques including physical examination, routine laboratory tests, ECG, exercise ECG, echocardiography, right and left catheterization, coronary angiography, left ventriculography, and right heart endomyocardial biopsy to rule out secondary causes of ventricular dysfunction (e.g., coronary artery disease, valvular or hypertensive heart disease). Endomyocardial biopsies were taken transvenously via the femoral approach from the right heart side of the intraventricular septum.

Sample Preparation and Immunohistologic Evaluation of Biopsies

Preparation of endomyocardial biopsies and immunohistologic staining was carried out as described elsewhere (2, 16, 17). The biopsy samples were classified as immunohistologically positive if the mean number of T lymphocytes exceeded 2.0 cells per high-power microscopic field (×400) (equivalent to 7 cells/mm^2) and, in addition, biopsy samples showed increased expression of histocompatibility antigens I or II or other adhesion molecules such as CD18, CD54, or CD29. The meaning of these immunologic markers for accurate diagnosis of cardiac inflammation has been discussed in detail elsewhere [2] (see also Kühl et al., this volume).

Selection of Patients for Immunosuppressive Treatment

Patients with clinically suspected DCM underwent biopsy and determination of right and left ventricular function during the initial examination. Most patients with globally depressed cardiac function (below 40%) were already being treated according to general guidelines with digitalis, diuretics, and ACE inhibitors at the time of their first physical examination. To exclude clinical and hemodynamic effects caused by a variation in medication or spontaneous remission of the infiltrative process, both immunohistologically negative and positive patients were treated with the above conventional therapy for an initial 6-month period. Drug dosage was individualized for each patient but kept constant during the study period. Patients with an ejection fraction below 35% additionally received Marcumar (phenprocoumon) (Quick 35 ± 5%) to prevent embolisms.

After 6 months patients underwent a follow-up biopsy and determination of ventricular function. They were required to have no significant impairment of ventricular function or of clinical symptoms and to have a follow-up biopsy that was immunohistologically positive according to the immunohistologic criteria given above. A change in hemodynamic indices was significant if the change exceeded 5% for EF and 3 mmHg for LVEDP.

Acute myocarditis according to the Dallas criteria was not seen in any of the initial or follow-up biopsies. All 20 patients with spontaneous remission of the inflammatory process (but persisting ventricular impairment) were kept on conventional therapy (see above) and taken as a control group for comparing their hemodynamic course with that of patients in the study group. The 29 patients with persisting cellular infiltrates but a lack of significant improvement in ventricular function or clinical symptoms became the study group for immunosuppressive treatment.

Treatment Protocol

Daily immunosuppressive treatment with 6-methylprednisolone was started at a dosage of 1 mg/kg body weight [18]. After 3 weeks the dose of corticoid was reduced by 20 mg and then similarly further reduced stepwise every second week until a maintenance level of 12 mg per day was reached. This low dose was maintained until week 24, when a repeat biopsy was taken and ventricular hemodynamic indices were reassessed.

Results

Spontaneous Resolution of the Inflammatory Process

After 6 months of conventional treatment with digitalis, diuretics, and ACE inhibitors, myocardial inflammation had resolved in 20 patients. These patients reported a significant clinical improvement in exercise capacity and reduction of cardiac symptoms according to the NYHA classification from 2.3 ± 1.0 to 1.7 ± 0.8. LVEDP decreased from 18.6 ± 8.1 mmHg to 11.8 ± 6.8 mmHg ($p < 0,05$). Other hemodynamic indices of the group as a whole did not change significantly (Table 1).

In 29 patients with an ongoing inflammatory process, both the NYHA classification (2.0 ± 0.9) and hemodynamic indices remained unchanged (Table 1).

Table 1. Hemodynamic data of 49 patients with dilated cardiomyopathy

	Conventional treatment				Immunosuppressive treatment (n = 29) Biopsy 3
	Inflammation resolved (n = 20)		Inflammation persisted (n = 29)		
	Biopsy 1	Biopsy 2	Biopsy 1	Biopsy 2	
LVEDP (mmHg)	18.2 ± 8.1	11.8 ± 6.8**	18.1 ± 8.9	18.8 ± 9.7	15.2 ± 8.8
PA (mmHg)	22.0 ± 7.5	16.0 ± 8.2	19.3 ± 9.5	18.6 ± 9.6	18.3 ± 6.9
EF (%)	33.0 ± 10.2	35.5 ± 17.1	35.0 ± 12.7	34.0 ± 12.7	43.9 ± 18.3*
EDVI (ml/m^2)	183 ± 81	178 ± 79	154 ± 48	155 ± 54	150 ± 20.1
ESVI (ml/m^2)	126 ± 66	126 ± 80	102 ± 46	99 ± 41	94 ± 69
SVI (ml/m^2)	57 ± 22	52 ± 10	51 ± 18	50 ± 18	54.9 ± 18

* $p < 0.01$; ** $p < 0.05$.
LVEDP, Left ventricular end-diastolic pressure; PA, mean pulmonary artery pressure; EF, ejection fraction; EDVI, end-diastolic volume index; ESVI, endsystolic volume index; SVI, stroke volume index.

Treatment with 5-Methylprednisolone

Immunohistologically, myocardial inflammation resolved in 20/29 patients (69%) (Table 2). CD3-positive inflammatory cells and the increased HLA expression normalized during therapy (Fig. 1). Macrophages did not change significantly, but it is known that 27E10-positive activated macrophages may be induced by cortisone treatment. Sixteen of the 20 patients (80%) with resolved cardiac inflammation reported an improvement in cardiac symptoms according to the NYHA classification, while none of the 9 patients who immunohistologically did not respond to therapy improved clinically. NYHA classification improved significantly ($p < 0.05$) from 2.9 (2.5–3.3) to 2.3 (2.0–2.6). A significant improvement was also seen in systolic cardiac function (EF,

Table 2. Immunohistologic data of 49 patients with dilated cardiomyopathy

	Conventional treatment				Immunosuppressive treatment (n = 29) Biopsy 3
	Inflammation resolved (n = 20)		Inflammation persisted (n = 29)		
	Biopsy 1	Biopsy 2	Biopsy 1	Biopsy 2	
Inflammation[a]	positive	negative	positive	positive	
Expression of:					
CD3	2.3 ± 1.3	0.7 ± 0.4*	3.1 ± 3.9	3.5 ± 3.2	1.3 ± 1.1*
CD4	1.3 ± 1.4	0.3 ± 0.3*	0.8 ± 0.5	1.3 ± 1.1	0.6 ± 0.7**
CD8	1.4 ± 0.7	0.4 ± 0.3*	1.1 ± 0.9	2.2 ± 0.7	0.7 ± 0.6*
Mac	1.5 ± 1.7	0.3 ± 0.3*	1.2 ± 1.0	1.1 ± 0.7	1.2 ± 1.1
HLA-DR	1.3 ± 0.5	1.0 ± 0.3	1.6 ± 0.6	1.7 ± 0.7	1.3 ± 0.4

[a] > 2.0 T lymphocytes per high-power field.

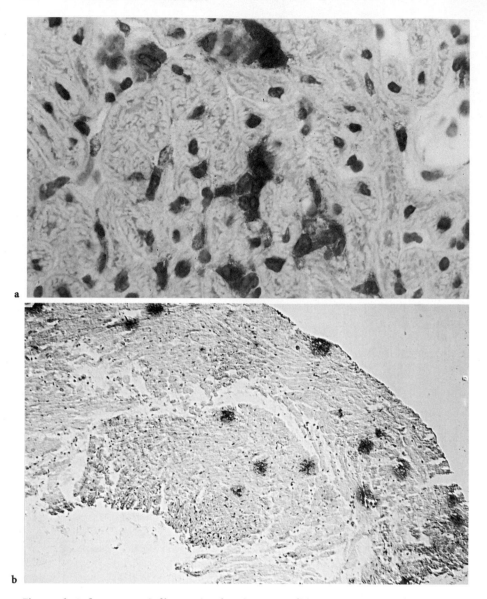

Fig. 1a–d. Inflammatory infiltrates in chronic myocarditis: **a** CD3-positive lymphocytes, **b** activated macrophages. **c, d** HLA-DR antigen expression in a CD3-positive biopsy before (**c**) and after (**d**) immunosuppressive therapy. Magnification: **a** ×400, **b–d** ×40

SVI, LVEDP) and in inflammatory infiltrates, while changes in other hemo-dynamic data (EDVI, ESVI, PA) did not reach the level of significance.

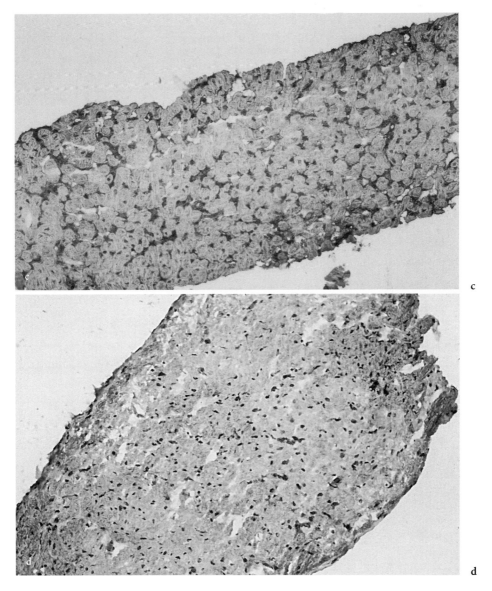

Fig. 1c,d

Discussion

Approaches to the understanding and treatment of chronic heart failure have undergone extensive development in the last 10 years or so. The identification of persisting viral mRNA in animal models and humans with myocarditis and

DCM and the immunohistochemical detection of an active inflammatory process in the myocardium of many of these patients has supported the idea that a postmyocarditic autoimmune process is responsible for the development and progression of DCM [19, 20]. This has led to the suggestion that the use of anti-inflammatory agents could be beneficial in preventing development and progression of the chronic immune process in a subgroup of patients with DCM.

Except for the recently published American Mycoarditis Trial which, however, relates to patients with acute myocarditis, no reports on randomized and controlled studies are available to provide information about the efficacy and safety of immunosuppressive treatment in humans [8]. The data from the myocarditis trial did not provide any evidence that immunosuppressive therapy has beneficial effects on ventricular contractility. The study group, however, was compared with a randomized control group of patients with acute myocarditis, which is known to be associated with spontaneous remission of the inflammatory process in a high percentage of patients. Spontaneous healing of myocarditis does not only occur at the very early phase of the disease, but is also seen at later stages. One must therefore assume that no positive therapeutic effect could be demonstrated because the effect of treatment was overlaid by improvement due to spontaneous healing of the inflammatory process. The results of this study should therefore not be applied to patients with a chronic persisting immune process.

The analysis of other reported data on treatment of myocarditis, originating from uncontrolled treatment studies, is limited by the differences in therapeutic regimens used and the lack of homogeneity of the patient groups studied, mostly due to the variety of diagnostic criteria used [21–25]. In most of these studies, myocarditis was histologically characterized according to the Dallas classification [26, 27]. However, it has by now become evident that conventional histologic analysis is not an appropriate method for the detection of chronic inflammation of the myocardium [2]. The histologic diagnosis requires the presence of infiltrating lymphocytes [27], but infiltrating cells, especially if not activated, are not necessarily representative of an ongoing immune process which affects the entire myocardium. Inaccurate diagnosis selects the wrong subgroup of patients for therapy. This might explain the poor response to immunosuppressive therapy reported in most published treatment trials.

Immunosuppressive treatment of patients with chronic myocarditis can only be successful if an active immunologic process has been identified at the time when treatment is started. Therefore, more sensitive and specific analytical methods should be used for the diagnosis of chronic myocarditis and the identification of the appropriate group of patients. Immunohistologic techniques have now been successfully introduced that more accurately identify cellular infiltrates in myocardial biopsies. When additional immune markers for the activity of the immune process are used, the diagnosis of inflammatory heart disease is markedly improved [2, 16, 17]. Our results show that, when only patients with an immunohistologically defined inflammatory process are treated with immunosuppressive drugs ventricular contractility and clinical symptoms are demonstrably improved and the cellular inflammation is eliminated from the myocardium. The treatment leads to a statistically significant improvement in clinical symptoms or ventricular function, and the improvement in systolic cardiac function far exceeds that seen in patients with spontaneous healing of chronic myocarditis.

Our findings differ significantly from those of others who were unable to demonstrate a clear improvement of ventricular function after corticoid treatment [8, 21–25]. In our opinion, this disparity results from differences in the selection of patients studied, due to inappropriate histologic diagnosis of the inflammatory process. The data in the present study show that immunosuppressive treatment of patients with clinically suspected DCM results in clinical, hemodynamic, and immunohistologic improvement in patients with an active, immunohistologically proven inflammatory process.

References

1. Report of the 1995 World Health Organization/International Society and Federation of Cardiology Task Force on The Definition and Classification of Cardiomyopathies (1996) Circulation 93: 841–842
2. Kühl U, Seeberg B, Noutsias M, Schultheiss H-P (1995) Immunohistochemical analysis of the chronic inflammatory process in dilated cardiomyopathy: Br Heart J 75: 295–300
3. Editorial (1990) Dilated cardiomyopathy and enteroviruses. Lancet 336: 971–973
4. Bowles NE, Ohlsen EGJ, Richardson PJ, Archard LC (1986) Detection of Cocksackie B-virus-specific RNA sequences in myocardial biopsy samples from patients with myocarditis and dilated cardiomyopathy. Lancet 1: 1120–1122
5. Grasso M, Arbusti E, Silini E, Diegoli M, Percivalle E, Ratti G, Bramerio M, Gavazzi A, Vigano M, Milanesi G (1992) Search for Coxsackie B3 RNA in idiopathic dilated cardiomyopathy using gene amplification by polymerase chain reaction. Am J Cardiol 69: 658–664
6. Kandolf R, Ameis D, Kirschner P, Canu A, Hofschneider P (1985) In situ detection of enteroviral genomes in myocardial cells by nucleic acid hybridization: an approach to the diagnosis of viral heart disease. Proc Natl Acad Sci 82: 4818–4822
7. Archard LC, Bowles NE, Cunningham L, Freeke CA, Olsen EG, Rose ML, Meany B, Why HJF, Richardson FJ (1991) Molecular probes for detection of persisting enterovirus infection of human heart and their prognostic value. Eur Heart J 12 (Suppl D): 56–59
8. Mason JW, O'Connel JB, Herskowitz A and the Myocarditis Treatment Trial Investigators (1994) A clinical trial of immunosuppressive therapy for myocarditis. N Engl J Med 321: 1061–1068
9. Schultheiss HP, Kühl U, Janda I, Schanwell M, Strauer BB (1992) Immunsuppressive Therapie der Myokarditis. Herz 17: 112–121
10. Ohlsen EGJ (1985) The problem of viral heart disease: how often do we miss it? Postgrad Med J 61: 479–480
11. Shanes JG, Ghali J, Billingham ME, Ferrans VJ, Fenoglio JJ, Edwards WD, Tsai CC, Saffitz JE, Isner J, Furner S, Subramanian R (1987) Interobserver variability in the pathologic interpretation of endomyocardial biopsy results. Circulation 75: 401–405
12. Hauck AJ, Kearney DL, Edwards WD (1989) Evaluation of postmortem endomyocardial biopsy specimen from 38 patients with lymphocytic myocarditis: implication for role of sampling error. Mayo Clin Proc 64: 1235–1245
13. Edwards WD, Holmes DR, Reeder GS (1982) Diagnosis of active lymphocytic myocarditis by endomyocardial biopsy. Quantitative criteria for light microscopy. Mayo Clin Proc 57: 419–425
14. Zee-Cheng CS, Tsai CC, Palmer DC, Codd JE, Pennington DG, Williams GA (1984) High incidence of myocarditis by endomyocardial biopsy in patients with idiopathic congestive cardiomyopathy. J Am Coll Cardiol 3: 63–70

15. Steenbergen C, Kolbeck PC, Wolfe JA, Anthony RM, Sanfilippo FP, Jennings RB (1986) Detection of lymphocytes in endomyocardium using immunohistochemical techniques. Relevance to evaluation of endomyocardial biopsies in suspected cases of lymphocytic myocarditis. J Appl Cardiol 1: 63–73
16. Kühl U, Noutsias M, Seeberg B, Schannwell M, Welp LB, Schultheiss HP (1994) Chronic inflammation in the myocardium of patients with clinically suspected dilated cardio-myopathy. J Card Failure 1: 13–27
17. Kühl U, Noutsias M, Seeberg B, Schannwell M, Welp LB, Schultheiss HP (1994) Chronic inflammation in dilated cardiomyopathy. J Heart Failure January : 231–245
18. Schultheiss HP, Kühl U, Janda I, Schanwell M, Strauer BB (1992) Immunsuppressive Therapie der Myokarditis. Herz 17: 112–121
19. Dec GW Jr, Palacios IF, Fallon JT, Aretz HT, Mills J, Mills DCS, Johnson RA (1985) Active myocarditis in the spectrum of acute dilated cardiomyopathies. N Engl J Med 312: 885–890
20. Quigley PJ, Richardson PJ, Meany BT et al . (1987) Longterm follow up of acute myo-carditis: correlation of ventricular function and outcome. Eur Heart J 8 [Suppl J]: 1303–1307
21. Jones SR, Herskowitz A, Hutchins G, Baughman KL (1987) Response to im-munosuppressive therapy in myocarditis with and without myocyte necrosis. Circulation 76 [Suppl IV]: 461
22. Parillo JE, Cunnion RE, Epstein SE et al. (1989) A prospective, randomized, controlled trial of prednisone for dilated cardiomyopathy. N Engl J Med 321: 1061–1068
23. Hosenpud JD, McAnulty JH, Niles NR (1985) Lack of objective improvement in ventricular systolic function in patients with myocarditis treated with azathioprine and prednisone. J Am Coll Cardiol 6: 217–222
24. Mason JW, Billingham ME, Ricci DR (1980) Treatment of acute inflammatory myocarditis assisted by endomyocardial biopsy. Am J Cardiol 45: 1037–1044
25. Latham RD, Mulrow JP, Virmani R, Robinowitz M, Moody JM (1989) Recently diagnosed idiopathic dilated cardiomyopathy: incidence of myocarditis and efficacy of prednisone therapy. Am Heart J 117: 876–882
26. Aretz HT, Billingham ME, Edwards WD, Factor S, Fallon JT, Fenoglio JJ Jr, Olsen EGJ, Schoen F (1986) Myocarditis: a histopathologic definition and classification. J Cardiovasc Pathol 1: 3–14
27. Aretz HT (1987) Myocarditis, the Dallas criteria. Human Pathol 18: 619–624

The Genetics of Dilated Cardiomyopathy

M.K. Baig, A.S. Coonar, J.H. Goldman, and W.J. McKenna

Dilated cardiomyopathy (DCM) is a heterogeneous condition, and probably encompasses a number of different disease entities which manifest similarly in their later stages as heart failure, but which are aetiologically distinct. The recent recognition of familial disease with mendelian inheritance implies the significant role of single genes in disease pathology, and thus provides an avenue to identify the molecular abnormality. Such molecular differences may in the future allow genetic classification of these disorders.

DCM may be idiopathic, familial, viral, immune, alcohol or otherwise toxic, or associated with recognised cardiovascular disease where the degree of myocardial dysfunction is not explained by the abnormal loading conditions or the extent of ischaemic damage. A cardiac phenotype identical to DCM is also seen in some patients with generalised myopathy, i.e., Duchenne, Becker, Myotonic dystrophy.

Dilated cardiomyopathy typically affects young men and frequently presents as end-stage heart failure. It is seen world-wide, but epidemiological information has been assessed only in a few countries. In the United States, clinical studies indicate a prevalence of 36 per 100,000 with an annual incidence of 5–8 per 100,000 (Codd et al. 1989). In Sweden an incidence of 5 per 100,000 has been reported from autopsy studies (Torp 1978). Similar numbers have been proposed for England and Germany; however, precise figures are not available. It is quite probable that the true incidence is underestimated by those figures, since DCM has a long preclinical phase during which patients are asymptomatic and in many cases the disorder may remain unrecognized altogether. (Gillum 1986; Codd et al. 1989). The diagnosis therefore is necessarily based on features that reflect advanced disease.

Patients normally present between 20 and 50 years of age, but children and the elderly may also be affected. The most common manifestation at the time of diagnosis is heart failure, frequently of an advanced type (New York Heart Association functional class III or IV).

In cases of more advanced heart failure systemic or pulmonary emboli may be the initial presentation. Atrial fibrillation and ventricular arrhythmias are

Department of Cardiological Sciences, St. George's Hospital Medical School, Cranmer Terrace, London SW17 ORE, UK

common. Rarely, syncope or sudden death may be seen as the initial manifestation, usually in association with histological or immunohistochemical
evidence of inflammation.

The diagnosis of idiopathic dilated cardiomyopathy requires exclusion of all
potentially reversible causes of left ventricular dysfunction, particularly excess
alcohol consumption, coronary heart disease and systemic hypertension
(Keeling and McKenna 1994; Keeling et al. 1995; Dec and Fuster 1995).

Clinical Genetics

X-linked, autosomal dominant and recessive as well as apparently true
sporadic cases have been identified. Initially, retrospective studies revealed a
predominantly X-linked pattern of inheritance, and whilst study of these families has provided an understanding of the molecular abnormality, the retrospective mode of pedigree acquisition necessarily underestimated the true
prevalence of familial disease. As more recent prospective studies have been
published, it seems clear that an important, and possibly predominant mode of
inheritance in DCM is likely to be autosomal dominant. Autosomal recessive
patterns of inheritance also have been described, but as is discussed below,
these may not have represented the true nature of inheritance, because of
phenotype underestimation in the relevant studies.

Recent prospective studies suggest that familial disease maybe present in at
least 20% of probands. In the Mayo Clinic study (Michels et al. 1992), families
of 59 consecutive unrelated DCM patients were screened for affected relatives.
DCM was diagnosed in 18 of 325 relatives (5.5%) from 12 families with a
familial prevalence of 20% (12/59). This study demonstrated the importance of
family screening; 83% of affected relatives were asymptomatic and would have
been missed by screening based on the presence of symptoms. In all cases a
mode of transmission most consistent with autosomal dominant inheritance
was determined. In the United Kingdom, Keeling et al. evaluated 40 families of
consecutive DCM probands (Keeling et al. 1995). 25/236 (10.6%) relatives from
ten families were identified as being affected with a familial prevalence of 25%
(10/40). Again, the main pattern of inheritance was determined to be autosomal dominant.

In both Michels and Keelings studies, 20%–25% of asymptomatic relatives
were found to have DCM; in addition, there were also a statistically significant
number of asymptomatic relatives in both studies, who had significant cardiac
structural or functional abnormalities. The most common of these abnormalities has been termed asymptomatic left ventricular enlargement, and may
represent an early stage of DCM. Therefore, the true prevalence of familial
disease may be considerably higher, and reliance on symptoms or observed
structural abnormalities alone to identify cases maybe inadequate. An autosomal dominant inheritance pattern suggests that in an individual pedigree the
disease is likely to be monogenic in aetiology. Therefore, the development of
molecular techniques may allow a more accurate level of diagnosis.

Molecular Genetics

Progress in the identification of the molecular abnormality in DCM may have been slower, in part be due to greater heterogeneity of aetiologies than is seen with other conditions (for example, hypertrophic cardiomyopathy). However, several abnormalities and some genes have been identified, and these are discussed below.

X-Linked DCM

Berko and colleagues (Berko and Swift 1987) described a five-generation pedigree of 63 persons. Affected males with DCM had early onset, rapid progression and severe disease in contrast to females with DCM who had later onset, slow progression, and milder disease. There was no male to male transmission and all affected females had sons who died of DCM. No patient had evidence of skeletal myopathy or neuromuscular disease though the affected males all had elevation in serum creatinine kinase level suggesting a process involving muscle damage. The consistently different pattern of disease by gender suggested a pattern of X-linked inheritance which suggested the role of mutations affecting either the X chromosome or mitochondrial genome.

Towbin et al. (1993), investigating two unrelated families identified linkage of X-linked DCM to Xp21, the site of the dystrophin gene. Abnormalities of cardiac dystrophin were shown by Western blotting with N-terminal dystrophin antibody, whereas skeletal muscle dystrophin was normal, suggesting primary involvement of the dystrophin gene with preferential involvement of cardiac muscle. The authors concluded that X-linked DCM was due to an abnormality within the centromeric half of the dystrophin gene region in the heart. This abnormality could be accounted for by a mutation in the 5' region of the dystrophin coding sequence preferentially affecting cardiac function, splicing abnormalities which resulted in an abnormal cardiac protein, or a cardiac-specific promoter mutation.

Subsequently Muntoni et al (Muntoni et al. 1993, 1995) showed in a large X-linked pedigree that a deletion removing the dystrophin muscle promoter, the first muscle exon and part of intron 1 caused a severe dilated cardiomyopathy with no associated skeletal muscle weakness. The presence of cardiac specific disease with certain mutations has also been described by Yoshida et al. (1993).

The determinants of whether a dystrophin mutation causes cardiomyopathy, skeletal myopathy or both are not yet fully known.

Because both the Becker and Duchenne type muscular dystrophies which arise from mutations in the dystrophin gene located at Xp21 have significant cardiac involvement, in a pattern similar to dilated cardiomyopathy, the identification of the causal gene in these diseases led to speculation that these mutations were also responsible for cases of idiopathic non-X-linked DCM. Dystrophin gene deletion analysis was performed by Michels et al. in 27 unselected DCM patients (Michels et al. 1993). No dystrophin gene defects were found, indicating that dystrophin mutations are probably a rare cause of dilated cardiomyopathy. A caveat is that increasing examination of the dystrophin gene has identified a larger number of small mutations than were previously thought to occur, i.e., missense rather than exonic. Application of more sophisticated techniques may yet identify a role for dystrophin mutations as a cause of sporadic idiopathic DCM.

Autosomal Dominant DCM

Four loci have been reported for the autosomal dominant form of disease.

1. In a large pedigree characterised by Graber (Graber et al. 1986) in whom dilated cardiomyopathy was associated with progressive cardiac conduction disease, Kass et al. (1994) demonstrated linkage of the disease locus to the locus 1p1-1q1.
2. Krajinovic studied a large six-generation kindred (Krajinovic et al. 1995) and two other families with an autosomal dominant pattern of transmission. All three families were unrelated and had identical clinical features. Linkage was found for chromosome 9q13-q22. The authors hypothesise as candidates the FRDA/FARR Friedreich ataxia gene, cAMP-dependent protein kinase and tropomodulin, a tropomyosin modulating protein.
3. Durand and colleagues studied a 46 member family with four generations and found linkage to 1q32 (Durand 1995). and suggested that the genes MEF-2D (myocyteenhancer factor 2D), FMOD (flavin-containing monooxygenase), PCMCA4, renin and the helix-loop helix DNA binding protein MYF-4 were candidate genes.
4. Linkage has also been identified in a family with dilated cardiomyopathy to the region 3p22–25 (Olson 1996). A number of candidate genes map to this locus including a G-protein (GNA12), calcium channel (CANCNLIA2), sodium channel (SCN5A), inositol triphosphate (ITPR1) and the gap junction connexin 45. Correlation of genetic and phenotypic data in this family suggests that sinus bradycardia may be an early clinical marker of disease manifestation. This pedigree has a similar phenotype (DCM with conduction disease) to the family characterised by Graber (Graber et al. 1986) which as discussed earlier mapped to chromosome 1p1-1q1 (Kass et al. 1994). This locus was specifically excluded in the pedigree studied by Krajinovic and hence this investigation further demonstrates genetic heterogeneity within DCM.

It has also been hypothesised that the myotin kinase gene may be a candidate for idiopathic DCM. Mutation in the CTGn region associated with the gene on 19q is associated with the development of dystrophia myotonica (DM). (Harley 1992; Buxton 1992; Aslandis 1992). The phenotype of DM includes cardiac failure, abnormalities of conduction, and arrhythmias. In patients with DM, variable penetrance, variable expression, and anticipation is recognised. Furthermore at a molecular level, tissue-specific mutation is recognised. It follows, therefore, that this gene is a good candidate for cases of idiopathic DCM, and is currently under review.

Autosomal Recessive DCM

True familial DCM occurring in an autosomal recessive inheritance pattern has been described only infrequently, and as yet no specific locus has been identified. In a study of 165 consecutive patients (Mestroni et al. 1990) inheritance was autosomal dominant in seven families, and recessive in four. Koike et al. (1987) in an investigation of the role of the HLA system identified a single family in which inheritance was most probably autosomal recessive. Goldblatt (1987) identified dilated cardiomyopathy occurring in three members of a consanguineous Madeira Portuguese family which followed a recessive pattern of inheritance.

As we now recognise a prolonged pre-symptomatic phase of DCM during which cardiac abnormalities may be present, it may be that apparently recessively inherited cases are not truly so if these pre symptomatic individuals are included. Thus the reports of recessive inheritance should be reviewed in the light of our current understanding of DCM, and as future diagnostic classification improves.

Summary

In summary, the genetic aetiology of dilated cardiomyopathy has clearly identified the role of the dystrophin gene. Four loci for autosomal dominant DCM have been identified, and candidate gene evaluation is underway. There is likely to be a monogenic answer in a subset of cases, but the heterogeneous nature of this disease suggests that multiple genes as well as other causes may become apparent. Current estimates of familial disease are likely to be underestimates. As new genetic diagnostic techniques are developed, our classification of DCM and our estimates of the prevalence of familial disease, are both likely to change.

References

Aslandis C (1992) Myotonic dystrophy. Nature 355: 548–551
Berko BAM, Swift M (1987) X-linked dilated cardiomyopathy. N Engl J Med 316: 1186–1191
Buxton J (1992) Detection of an unstable fragment of DNA specific to individuals with Myotonic dystrophy. Nature 355: (6360): 547–8
Codd MB, Sugrue DD, Gersh BJ, Melton LJ III (1989) Epidemiology of idiopathic dilated and hypertrophic cardiomyopathy: a population based study in Olmsted County, Minnesota, 1975–1984. Circulation 80: 564–572
Dec WG, Fuster V (1995) Idiopathic dilated cardiomyopathy. N Engl J Med 331: 1564–1575
Durand JB, Abchee AB, Roberts R (1995) Molecular and clinical aspects of inherited cardiomyopathies [Review]. Annals of Medicine 27(3): 311–7
Gillum RF (1986) Idiopathic cardiomyopathy in the United States 1970–1982. Am Heart J 111: 752–755
Goldblatt J (1987) Autosomal recessive inheritance of idiopathic dilated cardiomyopathy in a Madeira Portuguese Kindred. Clin Genet 31: 249–254
Graber HL, Unverferth DV, Baker PB, Ryan JM, Baba N, Wooley CF (1986) Evolution of a hereditary cardiac conduction and muscle disorder: a study involving a family with six generations affected. Circulation 74: 21–35

Harley G (1992) Myotonic dystrophy. Nature 355: 545–546

Kass S, MacRae C, Graber HL, Sparks EA, McNamara D, Boudoulas H, Basson CT, Baker P, Cody RJ, Fishman MC et al (1994) A gene defect that causes conduction system disease and dilated cardiomyopathy maps to chromosome 1p1-1q1. Nature Genet 7: 546–551

Keeling PJ, Gang Y, Smith G et al (1995) Familial dilated cardiomyopathy in the United Kingdom. Br Heart J 73: 417–721

Keeling PJ, McKenna WJ (1994) Clinical genetics of dilated cardiomyopathy. Herz 19: 91–96

Koike S, Kawa S, Yabu K, Endo R, Sasaki Y, Furta S, Ota M (1987) Familial dilated cardiomyopathy and human leucocyte antigen. A report of two family cases. J Heart Jpn 28: 941–945

Krajinovic M, Pinamonti B, Sinagra G, Vatta M, Severini GM, Milasin J, Falaschi A, Camerini F, Giacca M, Mestroni L, Group and the H. M. D. S. (1995) Linkage of familial dilated cardiomyopathy to chromosome 9 and the Heart Muscle Disease Study. Am J Hum Genet 57: 846–852

Mestroni L, Miani D, Di LA, Silvestri F, Bussani R, Filippi G, Camerini F (1990) Clinical and pathologic study of familial dilated cardiomyopathy. Am J Cardiol 65: 1449–1453

Michels VV, Moll PP, Miller FA et al (1992) The frequency of familial dilated cardiomyopathy in a series of patients with idiopathic dilated cardiomyopathy. N Engl J Med 326: 77–82

Muntoni F, Cau M, Ganau A et al (1993) Brief report: deletion of the dystrophin muscle-promoter region associated with X-linked dilated cardiomyopathy. N Engl J Med 329: 921–925

Muntoni F, Wilson L, Marrosu G, Marrosu MG, Cianchetti C, Mestroni L, Ganau A, Dubowitz V, Sewry C (1995) A mutation in the dystrophin gene selectively affecting dystrophin expression in the heart J Clin Invest 96: 693–699

Olson TM, Keating MT (1996) Mapping a cardiomyopathy locus to chromosome 3p 22–p25. Journal of Clinical Investigation 97(2): 528–32

Torp A (1978) Incidence of congestive cardiomyopathy. Postgrad Med J 54: 435–439

Towbin JA, Hejtmancik JF, Brink P (1993) X-linked dilated cardiomyopathy. Molecular genetic evidence of linkage to the Duchenne muscular dystrophy (dystrophin) gene at the Xp21 locus. Circulation 87: 1854–1865

Yoshida K, Ikeda S, Nakamura A, Kagoshima M, Takeda S, Shoji S, Yanagisawa N (1993) Molecular analysis of the Duchenne muscular dystrophy gene in patients with Becker muscular dystrophy presenting with dilated cardiomyopathy. Muscle Nerve 16: 1161–1166

Mechanisms of Allograft Rejection and Therapeutic Options

M. Hummel

Mechanisms of Allograft Rejection

Allograft rejection depends on the coordinated activation of alloreactive T cells and antigen-presenting cells, monocyte macrophages, dendritic cells, and B cells. Whereas acute rejection is a T-cell-dependent process, a broad array of effector mechanisms participate in the destruction of the allograft. Through the release of cytokines and cell-to-cell interactions, a diverse assembly of lymphocytes, including CD4+ T cells, CD8+ cytotoxic cells, antibody-forming B cells, and other proinflammatory leukocytes, are recruited into the anti-allograft response.

Antigen Recognition – T-Cell Activation

T-cell activation begins when T cells recognize intracellularly processed fragments of foreign, mostly major histocompatibility complex (MHC) proteins embedded in the groove of the MHC proteins expressed on the surface of the antigen-presenting cell [1–4, 5]. The T-cell antigen recognition complex is formed by the clonally variant immunoglobulin-like α and β peptide chains of the T-cell receptor which recognize the antigenic peptide in the context of MHC proteins and by the clonally invariant CD3 chains (γ, δ, ε and ζ) which initiate intracellular signals originating from antigenic recognition [4, 6].

Antigen recognition by T cells can occur either directly or indirectly. In the first instance, recipient T cells recognize donor antigenic peptides presented on the surface of donor antigen-presenting cells. In the second instance other T cells recognize the donor antigen only after it is processed and presented by the recipient antigen-presenting cells [7].

CD4 and CD8 proteins, expressed on reciprocal peripheral blood T-cell subgroups, bind to the monomorphic component of HLA class II and class I molecules, respectively (Fig. 1) [8]. Antigen recognition stimulates the redistribution of cell surface proteins and the clustering of the complex of T-cell antigen receptors and CD3 with the CD4 and CD8 antigen.

German Heart Institute Berlin, Augustenburger Platz 1, 13353 Berlin, Germany

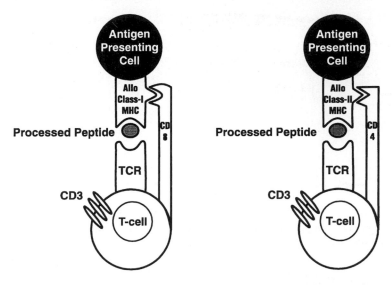

Fig. 1. Antigen presenting cell–T4/ T8 Cell interaction (*TCR*, T-cell receptor)

This multimeric complex includes additional signaling molecules, CD2 [9, 10], and CD5 [11] proteins, and functions as a unit in the stimulation of T-cell activation (Fig. 2). Upon stimulation with antigens, the CD3–T-cell antigen receptor complex, and the CD4 and CD8 proteins become physically associated, thereby activating several intracellular protein tyrosine kinases [4, 12].

A sequence of tyrosine phosphorylation and the generation of inositol triphosphate mobilizes intracellular bound calcium which synergistically promotes the sustained activation of protein C kinase and the expression of several

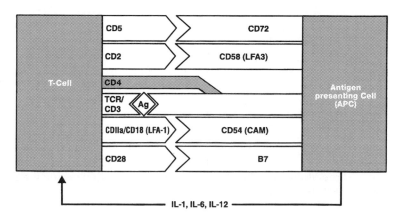

Fig. 2. T-cell–antigen presenting cell interaction. First and costimulating signals (*LFA*, lymphocyte function associated antigen; *TCR*, T-cell receptor; *CAM*, cellular adhesion molecule; IL, interleukin)

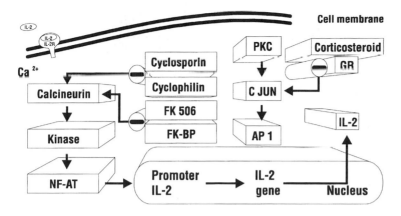

Fig. 3. T-cell activation – antigen presentation (*IL*, interleukin; *PKC*, protein kinase C; *GR*, glucocorticoid receptor; *FK-BP*, FK506 binding protein; *NF-AT*, nuclear factor of activated T cells)

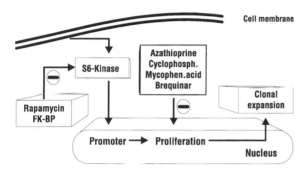

Fig. 4. T-cell activation – clonal expansion (*FK-BP*, FK506 binding protein)

nuclear regulatory proteins such as nuclear factor of activated T cells (NF–AT). This leads to the activation and expression of genes fundamental to T-cell growth [3, 4]. Calcineurin, a calcium- and calmodulin-dependent serine-threonine phosphatase, has recently been demonstrated to participate in signal transduction [13, 14]. The inhibition of the phosphatase activity of calcineurin by cyclosporine and tacrolimus appears to be central to their immunosuppressive activity (Figs. 3 and 4) [15, 16].

After T-cell activation which follows MHC-triggering, the expression of oncogenes (such as c-*fos*), interleukins (ILS, such as IL-2), receptors of IL-2 and IL-3, of DNA, and of very late antigens (VLA) occurs in a time-dependent manner. In vitro stimulation of T lymphocytes by foreign MHC causes an increase in the mRNA levels of these proteins.

T-Cell Activation/Anergy – Costimulatory Signals

It is important to note that in the absence of other signals, e.g., second or costimulatory signals, T-cell stimulation through the complex of T-cell antigen receptor and CD3 alone induces T-cell anergy or paralysis [19]. This may represent a therapeutic option for inducing tolerance in clinical transplantation (Fig. 5) [17, 18]. T-cell activation requires both antigenic and costimulatory signals engendered by cell–cell interactions among antigen-specific T cells and antigen-presenting cells [20].

Various interactions, especially of CD2–CD58 (LFA-3) and CD11a/CD18 with CD54 (intercellular adhesion molecule-(ICAM-1) and of CD5 with CD72 proteins and cytokines (IL-1 and IL-6), have an impact similar to such costimulatory signals [21]. These costimulatory signals depend on calcium and protein kinase C and are sensitive to cyclosporine A and tacrolimus (FK506) (Fig. 2) [14, 15].

Costimulatory signals induced by other cell-to-cell interactions, such as that of the B7 protein on antigen-presenting cells with the CD28 and CTLA-4 protein complexes, stimulate a T-cell costimulatory pathway which is independent of protein kinase C and calcium, and also leads to the stable transcription of the IL-2 gene, thus resulting in vigorous T-cell proliferation by IL-2 synthesis, the most important T cell growth factor involved in the allograft rejection process [17, 19, 22, 23]. This costimulatory signaling pathway is resistant to inhibition by cyclosporine and tacrolimus, but sensitive to rapamycin [24].

The stimulation of B cells also depends on the antigenic signal and a costimulatory signal. The antigenic signal is generated by the interaction between the specific antigen and the cell surface immunoglobulin. T-cell-derived cytokines (e.g. IL-2 and IL-4), or physical contact between T cells and B cells through specific pairs of receptors and coreceptors, or both, provide the signal or signals essential for B-cell stimulation [25].

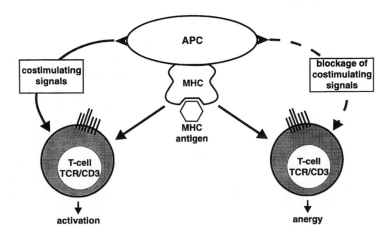

Fig. 5. T-cell activation – anergy pathways (*APC*, antigen-presenting cell; *MHC*, major histocompatibility complex; *TCR*, T-cell receptor)

After T cells are stimulated by an antigen (first signal) in combination with a costimulatory signal (second signal), i.e., IL-2 gene expression and IL secretion are induced, further T-cell proliferation is generated by the autocrine T cell stimulation of IL-2 binding to the IL receptor, which is expressed on the T cell surface [26, 27, 28]. This activation pathway leads to the expression of several DNA-binding proteins, including c-jun, c-fos, and c-myc, the activation of the S6 kinase, and the progression of the cell cycle through proliferation to clonal expansion [29]. In this later stage of T-cell activation, i.e., differentiation and proliferation, rapamycin and antimetabolite molecules, which inhibit DNA synthesis, can inhibit and reverse the process of allograft rejection (Fig. 4).

T-Cell Proliferation – Graft Destruction

The net consequence of T-cell proliferation and differentiation is the emergence of antigen-specific graft infiltration and of destructive T cells. These cells are capable of destroying the graft in combination with other activated inflammatory cells, such as macrophages, natural killer cells, and anti-donor antibodies produced by stimulated B cells. Moreover, cytokines can amplify the ongoing immune response by up-regulating the expression of human HLA and costimulatory molecules on graft parenchymal cells and antigen-presenting cells.

Invasion of the graft through the blood vessels is a very complex process which is triggered by an adhesion cascade. This leads to the transendothelial migration of activated and cytotoxic lymphocytes, starting with rolling of the lymphocytes over the endothelium surface and tethering via a selectin-mediated interaction (E-selectin, P-selectin, L-selectin). The latter activates signals to up-regulate integrin functions which are molecules of the immunoglobulin superfamily (ICAM, VLA). This subsequently leads to conformational changes which promote strong adhesion and flattening and finally transendothelial migration and chemotaxis [30, 31, 32].

Ultimately the allograft is destroyed by at least two mechanisms of T-cell mediated toxicity: by membranolysis mediated by lytic molecules, such as perforin and granzyme B (Fig. 6), and by apoptosis induced by surface FAS-like molecules which signal a process leading to DNA fragmentation (Fig. 7) [34].

Therapeutic Options

During the early days of organ transplantation, the first drugs proven effective for the prophylaxis and treatment of allograft rejection were corticosteroids and azathioprine, followed by antilymphocyte and antithymocyte globulins [35]. During the last decade, particularly within the last 5 years, an increasing number of potent immunosuppressants with different modes of action became available, either for investigational or for clinical use (Fig. 8).

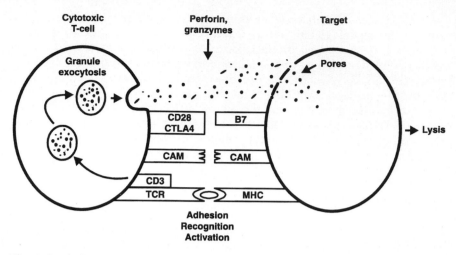

Fig. 6. Cytolysis. Two mechanisms of T-cell mediated cytotoxicity (*CAM*, cellular adhesion molecule; *MHC*, major histocompatibility complex; *TCR*, T-cell receptor; *CTLA*, cytotoxic T-cell antigen). (Adapted from [33])

Corticosteroids

Corticosteroids are very powerful immunosuppressive drugs which penetrate the cell membrane and bind to receptors of the glucocorticoid receptor family in the cytoplasm. This complex enters the cell nucleus after dissociation of the heat shock protein (HSP) 90.

The resulting dimeric transcription factors with a zinc finger structure recognize enhancer or negative regulatory elements on DNA and bind to the glucocorticoid response element (GRE) motif (GTACAnnnTGTTCT; n, any

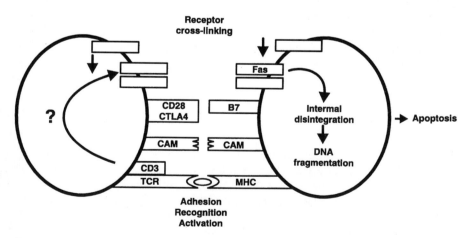

Fig. 7. Apoptosis. For abbreviations, see legend to Fig. 6. (Adapted from [33])

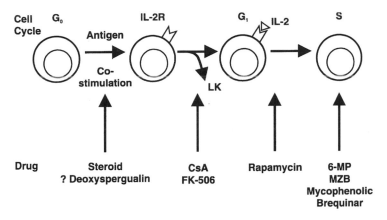

Fig. 8. Immunosuppressive drugs – site of action in the cell cycle (*IL*, interleukin; *LK*, lymphokine; *CsA*, cyclosporin A; *MZB*, mizoribine; *6-MP*, 6-mercaptopurine)

nucleotide). Sequences homologous to the GRE motif have been located in the promotor region of several cytokine genes, for example, IL-2 and interferon-γ, the products of which are involved in rejection processes. Corticosteroids inhibit T-cell proliferation, T-cell-dependent immunity, and the expression of cytokine genes (i.e. IL-1, IL-2, IL-6, interferon γ, and tumor necrosis factor α [36–39]. Because of their wide distribution and pleiotropic effects, these immunosuppressive drugs are unspecific and are associated with a wide spectrum of side effects.

Azathioprine

Azathioprine, a thioguanine derivative of mercaptopurine, is a prodrug which is metabolized by the liver to 6-thioguanine and inhibits the first enzyme of purine synthesis [40]. Administered alone, azathioprine is a relatively weak and unselective immunosuppressive drug which can be used only in combination with corticosteroids, cyclosporine, or tacrolimus to prevent allograft rejection. Although it effectively blocks the primary immune response, it is relatively ineffective in reversing ongoing acute rejection. Azathioprine is not cell specific and therefore causes dose-limited bone marrow suppression, gastrointestinal toxicity, sterility, hepatotoxicity, and acute pancreatitis.

Cyclosporine A and FK506 (Tacrolimus)

With the discovery of cyclosporine A in the late 1970s and of tacrolimus (FK506) a few years ago, two drugs with much more selective immunosuppressive activity became available for preventing allograft rejection. Both drugs dissect calcium and phosphokinase A-dependent activation leading to lym-

Immunophilins Drugs   Effector Proteins

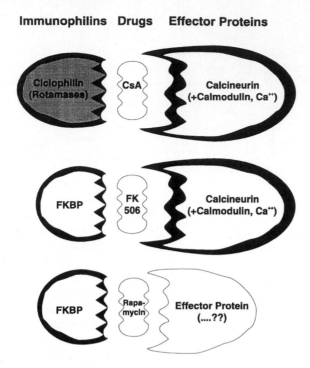

Fig. 9. Dual domain hypothesis for immunosuppresive compounds of microbial origin [*CsA*, cyclosporin A; *FKBP*, FK506 binding protein (poly-peptidyl-cis-trans-polymerases)]

phokine (IL-2) synthesis. Both drugs bind to immunophilins which are soluble cytosolic receptors [40]. The dual domain hypothesis considers the binding of cyclosporine A to cyclophilin and of tacrolimus to the FK506-binding protein (FKBP; Fig. 9). Both are parts of the calcineurin complex which is involved in the protein C kinase activation pathway. The recently developed immunosuppressant sirolimus (rapamycin) also binds to the FKBP. However, in contrast to cyclosporine A and tacrolimus (FK506), rapamycin can inhibit a Ca$^+$ -independent activation pathway during autocrine T cell activation when IL-2 has already been expressed.

To prevent allograft rejection, almost all immunosuppressive drug protocols include cyclosporine A (or tacrolimus). However, other immunosuppressive drugs have to be added since even maximum doses of cyclosporine A alone are incapable of preventing acute allograft rejection. FK506 is more potent than cyclosporine and reverses ongoing rejection more effectively, presumably by inhibiting cytokine synthesis in T cells infiltrating the allograft. However, it causes more toxic effects to the kidney and central nervous system than cyclosporine and is also probably diabetogenic [41].

Rapamycin (Sirolimus)

Rapamycin (sirolimus) is a macrolactam which was discovered nearly two decades ago during a screening of bacterial products for antifungal activity. Interest was renewed 13 years later when its structure was noted to be strikingly similar to that of the newly characterized FK506. Like FK506 it also binds to cytosolic FKBPs. However, unlike FK506 its immunosuppressive properties result from the inhibition of the growth factor-mediated cell cycle transition from G1 to S phase [42]. In animal models it has been demonstrated that rapamycin may be extremely effective in preventing antibody-mediated accelerated rejection and in prolonging allograft survival in previously sensitized cardiac transplant recipients [43, 44]. Moreover, its antiproliferative effect is not limited to lymphocytes (i.e., inhibition of IL-2-mediated T-cell activation); rapamycin also blocks the growth factor-stimulated mitogenesis of mesenchymal cells (Fig. 10) [46].

Mycophenolate Mofetil (RS 61443) and Mizoribine

In clinical trials mycophenolate mofetil (RS 61443) and mizoribine were found to be capable of suppressing the proliferation of activated T cells and B cells more selectively than azathioprine by inhibiting inosine monophosphate dehydrogenase and by suppressing de novo purine synthesis. The latter has been proven to be the main pathway of purine synthesis in lymphocytes, but not in endothelial cells or granulocytes. The side effects of mycophenolate mofetil are

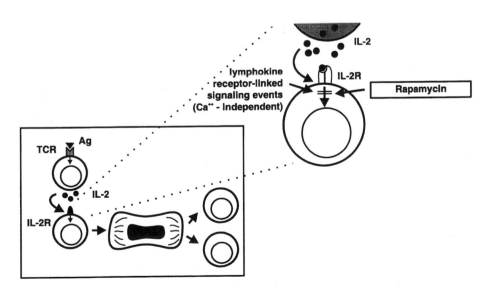

Fig. 10. Inhibition of T-cell proliferation after antigenic stimulus by rapamycin. For abbreviations, see legend to Fig. 2. (Adapted from [45])

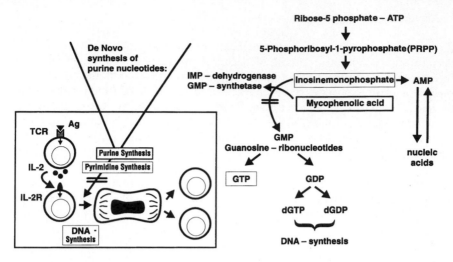

Fig. 11. Inhibition of T-cell proliferation after antigenic stimulus by mycophenol mofetil (RS 61443). (Adapted from [45])

limited to mild gastrointestinal disturbances. The incidence of infectious, renal, hepatic, and myelotoxic complications all remained unchanged compared with pre-treatment values (Fig. 11) [47].

Brequinar Sodium

Brequinar sodium and possibly leflunomide, which is used in clinical trials to treat rheumatic arthritis, act as relatively selective immunosuppressive drugs by inhibiting dihydroorotate dehydrogenase and thereby suppressing de novo pyrimidine synthesis, which is also a preferred pathway of lymphocytes but not of other fast growing cells for DNA synthesis. Brequinar sodium has been shown to be an effective inhibitor of cellular and humoral responses in animal models. The therapeutic window of this agent is much narrower than that of other antimetabolites and it is associated with myelotoxicity and gastro-intestinal disturbances at effective doses (Fig. 12) [48].

Leflunomide

Leflunomide, and isoxazole derivative, is one of the newest immunosuppressive agents. Contrary to cyclosporine and FK506, it prevents T-cell proliferation at a later stage than xenobiotic molecules, presumably by inhibiting cytokine-receptor-associated tyrosine kinases [49–51].

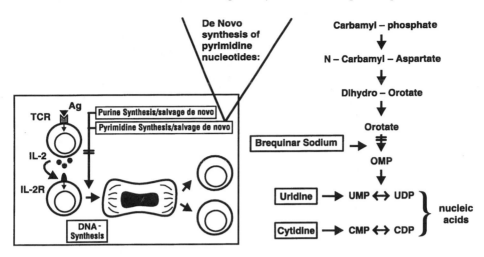

Fig. 12. Inhibition of T-cell proliferation after antigenic stimulus by brequinar sodium. (Adapted from [45])

Polyclonal and Monoclonal Antibodies

New concepts for a more selective immunosuppression and for the induction of temporary or permanent allograft tolerance are currently under development, namely a second generation of monoclonal antibodies. These antibodies would have an advantage over antilymphocyte or antithymocyte antibodies which unspecifically destroy all kinds of lymphocytes and T cells [52], whether activated or not. These newly developed antibodies are directed against defined epitope targets on cell surface receptors of antigen-presenting cells, T cells, and endothelial cells [53–55]. Since monoclonal antibodies directed against adhesion molecules can effectively block lymphocyte activation and lymphocyte adherence to the endothelium, they offer alternative strategies for inhibiting transplant rejection [56, 57]. Although monoclonal antibodies to single adhesion molecules such as ICAM-1 and lymphocyte function associated antigen-1 can prolong graft survival in experimental models and in transplant recipients, the most effective therapeutic strategy might use "cocktails" of antibodies against different adhesion molecules [58, 59].

   In contrast to the only clinically available anti-T-cell antibody OKT3 [60], some of these newly developed antibodies will be better adapted for human use with the advantage of a lower rate of sensitization and a much longer duration of action [61, 62].

Gene-Targeted Therapies and Xenotransplantation

In addition to the above-mentioned therapeutic possibilities for controlling allograft rejection, other new options have become available, including the possibility of xenotransplantation using gene-targeted therapies. Before xenotransplantation can become a viable alternative to allotransplantation, it will be necessary to modify donor cell surface proteins to overcome the as yet unsolved problem of hyperacute rejection. Such modifications are possible by breeding transgenic animals with genetic changes in complement inhibiting factors (decay-accelerating factor), terminal sugar transferase, and adhesion molecules, and by inhibiting endothelial cell activation mechanisms. An alternative approach would be to breed knock-out animals lacking MHC proteins, α-1,3 galactosyl transferase, and cellular adhesion molecules [63–68].

Another way to induce temporary or permanent tolerance in allogenic transplantation is to preoperatively present allogenic MHC genes in cells for antigen presentation. These models have already been tested in animals with MHC class I, MHC class II, adhesion molecules, and changes in the enhancement [69,70].

Recent experiments have shown long-lasting tolerance and persistently mixed chimerism in rodents that underwent transplantation at the same time that the marrow of both allogeneic (or xenogeneic) and syngeneic donors which was purged of T cells was transplanted into irradiated recipients.

Summary and Conclusion

Recently many mechanisms of complex immunologic events have been elucidated, beginning with allorecognition, lymphocyte activation, and differentiation, and followed by the interactions of antibodies and activated lymphocytes with the vascular endothelium and the subsequent cellular infiltration into the allograft resulting in inflammation and destruction of the allograft. These insights have led to a more rational use of well-known and newly identified and developed immunosuppressive drugs, thus yielding greater efficacy and fewer side effects after organ transplantation. Clinical and experimental experience with solid organ transplantation offers perspectives for the development of temporary or permanent tolerance induction strategies and for the use of xenografts to overcome the shortage of human donors.

A more detailed knowledge of the mechanisms of allograft recognition and of the effects of immunosuppressive drugs will also offer therapeutic options for other immunomodulated diseases, such as myocarditis, atherosclerosis, and skin and rheumatic disorders. In the near future there will be a variety of different options for inducing immunosuppression which may offer possibilities for individualized and adapted immunosuppressive or tolerance induction strategies.

References

1. Unanue ER, Cerottini J-C (1989) Antigen presentation. FASEB J 3: 2496–2502
2. Germain RN (1994) MHC-dependent antigen processing and peptide presentation: providing ligands for T lymphocyte activation. Cell 76: 287–299

3. Krensky AM, Weiss A, Crabtree G, Davis MM, Parham P (1990) T-lymphocyte-antigen interactions in transplant recipients. N Engl J Med 322: 510–517
4. Weiss A, Littman DR (1994) Signal transduction by lymphocyte antigen receptors. Cell 76: 263–274
5. Halloran PF, Broski AP, Batiuk TD, Madrenas J (1993) The molecular immunology of acute rejection: an overview. Transpl Immunol 1: 3–27
6. Clevers H, Alarcon B, Wileman T, Terhorst C (1988) The T cell receptor/CD3 complex: a dynamic protein ensemble. Annu Rev Immunol 6: 629–662
7. Shoskes DA, Wood KJ (1994) Indirect presentation of MHC antigens in transplantation. Immunol Today 15: 32–38
8. Miceli MC, Parnes JR (1991) The roles of CD4 and CD8 in T cell activation. Semin Immunol 3: 133–141
9. Suthanthiran M (1990) A novel model for the antigen-dependent activation of normal human T cells: transmembrane signaling by crosslinkage of CD3/T cell receptor-α/γ complex with the cluster determinant 2 antigen. J Exp Med 171: 1965–1979
10. Brown MH, Cantrell DA, Brattsand G, Crumpton MJ, Gullberg M (1989) The CD2 antigen associates with the T-cell antigen receptor CD3 antigen complex on the surface of human T lymphocytes. Nature 339: 551–553
11. Beyers AD, Spruyt LL, Williams AF (1992) Molecular associations between the T-lymphocyte antigen receptor complex and the surface antigen CD2, CD4, or CD8 and CD5. Proc Natl Acad Sci USA 89: 2945–2949
12. Klausner RD, Samelson LE (1991) T cell antigen receptor activation pathways: the tyrosine kinase connection. Cell 64: 875–878
13. O'Keefe SJ, Tamura J, Kincaid RL, Tocci MJ, O'Neill EA (1992) FK-506- and CsA-sensitive activation of the interleukin-2 promotor by calcineurin. Nature 357: 692–694
14. Clipstone NA, Crabtree GR (1992) Identification of calcineurin as a key signaling enzyme in T-lymphocyte activation. Nature 357: 695–697
15. Liu J, Farmer JD Jr, Lane WS, Friedman J, Weissman I, Schreiber SL (1991) Calcineurin is a common target of cyclophilin-cyclosporin A and FKBP-FK506 complex. Cell 66: 807–815
16. Frumann DA, Klee CB, Bierer BE, Burakoff SJ (1992) Calcineurin phosphatase activity in T lymphocytes is inhibited by FK 506 and cyclosporine A. Proc Natl Acad Sci USA 89: 3686–3690
17. Boussiotis VA, Gribben IG, Freeman GJ, Nadler LM (1994) Blockage of the CD28 costimulatory pathway: a means to induce tolerance. Curr Opin Immunol 6: 797–807
18. Lin H, Bolling SF, Linsley PS, Wei RQ, Gordon D, Thompson CB, Turka LA (1993) Long-term acceptance of major histocompatibility complex mismatched cardiac allografts induced by CTLA4Ig plus donor-specific transfusion. J Exp Med 178: 1801–1806
19. Schwartz RH (1993) T cell anergy. Sci Am 269: 62–73
20. Suthanthiran M (1993) Signaling features of T cells: implications for the regulation of the anti-allograft response. Kidney Int Suppl 43: S3–S11
21. Dustin ML, Springer TA (1989) T-cell receptor cross-linking transiently stimulates adhesiveness through LFA-1. Nature 341: 619–624
22. June CH, Lebetter JA, Linsley PS, Thompson CB (1990) Role of the CD29 receptor in T-cell activation. Immunol Today 11: 211–216
23. Linsley PS, Brady W, Urnes M, Grossmaire LS, Damle NK, Ledbetter JA (1991) CTLA-4 is a second receptor for the B cell activation antigen B7. J Exp Med 174: 561–569
24. Sigal NH, Lin CS, Siekierka JJ (1991) Inhibition of human T-cell activation by FK506, rapamycin and cyclosporin A. Transplant Proc 23 (Suppl 2): 1–5
25. Clark EA, Ledbetter JA (1994) How B and T cells talk to each other. Nature 367: 425–428
26. Smith KA (1988) Interleukin-2: inception, impact, and implications. Science 240: 1169–1176
27. Waldmann TA (1991) The interleukin-2 receptor. J Biol Chem 266: 281–284
28. Takeshita T, Asao H, Ohtani K et al (1992) Cloning of the γ chain of the human IL-2 receptor. Science 257: 379–382
29. Shibuya H, Yoneyama M, Ninomiya-Tsuji J et al (1992) IL-2 and EGF receptors stimulate the hematopoietic cell cycle via different signaling pathways: demonstration of the novel role of c-myc. Cell 70: 57–67

30. Bevilacqua MP (1993) Endothelial-leukocyte adhesion molecules. Annu Rev Immunol 11: 767–804
31. Tanaka Y, Adams DH, Shaw S (1993) Proteoglycans on endothelial cells present adhesion-inducing cytokines to leukocytes. Immunol Today 14: 111
32. Springer T (1994) Traffic signals for lymphocyte recirculation and leukocyte migration: the multistep paradigm. Cell 76: 301–314
33. Duquesnoy RJ, Demetris AJ (1995) Immunopathology of cardiac rejection. Curr Opin Cardiol 10: 195
34. Berke G (1994) The binding and lysis of target cells by cytotoxic lymphocytes: molecular and cellular aspects. Annu Rev Immunol 12: 735–773
35. White DJG (1993) Immunosuppression for heart transplantation. Br J Biomed Sci 50: 277–283
36. Knudsen PJ, Dinarello CA, Strom TB (1987) Glucocorticoids inhibit transcriptional and post-transcriptional expression of interleukin 1 in U937 cells. J Immunol 139: 4129–4134
37. Zanker B, Walz G, Wieder KJ, Strom TB (1990) Evidence that glucocorticoids block expression of the human interleukin-6 gene by accessory cells. Transplantation 49: 183–185
38. Arya SK, Wong-Staal F, Gallo RC (1984) Dexamethasone-mediated inhibition of human T cell growth factor and gamma-interferon messenger RNA. J Immunol 133: 272–276
39. Vacca A, Felli MP, Farina AR et al (1992) Glucocorticoid receptor-mediated suppression of the interleukin 2 gene expression through impairment of the cooperativity between nuclear factor of activated T cells and AP-1 enhancer elements. J Exp Med 175: 637–646
40. Bach J-F, Strom TB (1986) The mode of action of immunosuppressive agents. Research monographs in immunology, 2nd rev edn., Vol 9. Elsevier, Amsterdam pp 105–158
41. The U.S. Multicenter FK506 Liver Study Group (1994) A comparison of tacrolimus (FK506) and cyclosporine for immunosuppression in liver transplantation. N Engl J Med 331: 1110–1115
42. Morris RE (1994) Rapamycin for transplantation. In: Kupiec-Weglinski JW, Autin RG (eds) Medical Intelligence Unit: New immunosuppressive modalities and anti-rejection approaches in organ transplantation. Landes pp 43–63
43. Schmidbauer G, Hancock WW, Wasowska B, Badger AM, Kupiec-Weglinski JW (1994) Abrogation by rapamycin of accelerated rejection in sensitized rats by inhibition of alloantibody responses and selective suppression of intragraft mononuclear and endothelial cell activation, cytokine production, and cell adhesion. Transplantation 57: 933–941
44. Chen H, Luo H, Daloze P, Xu D, Shan X, St-Louis G, Wu J (1993) Long-term in vivo effects of rapamycin on humoral and cellular immune responses in the rat. Immunobiology 188: 303–315
45. Land W (1993) Neue Immunsuppressive Medikamente in der Organtransplantation – Chaos oder Fortschritt. In: Heidbreder E, Götz R, Heiland A (eds) Nierentransplantation, Immunsuppression, Nachsorge, Langzeitprobleme. Beck, Straubing
46. Cao W, Mohacsi P, Pratt R, Morris RE (1995) Effects of rapamycin on growth factor-stimulated vascular smooth muscle cell DNA synthesis: inhibition of bFGF and PDGF action and antagonism of rapamycin by FK506. Transplantation 59: 390–395
47. Kirklin JK, Bourge RC, Naftel DC, Morrow WR, Deierhoi MH, Kauffman RS, White-Williams C, Nomberg RI, Holman WL, Smith Jr DC (1994) Treatment of recurrent heart rejection with mycophenolate mofetil (RS-61443): initial clinical experience. J Heart Lung Transplant 13: 444–450
48. Nozaki S, Ito T, Kamiike W, Uchikoshi F, Yamamoto S, Nakata S, Shirakura R, Miyata M, Matsuda H, Stepkowski SM, Kahan BD (1994) Effect of brequinar sodium on accelerated cardiac allograft rejection in presensitized recipients. Transplant Proc 26: 2333–2335
49. Nair RV, Cao W, Morris RE (1995) Molecular mechanism of suppression of arterial thickening by leflunomide (LFM): demonstration of a direct antilymphoproliferative effect of murine smooth muscle cells (M-SMC) in vitro and antagonism of action by uridine (abstract). J Heart Lung Transplant 14: S54
50. Williams JW, Xiao F, Foster P, Clardy C, McChesney L, Sankary H, Chong AS-F (1994) Leflunomide in experimental transplantation: control of rejection and alloantibody pro-

duction, reversal of acute rejection, and interaction with cyclosporine. Transplantation 57: 1223–1231

51. Schreiber SL (1992) Immunophilin-sensitive protein phosphatase action in cell signaling pathways. Cell 70: 365–368
52. Norman DJ (1992) Antilymphocyte antibodies in the treatment of allograft rejection: targets, mechanisms of action, monitoring, and efficacy. Semin Nephrol 12: 315–324
53. Knight RJ, Kurrle R, McClain J et al (1994) Clinical evaluation of induction immunosuppression with murine IgG$_{2b}$ monoclonal antibody (BMA 031) directed toward the human α/β-T cell receptor. Transplantation 57: 1581–1588
54. Soulillou J-P, Cantarovich D, Le Mauff B et al (1990) Randomized controlled trial of a monoclonal antibody against the interleukin-2 receptor (33B3.1) as compared with rabbit antithymocyte globulin for prophylaxis against rejection of renal allografts. N Engl J Med 322: 1175–1182
55. Kirkman RL, Shapiro ME, Carpenter CB et al (1991) A randomized prospective trial of anti-Tac monoclonal antibody in human renal transplantation. Transplant Proc 23: 1066–1067
56. Orosz CG (1994) Lymphocyte-endothelial interactions and tolerance induction. Clin Transplant 8: 188–194
57. Paul LC, Davidoffr A, Benediktsson H, Issekutz TB (1993) The efficacy of LFA-1 and VLA-4 antibody treatment in rat vascularized cardiac allograft rejection. Transplantation 55: 1196–1199
58. Chavin KD, Qin L, Lin J, Yagita H, Bromberg JS (1993) Combined anti-CD2 and anti-CD3 receptor monoclonal antibodies induce donor-specific tolerance in a cardiac transplant model. J Immunol 151: 7249–7259
59. Nakakura EK, McCabe SM, Zheng B, Shorthouse RA, Scheiner TM, Blank G, Jardieu PM, Morris RE (1993) Potent and effective prolongation by anti-LFA-1 monoclonal antibody monotherapy of non-primarily vascularized heart allograft survival in mice without T-cell depletion. Transplantation 55: 412–417
60. Ortho Multicenter Transplant Study Group (1985) A randomized clinical trial of OKT3 monoclonal antibody for acute rejection of cadaveric renal transplants. N Engl J Med 313: 337–342
61. Queen C, Schneider WP, Selick HE et al (1989) A humanized antibody that binds to the interleukin 2 receptor. Proc Natl Acad Sci USA 86: 10029–10033
62. Gorman SD, Clark MR, Routledge EG, Cobbold SP, Waldhmann H (1991) Reshaping a therapeutic CD4 antibody. Proc Natl Acad Sci USA 88: 4181
63. Carrington CA, Richards AC, Cozzi E, Langford G, Yannoutsos N, White DJG (1995) Expression of human DAF and MCP on pig endothelial cells protect from human complement. Transplant Proc 27: 319–320
64. Cozzi E, Langford GA, Wright L, Tucker A, Yannoutsos N, Richards A, Rosengard A, Elsome K, Lancaster R, Whithe DJG (1995) Comparative analysis of human DAF expression in the tissues of transgenic pigs and man. Transplant Proc 27: 307–308
65. White DJF, Wallwork J (1993) Xenografting: probability, possibility, or pipe dream. Lancet 342: 879–880
66. McCurry KR, Kooyman DL, Diqmond LE, Byrne GW, Logan JS, Platt JL (1995) Transgenic expression of human complement regulatory proteins in mice result in diminished complement deposition during organ xenoperfusion. Transplantation 59: 1177–1182
67. Sandrin MS, McKenzie IF (1994) Gal alpha (1,3)Gal, the major xenoantigen(s) recognised in pigs by human natural antibodies. Immunol Rev 141: 169–190
68. Markmann JF, Campos L, Bhandoola A, Kim JL, Desai NM, Bassiri H, Claytor BR, Barker CF (1994) Genetically engineering grafts to study xenoimmunity: a role for indirect antigen presentation in the destruction of major histocompatibility complex antigen deficient xenografts. Surgery 116: 242–248
69. Tsuji K, Inoko H, Hagihara M, Shimura T, Sato T, Ando A (1993) Role of HLA-DP antigen in xenogeneic iso-skin grafts using transgenic mice. Transplant Proc 25: 136–137
70. Nishida Y, Kondo S, Miura Y, Iwata H, Isobe K (1993) Survival of syngeneic and allogenic grafted bone in transgenic mice. Biochem Biophys Res Comm 196: 1081–1085

Subject Index